Para and Adapted Sports Medicine

Editors

YETSA A. TUAKLI-WOSORNU
WAYNE DERMAN

PHYSICAL MEDICINE AND REHABILITATION CLINICS OF NORTH AMERICA

www.pmr.theclinics.com

Consulting Editor
SANTOS F. MARTINEZ

May 2018 • Volume 29 • Number 2

ELSEVIER

1600 John F. Kennedy Boulevard • Suite 1800 • Philadelphia, Pennsylvania, 19103-2899

http://www.theclinics.com

PHYSICAL MEDICINE AND REHABILITATION CLINICS OF NORTH AMERICA Volume 29, Number 2
May 2018 ISSN 1047-9651, ISBN 978-0-323-58372-5

Editor: Lauren Boyle
Developmental Editor: Meredith Madeira

Reprints. For copies of 100 or more of articles in this publication, please contact the Commercial Reprints Department, Elsevier Inc., 360 Park Avenue South, New York, NY 10010-1710. Tel.: 212-633-3874; Fax: 212-633-3820; E-mail: reprints@elsevier.com.

Physical Medicine and Rehabilitation Clinics of North America (ISSN 1047-9651) is published quarterly by Elsevier Inc., 360 Park Avenue South, New York, NY 10010-1710. Months of issue are February, May, August, and November. Business and Editorial Offices: 1600 John F. Kennedy Blvd., Suite 1800, Philadelphia, PA 19103-2899. Customer Service Office: 3251 Riverport Lane, Maryland Heights, MO 63043. Periodicals postage paid at New York, NY and additional mailing offices. Subscription price per year is $294.00 (US individuals), $571.00 (US institutions), $100.00 (US students), $351.00 (Canadian individuals), $752.00 (Canadian institutions), $210.00 (Canadian students), $427.00 (foreign individuals), $752.00 (foreign institutions), and $210.00 (foreign students). Foreign air speed delivery is included in all *Clinics* subscription prices. All prices are subject to change without notice. **POSTMASTER:** Send address changes to *Physical Medicine and Rehabilitation Clinics of North America*, Customer Service Office: Elsevier Health Sciences Division, Subscription Customer Service, 3251 Riverport Lane, Maryland Heights, MO 63043. **Customer Service: 1-800-654-2452 (US). From outside of the United States, call 314-447-8871. Fax: 314-447-8029. E-mail: JournalsCustomer Service-usa@elsevier.com (for print support); JournalsOnlineSupport-usa@elsevier.com (for online support).**

Physical Medicine and Rehabilitation Clinics of North America is indexed in *Excerpta Medica, MEDLINE/ PubMed (Index Medicus), Cinahl,* and *Cumulative Index to Nursing and Allied Health Literature.*

Contributors

CONSULTING EDITOR

SANTOS F. MARTINEZ, MD, MS
Diplomate of the American Academy of Physical Medicine and Rehabilitation, Certificate of Added Qualification Sports Medicine, Assistant Professor, Department of Orthopaedics, Campbell Clinic Orthopaedics, University of Tennessee, Memphis, Tennessee, USA

EDITORS

YETSA A. TUAKLI-WOSORNU, MD, MPH
Assistant Clinical Professor, Department of Chronic Disease Epidemiology, Yale School of Public Health, New Haven, Connecticut, USA; Physical Medicine and Rehabilitation Clinician, Yale Department of Orthopaedics and Rehabilitation, New Haven, Connecticut, USA; International Olympic Committee Working Group: Prevention of Harassment and Abuse in Sport, Lausanne, Switzerland; Welfare Officer, International Paralympic Committee Medical Committee, Bonn, Germany

WAYNE DERMAN, MBChB, MSc (Med) (Hons), PhD, FFIMS
Director, Institute of Sports and Exercise Medicine, Co-director, International Olympic Committee Research Centre, Pretoria, South Africa; Director, FIFA Medical Center of Excellence, Professor of Sport and Exercise Medicine, Department of Surgical Sciences, Division of Orthopaedic Surgery, Faculty of Medicine and Health Sciences, University of Stellenbosch, Stellenbosch, Cape Town, South Africa

AUTHORS

JASON BANTJES, D Lit et Phil
Alan J Flisher Centre for Public Mental Health, Department of Psychology, Stellenbosch University, Matieland, South Africa

EMMA M. BECKMAN, PhD
Associate Investigator, International Paralympic Committee Classification Research and Development Partnership (Physical Impairments), Senior Lecturer, School of Human Movement and Nutrition Sciences, The University of Queensland, Brisbane, Australia

ADAM W. BLEAKNEY, BS
University of Illinois at Urbana-Champaign, Urbana-Champaign, Illinois, USA

ELIZABETH BROAD, PhD, BSc, DipNutrDiet, MAppSc
Sport Performance, United States Olympic Committee (US Paralympics), Chula Vista, California, USA

BRENDAN BURKETT, PhD
Director, High Performance Sport, Professor in Sport Science (Biomechanics), Faculty of Science, Health, Education and Engineering, School of Health and Sport Sciences, University of the Sunshine Coast, Sippy Downs, Queensland, Australia

MARK J. CONNICK, PhD
Research Fellow, International Paralympic Committee Classification Research and Development Partnership (Physical Impairments), School of Human Movement and Nutrition Sciences, The University of Queensland, Brisbane, Australia

RORY A. COOPER, PhD
Director, Human Engineering Research Laboratories, VA Pittsburgh Healthcare System, University of Pittsburgh, Pittsburgh, Pennsylvania, USA

ROSEMARIE COOPER, MPT
Human Engineering Research Laboratories, VA Pittsburgh Healthcare System, University of Pittsburgh, Pittsburgh, Pennsylvania, USA

THERESA M. CRYTZER, DPT, ATP
Human Engineering Research Laboratories, VA Pittsburgh Healthcare System, University of Pittsburgh, Pittsburgh, Pennsylvania, USA

DANIEL DALY, PhD
Professor in Sport, Faculty of Kinesiology and Rehabilitation Sciences, KU Leuven, Heverlee, Belgium

WAYNE DERMAN, MBChB, MSc (Med) (Hons), PhD, FFIMS
Director, Institute of Sports and Exercise Medicine, Co-director, International Olympic Committee Research Centre, Pretoria, South Africa; Director, FIFA Medical Center of Excellence, Professor of Sport and Exercise Medicine, Department of Surgical Sciences, Division of Orthopaedic Surgery, Faculty of Medicine and Health Sciences, University of Stellenbosch, Stellenbosch, Cape Town, South Africa

BRAD E. DICIANNO, MD
Human Engineering Research Laboratories, VA Pittsburgh Healthcare System, University of Pittsburgh, Pittsburgh, Pennsylvania, USA

DAN DING, PhD
Human Engineering Research Laboratories, VA Pittsburgh Healthcare System, University of Pittsburgh, Pittsburgh, Pennsylvania, USA

MARK GENTRY, MA, MLS
Clinical Librarian, Cushing/Whitney Medical Library, Yale University, New Haven, Connecticut, USA

LARA GROBLER, PhD
Department of Sport Science, Faculty of Education, Institute of Sport and Exercise Medicine, Faculty of Health and Medical Sciences, Stellenbosch University, Cape Town, South Africa

MICHELLE GUERRERO, PhD
Student, Department of Kinesiology, University of Windsor, Windsor, Ontario, Canada

GEOFFREY V. HENDERSON, MD
University of Pittsburgh, Pittsburgh, Pennsylvania, USA

LUKE HOGARTH, PhD
Postdoc, School of Health and Sport Sciences, University of the Sunshine Coast, Sippy Downs, Queensland, Australia

P. DAVID HOWE, BSc, MA, PhD
Reader, Social Anthropology of Sport, School of Sport Exercise and Health Science, Loughborough University, Loughborough, United Kingdom

DINA CHRISTINA JANSE VAN RENSBURG, MBChB, MSc, MMed, MD
Section Sports Medicine, Faculty of Health Sciences and Sport, Exercise Medicine and Lifestyle Institute (SEMLI), University of Pretoria, Pretoria, South Africa

HANNAH JARVIS, PhD
Postdoc, HEAL Research Centre, Manchester Metropolitan University, Crewe, United Kingdom

DANIEL JENSEN, DPT
Assistant Professor, Department of Exercise Science, Black Hills State University, Spearfish, South Dakota

MARVIN KILIAN, MSc
PhD Candidate, Institute of Training Science and Sport Informatics, German Sport University, Cologne, Germany

NUWANEE KIRIHENNEDIGE, MS, RD, CSSD
Sport Performance, United States Olympic Committee (US Paralympics), Colorado Springs, Colorado, USA

JAMES KISSICK, MD, CCFP (SEM), Dip Sport Med
Department of Family Medicine, University of Ottawa Carleton University Sport Medicine Clinic, Ottawa, Ontario, Canada

ALICIA M. KOONTZ, PhD, RET
Human Engineering Research Laboratories, VA Pittsburgh Healthcare System, University of Pittsburgh, Pittsburgh, Pennsylvania, USA

ANDREI (V.) KRASSIOUKOV, MD, PhD, FRCPC
Division of Physical Medicine and Rehabilitation, Department of Medicine, Professor and Chair, International Collaboration on Repair Discoveries (ICORD), Blusson Spinal Cord Centre, University of British Columbia, GF Strong Rehabilitation Centre, Vancouver Coastal Health, Vancouver, British Columbia, Canada

DAVID LEGG, PhD
Chair and Professor, Department of Health and Physical Education, Mount Royal University, Calgary, Canada

JEFFREY MARTIN, PhD
Professor, Division of Kinesiology, Health and Sport Studies, Wayne State University, Detroit, Michigan, USA

EVGENY MASHKOVSKIY, MD, PhD
Associate Professor, Department of Sports Medicine and Medical Rehabilitation, Sechenov University, Moscow, Russia

CHRISTIANE MEHRKUEHLER, MSc
Masters Candidate, Faculty of Kinesiology and Rehabilitation Sciences, KU Leuven, Heverlee, Belgium

TAYLOR OTTESEN, BS
Department of Orthopaedics and Rehabilitation, Yale School of Medicine, New Haven, Connecticut, USA

CARL PAYTON, PhD
HEAL Research Centre, Manchester Metropolitan University, Crewe, United Kingdom

ELEANOR QUINBY, BS
University of Pittsburgh, Pittsburgh, Pennsylvania, USA

IAN RICE, PhD
University of Illinois at Urbana-Champaign, Urbana-Champaign, Illinois, USA

PHOEBE RUNCIMAN, BA (Hons), PhD
Division of Orthopaedic Surgery, Department of Surgical Sciences, Faculty of Medicine and Health Sciences, Institute of Sport and Exercise Medicine, Stellenbosch University, Stellenbosch, South Africa; International Olympic Committee Research Centre, South Africa

JACQUE SCARAMELLA, MS, RD, CSSD
Sport Performance, United States Olympic Committee (US Paralympics), Chula Vista, California, USA

MARTIN SCHWELLNUS, MBBCh, MSc, MD
Section Sports Medicine, Faculty of Health Sciences and Sport, Exercise Medicine and Lifestyle Institute (SEMLI), University of Pretoria, International Olympic Committee Research Centre, Pretoria, South Africa

CARLA FILOMENA SILVA, BA, BSc, MSc, PhD
Lecturer, Social Science of Sport, School of Science and Technology, Nottingham Trent University, Nottingham, United Kingdom

LESLIE SWARTZ, PhD
Department of Psychology, Stellenbosch University, Matieland, South Africa

KALAI TSANG, MS
Human Engineering Research Laboratories, VA Pittsburgh Healthcare System, University of Pittsburgh, Pittsburgh, Pennsylvania, USA

YETSA A. TUAKLI-WOSORNU, MD, MPH
Assistant Clinical Professor, Department of Chronic Disease Epidemiology, Yale School of Public Health, New Haven, Connecticut, USA; Physical Medicine and Rehabilitation Clinician, Yale Department of Orthopaedics and Rehabilitation, New Haven, Connecticut, USA; International Olympic Committee Working Group: Prevention of Harassment and Abuse in Sport, Lausanne, Switzerland; Welfare Officer, International Paralympic Committee Medical Committee, Bonn, Germany

SEAN M. TWEEDY, PhD
Principal Investigator, International Paralympic Committee Classification Research and Development Partnership (Physical Impairments), Associate Professor, School of Human Movement and Nutrition Sciences, The University of Queensland, Brisbane, Australia

PETER VAN DE VLIET, PhD
Medical and Scientific Department, International Paralympic Committee, Bonn, Germany

MATTHIAS WALTER, MD, PhD, FEBU
Faculty of Medicine, International Collaboration on Repair Discoveries (ICORD), University of British Columbia, Vancouver, British Columbia, Canada

NICK WEBBORN, MB BS, FFSEM, MSc
Clinical Professor, Centre for Sport and Exercise Science and Medicine (SESAME), University of Brighton, The Welkin, Eastbourne, United Kingdom; School of Sport and Service Management, University of Brighton, East Sussex, United Kingdom

Contents

> Paralympic athletes have unique preexisting medical conditions that predispose them to increased risk of illness, but data are limited to studies conducted during the last 3 Paralympic Games. This article reviews the epidemiology of illness (risk, patterns, and predictors) in Paralympic athletes and provides practical guidelines for illness prevention. The incidence rate of illness (per 1000 athlete-days) in Paralympic athletes is high in Summer (10.0–13.2) and Winter (18.7) Paralympic Games. The authors propose general and specific guidelines on preventative strategies regarding illness in these athletes.

> Sport-related injury patterns among Para athletes have been described with increasing frequency. This article summarizes musculoskeletal injuries in Para athletes. Seated Para athletes sustain upper extremity injuries more commonly; ambulant Para athletes frequently sustain lower extremity injuries. The upper extremity is the most commonly injured anatomic area in all Para athletes, unlike able-bodied athletes. Advanced age and spinal cord injury may increase the risk of upper extremity injury. Injury data for recreational and youth Para athletes are sparse. Summarizing current injury epidemiology data may help to accelerate the development of injury prevention strategies and lifetime injury models for Para athletes.

> Individuals sustaining a spinal cord injury (SCI) frequently suffer from sensorimotor and autonomic impairment. Damage to the autonomic nervous system results in cardiovascular, respiratory, bladder, bowel, and sexual dysfunctions, as well as temperature dysregulation. These complications not only impede quality of life but also affect athletic performance of individuals with SCI. This article summarizes existing evidence on how

of Para athletes with physical impairments. Development of classification systems based on scientific evidence has only recently been made possible by adoption of a statement of the purpose of classification by the International Paralympic Committee and its member organizations. Rigorous descriptive science can improve extant systems of classification, and a recently published study described a data-driven classification structure with validity superior to that of the extant system.

Swimming is one of the inaugural sports within the Olympic and Paralympic Games, the key difference between the Olympic and Paralympic games being the classification system. The aim of this study was to investigate how effective the current classification system creates clearly differentiated Paralympic competition classes, based on performance time for all swimming strokes and events. Based on the performance characteristics of swimmers within the current classification system, the relationship between impairment and swimming performance is inconsistent, potentially disadvantaging some athletes. Appropriate sports medicine tests are required for the development of an evidence-based swimming classification system.

Technologies capable of projecting injury and performance metrics to athletes and coaches are being developed. Wheelchair athletes must be cognizant of their upper limb health; therefore, systems must be designed to promote efficient transfer of energy to the handrims and evaluated for simultaneous effects on the upper limbs. This article is a brief review of resources that help wheelchair users increase physiologic response to exercise, develop ideas for adaptive workout routines, locate accessible facilities and outdoor areas, and develop wheelchair sports-specific skills.

Prostheses form an essential part of participation in sport and physical activity for athletes with lower or upper limb amputation. These prostheses come in the form of everyday non–sport-specific prostheses, as well as sport-specific prostheses designed to enable participation in specific sports. Sport-specific prostheses are designed to the requirements of the sport to facilitate the achievement of peak performance without causing significant risk of injury. This article addresses the various factors associated with participation in sport and physical activity for individuals with amputation, including the various prostheses for upper and lower limbs and prostheses for different sports.

This article reviews the literature on Para sport athletic identity and provides avenues for future research direction. First, the authors briefly describe the existing quantitative and qualitative research on Para sport athletic identity and, thereby, illustrate the complexities Para sport athletes experience regarding the way they describe their participation in competitive sport. Next, the authors describe how Para sport athletes with acquired permanent disabilities and congenital disabilities face similar, yet unique, identity-related challenges. Finally, the authors argue that future researchers should consider examining Para sport athletes' identity through narrative identity.

This article explores the significance of Para sport culture in highlighting an emancipatory understanding of difference and enhancing social empowerment. Disability studies are used to illuminate the influence of ableist ideology on people with impairments. Rather than being suppressed, difference should be recognized and valued in Para sport practices and ideologies, leading to a pluralist culture, in which farther and wider social emancipation can be grounded. Acceptance of difference is an absolute and essential precondition for Para sport cultures to promote positive social change for people with disabilities.

Medicine has played an integral role in both the inception and development of the Paralympic Games. Sports physicians are well positioned to continue to influence the development of the Paralympic Movement and to help focus the movement on its agenda to promote social inclusion. This article analyzes critically at some of the key challenges that the Paralympic Movement faces in its quest to promote social inclusion and considers the role of sports medicine in this process.

The Paralympic Games have an interesting history that began after World War II. The Games and Movement have been affected by and have had an impact on society and the larger able-bodied sport system. The future of the Games and Movement is also further affected by larger cultural shifts, and the Games themselves have potentially left lasting legacies for the host cities and persons with impairment worldwide.

PHYSICAL MEDICINE AND REHABILITATION CLINICS OF NORTH AMERICA

RELATED INTEREST

Orthopedic Clinics, October 2016 (Vol. 47, Issue 4)
Sports-Related Injuries
The Campbell Clinic, *Editor*

VISIT THE CLINICS ONLINE!
Access your subscription at:
www.theclinics.com

Foreword
Maximizing One's Potential

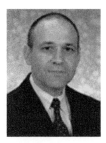

Santos F. Martinez, MD, MS
Consulting Editor

This issue of the *Physical Medicine and Rehabilitation Clinics of North America* is dedicated to all the volunteers, rehabilitation professionals, and organizations that have contributed to the evolvement of sports and exercise in this population. The rehabilitation and sports specialist, exercise physiologist, psychologist, and nutritionist all stand to become better informed regarding unique considerations when caring for these athletes. I commend the guest editors for their unique choice of authors, which additionally provides an international perspective. I hope it also serves as an incentive for the readers who have an interest in becoming more involved. Adapted sports exemplifies our ultimate objectives in rehabilitation. Maximizing ones capabilities rather than focusing on their limitations has always been a mantra in our field. The job does not stop with basic functional rehabilitation, but reintroduces missing components such as exercise and competition, which contribute to a better and healthier quality of life. Let these athletes serve as an inspiration for us all.

Santos F. Martinez, MD, MS
American Academy of Physical Medicine
and Rehabilitation
Campbell Clinic Orthopaedics
Department of Orthopaedics
University of Tennessee
Memphis, TN 38104, USA

E-mail address:
smartinez@campbellclinic.com

Phys Med Rehabil Clin N Am 29 (2018) xv
https://doi.org/10.1016/j.pmr.2018.02.002
1047-9651/18/© 2018 Published by Elsevier Inc.

Preface

Contemporary Medical, Scientific & Social Perspectives on Para Sport

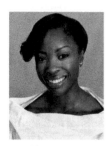 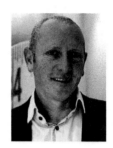

Yetsa A. Tuakli-Wosornu, MD, MPH

Wayne Derman, MBChB, MSc (Med) (Hons), PhD, FFIMS

Editors

Language and culture are interdependent. One is a reflection of the other. Over the past few decades, the popular and scientific language used to describe "Para sport" has changed dramatically, signifying society's evolving understanding of sport for individuals with impairment. "Disabled sport," "disability sport," and "adapted/adaptive sport" remain among the more common descriptors, while the term "handicapped sport" has all but disappeared from modern literature. In 2016, the International Paralympic Committee encouraged the use of the terms Para sport and Para athlete (capital "P," no hyphen), a reflection perhaps of the rising sociocultural status that sport for persons with impairment holds.

We perceive a meaningful distinction between the terms *Para* and *adapted*. "Para," a standalone prefix meaning "at or to one side of, beside, side by side," connotes objects, activities, or fields similar to but distinct from the base word (ie, paralegal). While "adapted sport" connotes sport that has been modified from its original form (ie, wheelchair tennis), "Para sport" encompasses all independent, self-governing sports for persons with impairment, whether or not an able-bodied equivalent exists (ie, goalball). This issue is dedicated to Para *and* adapted sport.

For the athletes and communities in which they play, Para sport matters. The physical and mental health benefits of sport for persons with intellectual and/or physical impairment are well documented. Furthermore, Para sport offers public health and social scientists a platform for discussing and developing modern social inclusion programming in both resource-rich and resource-scarce settings. At all levels of competition, from youth to recreational to collegiate to elite, Para sport is a powerful, positive tool for individuals, families, and communities.

Phys Med Rehabil Clin N Am 29 (2018) xvii–xviii
https://doi.org/10.1016/j.pmr.2018.02.001
1047-9651/18/© 2018 Published by Elsevier Inc.

pmr.theclinics.com

At the elite level, Para sport has increased in popularity and visibility. With 4302 athletes, the London 2012 Paralympic Games ushered in a watershed change in public perception and commercial appeal of Para sport. Brands looked beyond disability and bought into high-performance sport with a diverse and inclusive image. London had a global television audience of 3.8 billion viewers in 115 countries and was hailed as the "greatest Paralympic Games ever." Sochi 2014 and Rio 2016 continued the trend: Rio received an unprecedented 116 hours of television coverage in the United States and included 4378 athletes.

While its commercial success has been meteoric, developments in Para sport science and medicine may not be as public. In recent years, there has been a significant increase in the knowledge and research related to the science, medicine, and technology of Para sport. This increase is reflected in the current publication. Our goal with this issue of *Physical Medicine and Rehabilitation Clinics of North America* is to present a wide-reaching, contemporary overview of Para sport through the lens of clinical, physiologic, public health, social, and technological science, building on J. Bergeron's original *Physical Medicine and Rehabilitation Clinics of North America* article, "Athletes with Disabilities" (February 1999). Our hope is that the entire *Physical Medicine and Rehabilitation Clinics of North America* audience, a diverse cadre of function-focused clinicians and scientists, will find something that speaks directly to their practice, passion, and purpose.

With great enthusiasm, we thank all of the international experts who have contributed and wish you, the audience, a pleasant read. We hope this issue of *Physical Medicine and Rehabilitation Clinics of North America* ignites a new passion for the exciting and diverse field of Para and adapted sport.

Yetsa A. Tuakli-Wosornu, MD, MPH
Department of Chronic Disease Epidemiology
Yale School of Public Health
60 College Street
New Haven, Connecticut 06511, USA

Wayne Derman, MBChB, MSc (Med) (Hons), PhD, FFIMS
Institute of Sports and Exercise Medicine
International Olympic Committee Research Centre–South Africa
FIFA Medical Center of Excellence
Division of Orthopaedic Surgery
Faculty of Medicine and Health Sciences
University of Stellenbosch
PO Box 19063
Francie Van Zijl Drive
Rylaan, Tygerberg 7505, South Africa

E-mail addresses:
yetsa.tuakli-wosornu@yale.edu (Y.A. Tuakli-Wosornu)
ewderman@iafrica.com (W. Derman)

Illness Among Paralympic Athletes

Epidemiology, Risk Markers, and Preventative Strategies

Dina Christina Janse Van Rensburg, MBChB, MSc, MMed, MD[a],*,
Martin Schwellnus, MBBCh, MSc, MD[a,b],
Wayne Derman, MBChB, MSc (Med) (Hons), PhD, FFIMS[b,c],
Nick Webborn, MB BS, FFSEM, MSc[d]

KEYWORDS

- Paralympic • Athletes • Illness • Epidemiology • Risk markers • Prevention

KEY POINTS

- Paralympic athletes have a documented risk of contracting an illness at times of key sporting events, such as the Paralympic Games.
- Illness patterns are consistent for the Summer and Winter Paralympic Games, mainly affecting the respiratory, dermatologic, and digestive systems.
- Data are limited on identifying potential risk markers for illness, but there are data that show that sporting code (specifically athletics) may be an important extrinsic risk marker for illness.
- Current available studies suggest that age and sex are not accountable as risk markers.

INTRODUCTION

The Paralympic movement, through its International Paralympic Committee (IPC) Medical Code, is committed to ensure athlete health, and the IPC encourages all initiatives and measures to minimize the risk of injury and illness in Paralympic athletes (https://www.paralympic.org/ice-hockey/athletes/health; accessed 25 August 2017).

[a] Section Sports Medicine, Faculty of Health Sciences and Sport, Exercise Medicine and Lifestyle Institute (SEMLI), University of Pretoria, Sports Campus, Burnett Street, Hatfield, Pretoria 0020, South Africa; [b] International Olympic Committee (IOC) Research Centre, Sports Campus, Burnett Street, Hatfield, Pretoria 0020, South Africa; [c] Faculty of Medicine and Health Sciences, Institute of Sport and Exercise Medicine (ISEM), Stellenbosch University, Francie van Zijl Drive, Tygerberg, 7505 Cape Town, South Africa; [d] Centre for Sport and Exercise Science and Medicine (SESAME), University of Brighton, The Welkin, Carlisle Road, Eastbourne BN20 7SN, UK
* Corresponding author.
E-mail address: Christa.JanseVanRensburg@up.ac.za

Phys Med Rehabil Clin N Am 29 (2018) 185–203
https://doi.org/10.1016/j.pmr.2018.01.003
1047-9651/18/© 2018 Elsevier Inc. All rights reserved.
pmr.theclinics.com

One of these initiatives is to conduct injury and illness epidemiologic studies during the Paralympic Games in order to identify the patterns of injury and illness as well as identify risk factors associated with injury and illness. Such epidemiologic studies have been conducted for injuries since 2002 at the Winter Paralympic Games,[1-3] and from 2012 for injury[4,5] and illness at the Summer[4,6] and Winter Paralympic Games.[3] Although the injury profile of Paralympic athletes has been better studied,[1-5] the literature on the illness profiles is limited to studies conducted at the London 2012 Summer Paralympic Games, the Sochi 2014 Winter Paralympic Games, and the Rio 2016 Summer Paralympic Games.[3,4,6] Data from these studies can be used to design preventative strategies to reduce the risk of injury and illness in order to protect the health of Paralympic athletes.

Until recently, studies focused mostly on injury and injury prevention. However, illness is at least as important as injury, because it not only affects the athlete during the competition period but also has a potential long-term effect on the health of the athlete after the competition period.[4,7-9] Paralympic athletes, in contrast to Olympic athletes, potentially have a range of preexisting medical conditions, and these athletes therefore face unique medical problems, such as autonomic dysfunction, neurogenic bladder, neurologic disorders, premature osteoporosis, and stump socket interface complications, that can predispose them to an increased risk of further illness.[1,10,11]

The aim of this article is to review illness in Paralympic athletes in the following 3 aspects: (1) the risk of illness, (2) patterns of illness, and (3) possible predictors of illness in Paralympic athletes that may predispose them to illness before, during, and after competitions. Finally, the authors also want to suggest practical guidelines for the prevention of illness in Paralympic athletes.

METHODOLOGY

A literature search was conducted to source published information on (1) the risk of illness, (2) patterns of illness, and (3) possible predictors of illness in Paralympic athletes. The authors' search strategy to obtain relevant peer-reviewed publications was based on the methodology used in systematic reviews. A search was conducted on PubMed, CINAHL, Google Scholar, and SPORTDiscus databases, using the following keywords in different combinations: Paralympic, impairment, disability, illness, prevention of illness, medical conditions, international sporting events, and athletes. The authors included only publications in English and studies that involved human participants. After removing duplicates, the initial search revealed 66 publications. A further 21 publications were sourced from the reference lists of the reviewed publications. Two researchers (D.C.J.v.R. and M.S.) then independently reviewed the abstracts from these 87 publications, using the following inclusion criteria for studies in this article:

- Studies involving Paralympic athletes of all levels (recreational to elite) and sports;
- Studies involving a Paralympic Games setting;
- Studies where a specific definition of illness was included and explained.

For uniformity in reporting, the authors only used publications that defined illness as "any athlete requiring medical attention, regardless of the consequences with respect to absence from competition *or training*." A medical illness was specifically defined as "any newly acquired illness as well as exacerbations of pre-existing illness that occurred during training and/or competition or during or immediately before the Winter/Summer Paralympic Games."[3,6,12,13] The final number of studies included in this narrative review of the risk of illness, patterns of illness, and possible predictors of illness in Paralympic athletes was 3. From the initial search (87 publications), all publications that related to the unique medical problems suffered by Paralympic athletes (12 publications), as well as those publications referring to general preventative measures (8 publications), were included for the final part of this article.

RISK OF ILLNESS IN PARALYMPIC ATHLETES
Incidence Rate and Incidence Proportion of Illness in Paralympic Athletes Versus Olympic Athletes

The incidence of illness (incidence rate [IR]) (per 1000 athlete-days) and the incidence proportion of illness (IP) (% of all athletes with illness during the Games) in Paralympic athletes compared with Olympic athletes competing in both the Summer and the Winter Games are presented in **Table 1**. The first main observation from this table is that the IR in Paralympic athletes during the Summer Games varies from 10.0 to 13.2 (Rio 2016 Paralympic Games and London 2012 Paralympic Games). This finding implies that in a team of 100 athletes, the team physician will consult with about one ill athlete each day. A second observation is that in Paralympic athletes the IR is significantly higher in the Winter Games (Sochi 2014) (18.7; 95% confidence interval [CI], 15.1–23.2) compared with both the London (13.2; 95% CI, 12.2–14.2) and the Rio (10.0; 95% CI, 9.2–10.9) Summer Games.

A further observation is that the IP of illness is almost twice as high in Paralympic compared with Olympic athletes, and this is evident in both the Summer (Paralympic = 12.4%–14.2%; Olympic = 5%–7%) and the Winter Games (Paralympic = 17.4%; Olympic = 9%). Therefore, these data indicate that Paralympic athletes are at higher risk of contracting an illness during the Winter, compared with the Summer Games, and that Paralympic athletes are at higher risk of illness compared with Olympic athletes.

Incidence of Illness in Paralympic Athletes in Different Organ Systems

The IR and IP of illness in Paralympic athletes in different organ systems during the Summer and Winter Paralympic Games are represented in **Table 2**. The main observation is that the IR of illness in Paralympic athletes is consistently highest in the respiratory system, followed by skin and subcutaneous tissue, gastrointestinal tract (GIT), and genitourinary tract (GUT). In both the Summer and Winter Paralympic Games, illness was most common in the respiratory system. However, the authors note that during the Summer Paralympic Games there was a higher incidence of skin, nervous system, and ear, nose, and throat involvement compared with the Winter Paralympic Games, whereas mental illness and eye involvement were more common in the Winter Paralympic Games (see **Table 2**). Therefore, the overall pattern of illness affecting the different organ systems in Paralympic athletes during competition shows a very consistent pattern (respiratory, dermatologic, and digestive being the most common), but there are small differences in illness affecting organ systems during the Summer Games versus the Winter Games.

RISK MARKERS FOR ILLNESS IN PARALYMPIC ATHLETES

The identification of risk markers for illness is a key element in the development of any intervention strategy for illness. However, from the authors' literature search, to date, there are very limited data on extrinsic (precompetition vs competition period, sport code, medication, and other) and intrinsic (age, sex, and other) risk markers for illness in Paralympic athletes. Indeed, the authors are only aware of 4 epidemiologic studies wherein risk markers for illness in Paralympic athletes were explored.[3,6,12,13] In 3 of

Table 1
The number of athletes, athlete-days, number of illnesses, incidence proportion, and incidence (per 1000 athlete-days) of illness in the Summer and Winter Paralympic and Olympic Games

			Athletes	Athlete-Days	No. of Illnesses	No. of Athletes with Illness	IP (% Athletes with Illness)	IR/1000 Athlete-Days	IR 95% CI
Summer Games	Paralympic Games	London	3565	49,910	657	505	14.2	13.2	12.2–14.2
		Rio	3657	51,198	511	454	12.4	10.0	9.2–10.9
	Olympic Games	London	10,568	179,656[a]	758	—	7.2	4.2[b]	—
		Rio	11,274	191,658[a]	613	587	5.4	3.2[b]	—
Winter Games	Paralympic Games	Sochi (Winter)	547	6564	123	95	17.4	18.7	15.1–23.2
	Olympic Games	Sochi (Winter)	2780	50,040[a]	249	—	8.9	5.0[b]	—

[a] Estimated athlete-days (calculated as the total quantity of participating athletes multiplied by the number of days at the games. *Limitation:* assumption that all athletes were present for all days).
[b] Estimated IR.
Data from Refs.[3,6,8,13–15]

these studies,[3,12,13] only univariate analysis was performed, and in only one study,[6] a regression model was applied to identify independent risk markers for illness in Paralympic athletes. Therefore, although data to identify risk markers for illness are very limited, the authors review the evidence for these risk markers accordingly.

Extrinsic Risk Markers for Illness in Paralympic Athletes

Precompetition versus competition period

Evaluation of precompetition versus competition illness allows an indirect evaluation of the health status of athletes arriving in the Games setting. In one study during the 2010 Winter Paralympic Games, 2717 medical encounters were recorded (657 athletes, 682 International Federation/National Paralympic Committee officials, 57 IPC officials, 1075 workforce, 8 media, 127 spectators, and 111 others). The investigators reported a higher incidence of medical encounters during the competition period.[16] However, because there was no distinction made between nonathletes and athletes, or between injury and illness, the precompetition or competition periods could not be identified as extrinsic risk markers for illness from this study. In contrast, data from 2 recent prospective studies during the Summer Paralympic Games showed no difference in the IR of illness (per 1000 athlete-days) between the precompetition (London 2012, IR 14.6; 95% CI 12.4–17.1; Rio 2016, IR 9.6; 95% CI 7.9–11.6) versus the competition period (London 2012, IR 12.8; 95% CI 11.7–17.1; Rio 2016, IR 10.1; 95% CI 9.2–11.1).[6,13] Therefore, the precompetition versus the competition period does not appear to be extrinsic risk markers for illness in Paralympic athletes.

Sport code

The IR of illness per 1000 athlete-days as well as the IP of illness in Paralympic athletes per Summer sport codes is summarized in **Table 3**. Reviewing the univariate data available from 2 datasets, the risk of illness differed between sporting codes. In London 2012, equestrian sports (20.7), powerlifting (15.8), athletics (15.4), and table tennis

Table 2
The number, percentage of all illnesses, incidence proportion of illness, and incidence rate (per 1000 athletes) of illness in different organ systems in Paralympic athletes during the Summer and Winter Paralympic Games

| | Summer Paralympic Games | | | | | | | | Winter Paralympic Games | | | |
| | London 2012 | | | | Rio 2016 | | | | Sochi 2014 | | | |
	N[a]	%	IP	IR	N[a]	%	IP	IR	N[a]	%	IP	IR
Respiratory	180	29	27.4	3.6	167	33	4.4	3.3	37	30	5.5	5.6
Skin and subcutaneous	120	20	18.3	2.4	91	18	2.4	1.8	16	13	2.4	2.4
Digestive	95	15	14.5	1.9	66	13	1.8	1.3	16	13	2.6	2.4
Genitourinary	56	9	8.5	1.1	55	11	1.5	1.1	8	7	1.5	1.2
Nervous	63	10	9.6	1.3	21	4	0.5	0.4	—	0	—	—
Mental and behavior	7	1	1.1	0.1	19	4	0.5	0.4	8	7	1.5	1.2
Ears and mastoid	44	7	6.7	0.9	15	3	0.4	0.3	—	0	—	—
Eye and adnexa	25	4	3.8	0.5	13	3	0.4	0.3	18	15	3.1	2.7
Circulatory	3	0	0.5	0.1	12	2	0.3	0.2	—	0	—	—

Abbreviations: %, % of illness in organ systems; N, number of illnesses.
[a] Illness in other systems were not included (London, n = 64; Rio, n = 52; Sochi, n = 20).
Data from Refs.[3,6,13]

Table 3
The number of illnesses, percentage of total number of illnesses, incidence proportion, and incidence rate of illness in different Summer Paralympic sporting codes

Summer Paralympic Sporting Code	London 2012				Rio 2016			
	Total Number of Athletes Competing in the Sport Code	Total Number of Illnesses in the Sport Code	IP in the Sport Code	IR in the Sport Code	Total Number of Athletes Competing in the Sport Code	Total Number of Illnesses in the Sport Code	IP in the Sport Code	IR in the Sport Code
Archery	128	20	15.6	11.2	113	14	10.6	8.9
Athletics	977	210	21.5	15.4	894	129	12.9	10.3
Boccia	98	16	16.3	11.7	99	17	16.2	12.3
Canoe	$	$	$	$	52	10	17.3	13.7
Cycling (track and road)	—	—	—	—	204	30	13.2	10.5
Cycling—road	182	36	19.8	14.1	—	—	—	—
Cycling—track	92	16	17.4	12.4	—	—	—	—
Equestrian	69	20	29	20.7	71	9	11.3	9.1
Football, 5-a-side	70	8	11.4	8.2	70	4	5.7	4.1
Football, 7-a-side	96	3	3.1	2.2	112	5	4.5	3.2
Goalball	110	13	11.8	8.4	102	8	7.8	5.6
Judo	115	15	13	9.3	115	6	5.2	3.7
Powerlifting	163	36	22.1	15.8	141	16	9.9	8.1

Rowing	91	18	19.8	14.1	88	12	13.6	9.7
Sailing	70	13	18.6	13.3	76	12	13.2	11.3
Shooting	33	2	6.1	4.3	130	22	16.9	12.1
Sitting volleyball	154	22	14.3	10.2	127	14	10.2	7.9
Swimming	499	91	18.2	13	492	87	15.4	12.6
Table tennis	226	48	21.2	15.2	223	29	12.1	9.3
Triathlon	$	$	$	$	58	4	6.9	4.9
Wheelchair basketball	202	40	19.8	14.1	228	40	14.5	12.5
Wheelchair fencing	95	16	16.8	12	72	15	15.3	14.9
Wheelchair rugby	79	12	15.2	10.8	96	18	15.6	13.4
Wheelchair tennis	106	20	18.9	13.5	94	10	7.4	7.6

Abbreviation: $, sport code only included from 2016.

Data from Schwellnus M, Derman W, Jordaan E, et al. Factors associated with illness in athletes participating in the London 2012 Paralympic Games: a prospective cohort study involving 49,910 athlete-days. Br J Sports Med 2013;47(7):433–40; and Derman W, Schwellnus MP, Jordaan E, et al. Sport, sex and age increase risk of illness at the Rio 2016 Summer Paralympic Games: a prospective cohort study of 51,198 athlete days. Br J Sports Med 2018;52(1):17–23.

(15.2) had higher crude unadjusted IR of illness compared with all other sports. In Rio 2016, wheelchair fencing (14.9), swimming (12.6), and wheelchair basketball (12.5) were the sporting codes with the highest IR. However, multivariate regression analysis was only performed on the London 2012 data, and this showed that only athletics (adjusted for gender and age) was associated with a higher risk of illness compared with other sporting codes ($P = .01$). Therefore, Paralympic athletes participating in athletics during the Summer Paralympic Games appear to be more susceptible to illness compared with other sporting codes. However, this conclusion is based on only a single study wherein sporting code, as a risk marker for illness, was assessed using multivariate analysis.

The IR of illness per 1000 athlete-days as well as the IP of illness in Paralympic athletes per Winter sport codes is summarized in **Table 4**. During the Sochi 2014 Winter Paralympic Games, the IR of illness was similar in 4 sporting categories. Again, based on very limited data, sporting code is not an independent risk marker for illness in Winter Paralympic athletes.

Other possible extrinsic risk markers for illness

It is well recognized that there are many more risk markers (travel, training load, competition load, nutrition, personal habits, and so forth) that may contribute to increased risk of illness in elite athletes, and these risk markers were recently reviewed.[17] However, these markers have not been researched in Paralympic athletes. It would be reasonable to assume that extrinsic risk markers for illness in elite Olympic athletes, such as training load, travel, and change of environment, would be equally applicable to Paralympic athletes.

Presently, data indicate that high absolute training and competition loads are associated with an increased risk of illness in subelite and recreational athletes (J-shaped curve), but are not related to increased risk of illness in elite athletes (S-shaped curve).[17] It has been suggested that training monotony is a possible risk marker for increased risk of illness. In elite cross-country skiers, there was a lower risk of illness in the period when little changes were added to training load,[18] but this finding could not be reproduced in a group of 32 rugby league players whereby training monotony was associated with a higher risk of illness.[19] The relationship between training load and illness in Paralympic athletes requires further study. Competition load has also been associated with increased risk of illness,[20] but this has not yet been studied systematically in Paralympic athletes.

Table 4
The number of illnesses, percentage of total number of illnesses, incidence proportion, and incidence rate of illness in different Winter Paralympic sporting codes

Winter Paralympic Sporting Code	Total Number of Athletes Competing in the Sport Code	Total Number of Illnesses in the Sport Code	IP in the Sport Code	IR in the Sport Code
Alpine skiing/ snowboarding	219	51	18.7	19.4
Cross-country skiing/ biathlon	149	30	16.1	16.8
Ice sledge hockey	129	30	14	19.4
Wheelchair curling	50	12	24	20

Data from Derman W, Schwellnus MP, Jordaan E, et al. The incidence and patterns of illness at the Sochi 2014 Winter Paralympic Games: a prospective cohort study of 6564 athlete days. Br J Sports Med 2016;50(17):1064–8.

The modern-day Paralympic athlete needs to travel globally, often across multiple time zones to compete. A study by Schwellnus and colleagues[20] showed that elite able-bodied athletes traveling to international destinations crossing more than 5 time zones distant from their home country have a potential 2 to 3 times increased risk of all illness, in comparison to return to home travel. The same pattern was seen for respiratory tract illness, GIT illness, and all infective illness. Thus, an increase in the incidence of illness may also be associated with the distant destinations rather than with travel per se. In another prospective study, international travel was also reported as an independent risk factor for illness among elite cross-country skiers.[18] Changes in environmental conditions (eg, temperature, humidity, climate, altitude, pollution, and pollens), nutrition and exposure to diverse cultures, populations, and pathogens could all be involved.[20] Winter Paralympic Games compared with Summer Paralympic Games may also be associated with an increased risk of illness because of weather conditions and seasonal change. The relationship between international travel and changes in environmental conditions as risk markers for illness in Paralympic athletes requires further investigation.

Finally, other extrinsic risk markers for illness in Paralympic athletes, such as nutrition and personal habits, have not been studied. These other extrinsic risk markers are important and should also be further investigated.

Intrinsic Risk Markers for Illness in Paralympic Athletes

Age
Crude unadjusted IRs of illness in the Sochi 2014 Winter Paralympic Games and the Rio 2016 Summer Paralympic Games indicate that older athletes (older than 35 years) had a higher IR of illness compared with younger athletes (Sochi 2014, IR 22.6; 95% CI, 16.0–31.9; Rio 2016, IR 11.8; 95% CI, 10.3–13.4).[3,13] However, adjusted IRs from the London 2012 Summer Paralympic Games did not confirm that the older Paralympic athlete is at higher risk of illness.[6]

Sex
Sex does not appear to be an intrinsic risk marker for illness in Paralympic athletes. In the London 2012 Summer Paralympic Games, adjusted IRs of illness in female and male Paralympic athletes were not different.[6] Similarly, crude unadjusted IRs of illness were similar in female and male Paralympic athletes during the Sochi 2014 Winter Paralympic Games (women, IR 18.1; 95% CI, 11.6–28.3; men, IR 18.9; 95% CI, 14.9–24.2).[3] However, in the Rio 2016 Summer Paralympic Games, Derman and colleagues[13] reported that women had a higher risk of illness compared with men (women, IR 11.1; 95% CI, 9.7–12.7: men, IR 9.3, 95% CI, 8.3–10.4), but these were crude unadjusted IRs. Therefore, the authors conclude that sex is not an intrinsic risk factor for illness in Paralympic athletes, but this also requires further research.

Other possible intrinsic risk markers for illness in Paralympic athletes
There are other potential intrinsic risk markers for illness in Paralympic athletes, including impairment type, underlying unique medical problems in Paralympic athletes, and others. In general, research to identify these as independent intrinsic risk markers for illness is very limited.

Impairment type
Although the classification system has recently been changed, literature identified for this review reported data based on the previous system, that is, spinal cord–related injury (SCI), amputation or limb deficiency, cerebral palsy, les autres (all others), visual impairment, and intellectual impairment.[10] There are data suggesting that the type of

impairment is an intrinsic risk marker for illness in Paralympic athletes. For the London 2012 Summer Paralympic Games, the highest proportion of illness was reported in athletes with SCI (115 illnesses; 29.9% of all illnesses) followed by athletes with amputation or limb deficiency (102 illnesses; 26.5% of all illnesses) and athletes with visual impairment (81 illnesses, 21% of all illnesses). Similarly, in the Rio 2016 Summer Paralympics Games, athletes with SCI had the highest proportion of illnesses (162 illnesses, 31.7% of all illnesses), followed by athletes with limb deficiency (118 illnesses, 23.1% of all illnesses), and central neurologic injury (79 illnesses, 15.5% of all illnesses) (**Table 5**). The major limitations of these data are that there was no control group of uninjured athletes for the various impairment types. Therefore, true IR, and adjusted IR, could not be reported. The above limitations are important areas for further research so that targeted prevention program for illness prevention in higher risk groups can be developed and implemented.

Underlying unique medical conditions in Paralympic athletes

Various impairment types are associated with unique and preexisting medical conditions. Most of these medical conditions are associated with comorbidities and therefore are potentially associated with a higher risk of illness.[4] Some of the unique

Table 5
The total number of reported illnesses (on the WEB-IISS)[a], and the percentage of illnesses by impairment type during the Summer Paralympic Games

	London 2012 (WEB-IISS Data)		Rio 2016 (WEB-IISS Data)	
	Total Number of Illnesses	% of Total Number of Illnesses	Total Number of Illnesses	% of Total Number of Illnesses
Spinal cord injury	115	29.9	162	31.7
Limb deficiency (amputation, dysmelia, congenital deformity)	102	26.5	118	23.1
Central neurologic injury (cerebral palsy, traumatic brain injury, stroke, other neurologic impairment)	38	9.9	79	15.5
Visual impairment	81	21	62	12.1
Intellectual impairment	10	2.6	27	5.3
Les autres (nonspinal poliomyelitis, ankylosis, leg shortening, joint movement restriction, nerve injury resulting in local paralysis)	39	10.1	13	2.5
Other	—	—	31	6.1
Unknown	—	—	6	1.2
Short stature	—	—	13	2.5

[a] WEB-IISS (web-based injury and illness surveillance system) a previous classification system used to conform as per reported in the identified publications.

Data from Derman W, Schwellnus M, Jordaan E. Clinical characteristics of 385 illnesses of athletes with impairment reported on the WEB-IISS system during the London 2012 Paralympic Games. PM R 2014;6(8 Suppl):S23–30; and Derman W, Schwellnus MP, Jordaan E, et al. Sport, sex and age increase risk of illness at the Rio 2016 Summer Paralympic Games: a prospective cohort study of 51,198 athlete days. Br J Sports Med 2018;52(1):17–23.

Table 6
Unique medical conditions (including mechanisms and pathophysiology) in Paralympic athletes that may predispose to illness risk

Impairment Type	Illness Risk	Mechanism/Pathophysiology	Preventative Measures
Spinal cord injury	Heat illness/hypothermia	Altered regulation of body temperature: Loss of ANS if level >T8 Loss of mechanisms such as sweating and shivering Medication use Loss of sensation	Prevent dehydration and heat illness Use of cooling vests, water sprays, cooling fans (combined with wetted hair and head) Emersion of hands and wrists in cold water Nutritional interventions Appropriate clothing Proper hydration
	Urinary tract infection	Neurogenic bladder: Dehydration Incomplete voiding Increased pressure Catheter use Poor hand hygiene	Good hand hygiene & sanitation Regular bladder emptying Antiseptic catheterization Routine (daily) urine dipstick monitoring If asymptomatic: routine treatment with antibiotics not recommended (many SCI patients have culture bacteriuria) If symptomatic: antibiotic course for 10–14 d
	Renal calculi	Neurogenic bladder: Dehydration Incomplete voiding Increased pressure	Proper hydration Regular bladder emptying
	Constipation	Bowel mobility is compromised	Nutritional intervention (eg, dried fruit and increased fiber) Proper hydration
	CV stressors	Restricted potential for improvement in cardiac output & Vo_{2max} (excess CV strain) Lesion around T1-4 will limit HR to 110–130 Resting heart rate is decreased Stroke volumes is lowered at rest and during exercise	Wear heart rate monitors Manage training and competition load

(continued on next page)

Table 6
(continued)

Impairment Type	Illness Risk	Mechanism/Pathophysiology	Preventative Measures
	Life-threatening conditions in the CNS (cerebral hemorrhage, seizures), CV (arrhythmias, myocardial ischemia), and pulmonary (edema) systems	Autonomic dysreflexia Injury usually at or >T6 level Sympathetic pathway blocked Hypertension Vagal nerve activity (HR substantially lower)	Avoid triggers (bladder distension, urinary tract infections, catheter blocks, noxious stimuli) Education (bowel and bladder maintenance, skin care) Do not allow training or competition in a boosted state (IPC)
	Pressure ulcers (sores)	Extrinsic risk factors (pressure, shear, friction, immobility, and moisture) Intrinsic risk factors (condition of the patient, such as sepsis, local infection, decreased autonomic control, altered level of consciousness, increased age, vascular occlusive disease, anemia, malnutrition, sensory loss, spasticity, and contractures)	Skin care
	Premature osteopenia/osteoporosis	Disuse Neural factors	Mechanical stimulus to bones of lower limb Nutritional interventions, for example, calcium supplements, vit. D Consider medication (calcitonin, bisphosphonates) Care with transfer from chair
Cerebral palsy	Convulsive disorders	Underlying abnormality Triggers (dehydration, emotional stress, hypoglycemia, hyperventilation, electrolyte imbalances)	Increased lactic acid (lowered pH) stabilizes membranes and lower risk of seizures (aerobic exercise) Prevent triggers (dehydration, emotional stress, hypoglycemia, hyperventilation, electrolyte imbalances) Compliance with antiseizure medication
	Predisposition for musculoskeletal injury	Increased muscle tone Altered biomechanical stresses	Focus strength training on extension exercise (flexion often dominates) Physical therapy with special attention to stretching

Group	Condition/Diagnosis	Description	Management/Prevention
Amputees	Heat illness/hypothermia	Altered regulation of body temperature Loss of body surface	Prevent dehydration and heat illness Use of cooling vests, water sprays, ice slush ingestion, cooling fans (combined with wetted air and head) Emersion of hands and wrists in cold water Nutritional requirements Appropriate clothing
	Infections (stump)	Chafing of stump	Well-fitted prosthesis and socket Silicone lining Appropriate skin care (talcum powder/cool clothing) Appropriate rest and recovery of stump Daily stump skin inspection
	Choke syndrome	Venous return from the stump is impaired, allowing for lymphatic and venous pooling in surrounding soft tissue	Daily assessment of stump Correct use of liners for compression
	Phantom limb pain		Good pain management, advanced management with respect to psychological and physiotherapeutic interventions, for example, cognitive behavioral therapy, mindfulness interventions, and mirror therapy
	Recurrence of malignancy		Screening
Les autres	Diverse diagnosis	For example, multiple sclerosis: increased risk of exacerbation by • Overfatigue • Increased core temperature	Participate in water sports
Visually impaired	Sleep patterns		Education Choice of accommodation area
Intellectually impaired	For example, Down syndrome	Concern is cervical instability/heart defects	Comprehensive preparticipation evaluation

Abbreviations: ANS, autonomic nervous system; CNS, central nervous system; CV, cardiovascular; HR, heart rate.
Data from Refs. [6,10,11,21–29]

medical conditions in Paralympic athletes from various impairment categories are summarized in **Table 6**.

Of particular interest is a recent study in which a high prevalence of cardiovascular abnormalities was reported in Paralympic athletes. In a group of Italian athletes (n = 267) that were studied between 2000 and 2012, structural cardiac abnormalities (cardiomyopathy, aorta root dilatation, and valvular disease) were reported in 33 athletes (12%), and arrhythmogenic cardiac disease was identified in 9 athletes (3.4%).[30] Underlying cardiovascular disease may therefore also predispose these athletes to a risk of an acute event.[30] In addition, a reasonably high prevalence of coronary risk factors (systemic hypertension, family history of premature coronary heart disease, smoking, elevated triglycerides, high cholesterol, diabetes, and obesity) was reported in a small cohort of Brazilian Paralympic athletes (79 athletes).[31]

In one study, chronic medication use, as part of the management of these underlying medical conditions, was documented in Paralympic athletes. The major groups of medicines used by Paralympic athletes include central nervous system drugs, antihypertensives, antithrombotics, cholesterol-lowering drugs, and bronchodilators.[22] Chronic medication use carries a risk of side effects that may compromise the athlete's health. The additional intake of pain medication may further burden the Paralympic athlete's health.

PREVENTATIVE STRATEGIES TO DECREASE RISK OF ILLNESS IN PARALYMPIC ATHLETES
General Preventative Strategies

The general preventative strategies to reduce the risk of illness in elite athletes have recently been reviewed.[17] It is reasonable to assume that these measures are equally applicable to Paralympic athletes and can therefore be applied in these athletes. In **Box 1**, the authors suggest general preventative strategies to limit illness in Paralympic athletes, which they adapted from the recently reviewed strategies for able-bodied athletes.[17]

Specific Preventative Strategies

However, in Paralympic athletes, there is an additional layer of medical complexity that is related to the considerable structural and anatomic differences in athletes with disabilities.[28,29] Therefore, specific medical considerations and related preventative strategies to reduce the risk of illness in Paralympic athletes are important. The authors therefore suggest specific preventative strategies for these unique medical conditions in Paralympic athletes (see **Table 6**).

Finally, regular periodic health assessments (PHA) are essential and should include a baseline and frequent functional reviews. Information on health conditions, medication use, and immunization is important. In this process, the team physician can identify conditions that may require close supervision during training or even need further evaluation before the athlete is cleared for participation.[3,28,29,32]

SUMMARY

Paralympic athletes have a documented risk of contracting an illness at times of key sporting events, such as the Paralympic Games. In this article, the authors identify that Paralympic athletes have a significantly higher likelihood of becoming ill in the Winter Games compared with the Summer Games. Furthermore, illness patterns are consistent for the Summer and Winter Paralympic Games, mainly affecting the respiratory, dermatologic, and digestive systems. Data are limited on identifying potential risk

Box 1
General guidelines for illness prevention in Paralympic athletes

A. Infective illness (referring mostly to respiratory and GIT)
  Athletes are advised to:
  a. Minimize contact with infected people, young children, animals, and contagious objects;
  b. Avoid crowded areas and shaking hands and minimize contact with people outside the team and support staff;
  c. Keep a distance to people who are coughing, sneezing, or have a "runny nose," and, when appropriate, wear (or ask them to wear) a disposable mask;
  d. Cough or sneeze on to the elbow and not on the hands—always clean the hands and nose after sneezing or coughing;
  e. Wash hands regularly and effectively with soap and water, especially before meals, and after direct contact with potentially contagious people, animals, blood, secretions, public places, and bathrooms;
  f. Use disposable paper towels and limit hand to mouth/nose contact when suffering from upper respiratory symptoms or gastrointestinal illness (putting hands to eyes and nose is a major route of viral self-inoculation);
  g. Carry insect repellent, antimicrobial foam/cream, or alcohol-based hand washing gel with them;
  h. Do not share drinking bottles, cups, cutlery, towels, and so forth, with other people;
  i. Choose beverages from sealed bottles, avoid raw vegetables and undercooked meat, wash and peel fruit before eating, while competing or training abroad.
  Medical staff is advised to:
  a. Screen for airway inflammation disturbances (asthma, allergy, and other inflammatory airway conditions);
  b. Arrange for single-room accommodations during tournaments for athletes with heavy competition load or known susceptibility to respiratory tract infections, or high-performance priority athletes;
  c. Consider protecting the airways of athletes from being directly exposed to very cold (<0°C) and dry air during strenuous exercise by using a facial mask;
  d. Update athletes and support staff on vaccines needed at home and for foreign travel and take into consideration that influenza vaccines take 5 to 7 weeks to take effect; intramuscular vaccines may have a few small side effects; vaccinations are performed preferably out of season; and avoid vaccinating just before competitions or if symptoms of illness are present;
  e. Consider zinc lozenges (high ionic zinc content) at the onset of upper respiratory symptoms, because there is some evidence that the number of days with illness symptoms can be reduced.
  f. Measure and monitor for early signs and symptoms of illness:
    i. On-going illness (and injury) surveillance systems should be implemented in all sports;
    ii. Athletes should be monitored, using sensitive tools, for subclinical signs of illness, such as nonspecific symptoms and signs, or selected special investigations;
    iii. Athletes should be monitored for overt symptoms and signs of illness.
  The athlete support team can:
  a. Consider to advise athletes to ingest probiotics, such as Lactobacillus probiotics on a daily basis;
  b. Consider advising athletes on the regular consumption of fruits and plants, polyphenol supplements (eg, quercetin), or foodstuffs (eg, nonalcoholic beer and green tea) that may reduce risk of illness.

B. Travel issues
  Environmental conditions:
  Take into consideration:
  a. Temperature changes;
  b. Destination altitude;
  c. Humidity;
  d. Atmospheric pollution;
  e. Aero allergen exposure;
  f. Different strains of pathogenic organisms.

Jet lag and travel fatigue:

Depending on east-bound or west-bound flight, the guidelines will differ:

a. Nonpharmacologic management:

  i. Preadaptation;

  ii. Bright light therapy making use of blue light exposure, amber lenses, and natural light. Exposure in late evening delays and exposure in the morning advances the body clock;

  iii. Sleep patterns based on flight schedule, power naps, sleep and wake times, and sleep hygiene;

  iv. Dietary regimens should be adapted to avoid alcohol at all times and caffeine at nighttime. Timing of the meal seems to be more important than the type of the meal;

  v. Exercise cannot reliably shift circadian rhythms but may maintain arousal levels. Change the training routine not to coincide with the circadian nadir (2–4 AM) at the departure zone.

b. Pharmacologic management:

  i. Melatonin can be used as a chrono-biotic (phase shifter) and chrono-hypnotic (sleep initiator). Product quality may be a concern;

  ii. Sleeping tablets (short acting) are recommended in athletes with persistent insomnia that have tolerated it before;

  iii. Stimulants are banned substances but can be considered in team management for daytime sleepiness.

Deep vein thrombosis:

1. Prevention:

  a. Compression hose;

  b. Hydration strategy;

  c. Avoid periods of prolonged immobility.

  d. Consider anticoagulant prophylaxis in athletes with high-risk medical conditions;

2. Monitoring after arrival:

  a. Educate about symptoms and signs after arrival;

  b. Recommend self-check for calf swelling/redness and report early;

C. Training and competition load management

General recommendations may include:

a. Very high loads can have either positive or negative influences on risk of illness in athletes, with the athlete's level of competition (elite), load history (chronic load), and intrinsic risk factor profile being important;

b. Athletes should have a detailed individualized training and competition plan, including postevent recovery measures (encompassing nutrition and hydration, sleep, and psychological recovery);

c. The training load is monitored using measurements of external and internal load;

d. Training load is managed by adopting the following principles:

  i. Changes in training load should be individualized because there are large intraindividual and interindividual variances in the timeframe of response and adaptation to load;

  ii. Changes in training load should be in small increments, with data (from the injury literature) indicating that weekly increments should be less than 10%;

e. The competition load is monitored and managed;

f. Variation in an athlete's psychological stressors should guide the prescription of training and/or competition loads;

g. It is recommended that coaches and support staff schedule adequate recovery, particularly after intensive training periods, competitions, and travel, including nutrition and hydration, sleep and rest, active rest, relaxation strategies, and emotional support;

h. Sports governing bodies have the responsibility to consider the competition load and hence the health of the athletes when planning their event calendars. This responsibility requires increased coordination between single-sport and multisport event organizers, and the development of a comprehensive calendar of all international sports events;

i. Psychological load management:
   i. Develop resilience strategies that help athletes understand the relationship between personal traits, negative life events, thoughts, emotions, and physiologic states, which, in turn, may help them minimize the impact of negative life events and the subsequent risk of illness;
   ii. Educate athletes in stress management techniques, confidence building, and goal setting, optimally under supervision of a sport psychologist, to help minimize the effects of stress and reduce the likelihood of illness;
   iii. Reduce training and/or competition loads and intensities to mitigate risk of illness for athletes who appear unfocused as a consequence of negative life events or ongoing daily hassles;
   iv. Implement periodic stress assessments (eg, hassle and uplift scale, Life Events Survey for Collegiate Athletes) to inform adjustment of athletes' training and/or competition loads. An athlete who reports high levels of daily hassle or stress could likely benefit from reducing the training load during a specified time period to prevent potential fatigue, illness, or burnout.

Adapted from Schwellnus M, Soligard T, Alonso JM, et al. How much is too much? (Part 2) International Olympic Committee consensus statement on load in sport and risk of illness. Br J Sports Med 2016;50(17):1049–50; with permission.

markers for illness, but there are data that show that sporting code (specifically athletics) may be an important extrinsic risk marker for illness. Current available studies suggest that age and sex are not accountable as risk markers. However, the type of impairment (eg, SCI and athletes with limb deficiencies) as well as the unique underlying medical problems (eg, neurogenic bladder) may be contributing factors. The authors recommend preventative strategies (general and specific) that take all these factors into account and also suggest that a PHA should be mandatory in all Paralympic athletes.

ACKNOWLEDGMENTS

The authors recognize Madeleen Scheepers for assistance with the referencing and Audrey Jansen van Rensburg for formatting of tables and assistance with the literature search.

REFERENCES

1. Webborn N. The disabled athlete. In: Brukner P, Khan K, editors. Clinical sports medicine. New York: McGraw-Hill; 2006. p. 778–86.
2. Webborn N, Willick S, Emery CA. The injury experience at the 2010 Winter Paralympic Games. Clin J Sport Med 2012;22(1):3–9.
3. Derman W, Schwellnus MP, Jordaan E, et al. The incidence and patterns of illness at the Sochi 2014 Winter Paralympic Games: a prospective cohort study of 6564 athlete days. Br J Sports Med 2016;50(17):1064–8.
4. Derman W, Schwellnus M, Jordaan E, et al. Illness and injury in athletes during the competition period at the London 2012 Paralympic Games: development and implementation of a web-based surveillance system (WEB-IISS) for team medical staff. Br J Sports Med 2013;47(7):420–5.
5. Willick SE, Webborn N, Emery C, et al. The epidemiology of injuries at the London 2012 Paralympic games. Br J Sports Med 2013;47(7):426–32.
6. Schwellnus M, Derman W, Jordaan E, et al. Factors associated with illness in athletes participating in the London 2012 Paralympic Games: a prospective cohort study involving 49,910 athlete-days. Br J Sports Med 2013;47(7):433–40.

7. Derman W. Profile of medical and injury consultations of Team South Africa during the XXVIIIth Olympiad, Athens 2004. SAJSM 2008;20(3):72–6. Available at: https://www.ajol.info/index.php/sasma/article/view/31931. Accessed February 5, 2018.

8. Engebretsen L, Soligard T, Steffen K, et al. Sports injuries and illnesses during the London Summer Olympic Games 2012. Br J Sports Med 2013;47(7):407–14.

9. Mountjoy M, Junge A, Alonso JM, et al. Sports injuries and illnesses in the 2009 FINA World Championships (aquatics). Br J Sports Med 2010;44(7):522–7.

10. Webborn N, Van de Vliet P. Paralympic medicine. Lancet 2012;380(9836):65–71.

11. Miller SL. Medical aspects of Paralympic sport. SportEX Medicine 2009;(42).

12. Derman W, Schwellnus M, Jordaan E. Clinical characteristics of 385 illnesses of athletes with impairment reported on the WEB-IISS system during the London 2012 Paralympic Games. PM R 2014;6(8 Suppl):S23–30.

13. Derman W, Schwellnus MP, Jordaan E, et al. Sport, sex and age increase risk of illness at the Rio 2016 Summer Paralympic games: a prospective cohort study of 51,198 athlete days. Br J Sports Med 2018;52(1):17–23.

14. Soligard T, Steffen K, Palmer D, et al. Sports injury and illness incidence in the Rio de Janeiro 2016 Olympic Summer Games: a prospective study of 11 274 athletes from 207 countries. Br J Sports Med 2017;51(17):1265–71.

15. Soligard T, Steffen K, Palmer-Green D, et al. Sports injuries and illnesses in the Sochi 2014 Olympic Winter Games. Br J Sports Med 2015;49(7):441–7.

16. Taunton J, Wilkinson M, Celebrini R, et al. Paralympic medical services for the 2010 Paralympic Winter Games. Clin J Sport Med 2012;22(1):10–20.

17. Schwellnus M, Soligard T, Alonso J-M, et al. How much is too much? (Part 2) International Olympic Committee consensus statement on load in sport and risk of illness. Br J Sports Med 2016;50(17):1043–52.

18. Svendsen IS, Taylor IM, Tønnessen E, et al. Training-related and competition-related risk factors for respiratory tract and gastrointestinal infections in elite cross-country skiers. Br J Sports Med 2016;50(13):809–15.

19. Thornton HR, Delaney JA, Duthie GM, et al. Predicting self-reported illness for professional team-sport athletes. Int J Sports Physiol Perform 2016;11(4):543–50.

20. Schwellnus MP, Derman WE, Jordaan E, et al. Elite athletes travelling to international destinations >5 time zone differences from their home country have a 2–3-fold increased risk of illness. Br J Sports Med 2012;46(11):816–21.

21. Johnson B, Mushett C, Richter K, et al. Sport for athletes with physical disabilities: injuries and medical issues. Decatur (GA): BlazeSports America; 2004.

22. Tsitsimpikou C, Tsiokanos A, Tsarouhas K, et al. Medication use by athletes at the Athens 2004 Summer Olympic Games. Clin J Sport Med 2009;19(1):33–8.

23. Halpern BC, Bochm R, Cardone DA. The disabled athlete. Principles and practice of primary care sports medicine. Philadelphia: Lippincott Williams & Wilkins; 2001. p. 115–32.

24. Garcia Leoni M, Esclarin De Ruz A. Management of urinary tract infection in patients with spinal cord injuries. Clin Microbiol Infect 2003;9(8):780–5.

25. Jiang S-D, Dai L-Y, Jiang L-S. Osteoporosis after spinal cord injury. Osteoporos Int 2006;17(2):180–92.

26. Maimoun L, Fattal C, Micallef J, et al. Bone loss in spinal cord-injured patients: from physiopathology to therapy. Spinal Cord 2006;44(4):203.

27. Moran de Brito C, Battistella L, Saito E, et al. Effect of alendronate on bone mineral density in spinal cord injury patients: a pilot study. Spinal Cord 2005;43(6):341.

28. Klenck C, Gebke K. Practical management: common medical problems in disabled athletes. Clin J Sport Med 2007;17(1):55–60.

29. Hawkeswood JP, O'Connor R, Anton H, et al. The preparticipation evaluation for athletes with disability. Int J Sports Phys Ther 2014;9(1):103.

30. Pelliccia A, Quattrini FM, Squeo MR, et al. Cardiovascular diseases in Paralympic athletes. Br J Sports Med 2016;50(17):1075–80.

31. Salvetti X, de Mello M, da Silva A. Coronary risk in a cohort of Paralympic athletes. Br J Sports Med 2006;40(11):918–22.

32. Gawroński W, Sobiecka J. Medical care before and during the Winter Paralympic Games in Turin 2006, Vancouver 2010 and Sochi 2014. J Hum Kinet 2015;48(1):7–16.

Acute and Chronic Musculoskeletal Injury in Para Sport: A Critical Review

Yetsa A. Tuakli-Wosornu, MD, MPH[a],*,
Evgeny Mashkovskiy, MD, PhD[b], Taylor Ottesen, BS[c],
Mark Gentry, MA, MLS[d], Daniel Jensen, DPT[e],
Nick Webborn, MB BS, FFSEM, MSc[f]

KEYWORDS

- Injury epidemiology • Musculoskeletal injury • Paralympic sport • Para athlete
- Review

KEY POINTS

- Seated Para athletes sustain upper extremity injuries more commonly, whereas ambulant Para athletes frequently sustain lower extremity injuries.
- The upper extremity is the most commonly injured area in all Para athletes, unlike able-bodied athletes for whom lower extremity injuries predominate.
- Minor soft tissue injuries are the most common injuries among Para athletes, similar to injury patterns observed among able-bodied athletes.
- Football 5-a-side, powerlifting, Goalball, Wheelchair fencing, and Wheelchair rugby are the highest risk summer sports; ice hockey, alpine skiing, and snowboarding are the highest-risk winter Paralympic sports.
- Compared with elite Para athletes, recreational and youth Para athletes remain under-studied in the literature.

The authors have nothing to disclose.
[a] Department of Chronic Disease Epidemiology, Yale School of Public Health, 60 College Street, New Haven, CT 06510, USA; [b] Department of Sports Medicine and Medical Rehabilitation, Sechenov University, 2-4 Bolshaya Pirogovskaya Street, Moscow 119991, Russia; [c] Department of Orthopaedics and Rehabilitation, Yale School of Medicine, 47 College Street, New Haven, CT 06511, USA; [d] Cushing/Whitney Medical Library, Yale University, 333 Cedar Street, New Haven, CT 06510, USA; [e] Department of Exercise Science, Black Hills State University, 1200 University Street, Spearfish, SD 57799, USA; [f] Centre for Sport and Exercise Science and Medicine (SESAME), School of Sport and Service Management, University of Brighton, Mithras House Lewes Road, Brighton BN2 4AT, UK
* Corresponding author.
E-mail address: yetsa.tuakli-wosornu@yale.edu

Phys Med Rehabil Clin N Am 29 (2018) 205–243
https://doi.org/10.1016/j.pmr.2018.01.014
1047-9651/18/© 2018 Elsevier Inc. All rights reserved.

INTRODUCTION

Congenital and acquired disabilities increase the baseline risk of lifestyle-related disease[1]: obesity and its attendant medical comorbidities are nearly 4 times higher among those with disabilities compared with the general population.[2,3] Physical activity and sport are thus important preventive health strategies for persons with impairment.[4] The term 'Para athlete' is the International Paralympic Committee's (IPC) general term for sportspersons with impairment, and signifies athletes who compete at all levels. Similarly, the term 'Para sport' encompasses both recreational and elite levels of competition. In contrast, the terms 'Paralympian' and 'Paralympic sport' connote the highest level of international competition, the Paralympic Games. Thus, Paralympians are a subset of Para athletes who have competed at the Paralympic Games. Over the past decade, sport for Para athletes has increased in popularity and visibility.[5,6] Like their able-bodied counterparts, Para athletes may enjoy the well-documented health benefits of increased physical activity.[1,7–13] Sport has a particularly positive impact on mental health indices for athletes with impairment, including life purpose, self-acceptance, and autonomy; it also decreases health care costs.[14,15]

All sports carry an inherent risk of injury and this is no different for Para sport.[16,17] Musculoskeletal injury epidemiology among Para athletes is similar to able-bodied sports injury patterns; for example, strains, sprains, contusions, and lacerations are most common.[18–22] However, the biomechanics of Para athlete injury are Para sport specific and relate to impairment, level of competition, mechanism, anatomic area, and equipment-specific factors.[23–28]

The aim of this critical review is to summarize current literature on the epidemiology of musculoskeletal injuries in Para athletes, and to discuss apparent research gaps.[29–31]

METHODS

Five electronic databases were searched between May 31 and June 21, 2017, for relevant articles: Ovid Medline (1946 to June Week 2, 2017), Ovid Medline In Process & Other Non-Indexed Citations, Ovid Embase (1974–2017 June 15), Cumulative Index to Nursing and Allied Health (CINAHL), and Web of Science. Controlled vocabulary and free text terms were used. The Yale MeSH Analyzer (http://mesh.med.yale.edu) was used in the initial stages of strategy formulation to harvest controlled vocabulary and keyword terms from highly relevant, known articles. The search strategy for Ovid MEDLINE is documented in Appendix 1.

Inclusion criteria were (a) written in the English language, (b) published in a peer-reviewed journal or book between January 1975 and June 2017, (c) inclusive of athletes with impairment participating in recreational or elite Para sports, and (d) describe sports-related injury/injuries to the musculoskeletal system including acute traumatic and/or chronic overuse injury to the appendicular and/or axial skeleton. Exclusion criteria were (a) not written in English, (b) not inclusive of athletes with impairment, (c) focused on injury/pathology unrelated to sports, and (d) review(s).

Before the removal of duplicate articles, the search yielded a total of 993 citations. This was reduced to 871 after the removal of duplicate records using the duplicate detection function of EndNote X7. Citations with abstracts were ingested into Covidence, a screening and data extraction tool. Two screeners selected 174 records for full-text review, and 47 citations were selected based on predefined inclusion/exclusion criteria (**Fig. 1**).

A number of analyses used retrospective data within a cross-sectional study design. For example, a cohort of athletes competing at a single tournament may have been asked to report demographic data, describe their impairment(s), and recall past

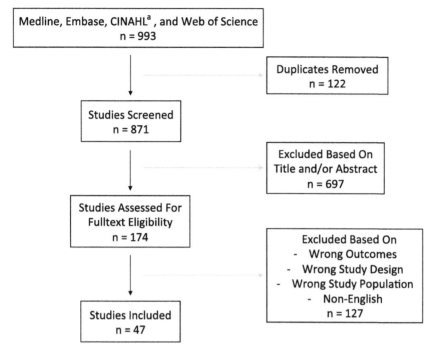

Fig. 1. Summary of search results. ᵃ Cumulative index to nursing and allied health.

musculoskeletal injuries in a single survey administered at a single point in time. In these instances, for the sake of consistency, we have designated these studies 'cross-sectional,' which refers to the study design. **Table 1** summarizes the study characteristics for all full-text articles included in the review.

RESULTS
Summary of Search Results

Eligible impairment categories
Historically, the IPC organized athlete impairment categories in the same way a clinician might, by diagnosis: spinal cord–related disability, cerebral palsy, amputee or limb deficiency, and visual impairment. Athletes with physical impairments not fitting these categories were classified as *Les Autres* (the others [French]). Athletes with an intellectual impairment were later included as well.[32,33] Recently, the impairment classification system was revised; categories now reflect the impact of the impairment on sport-specific function and are summarized in **Table 2**.[34]

   In the literature, sport-related injury patterns have been organized by impairment type, sport, and/or season (summer vs winter), among other factors. This discussion refers to updated impairment categories as often as possible, and organizes sport-related injury epidemiology by season.

General injury trends in summer and winter Para sports
During both summer and winter sports, seated Para athletes generally sustain upper limb injuries more commonly, whereas ambulant Para athletes frequently sustain lower extremity injuries (**Fig. 2**).[26,29,35,36] The upper extremity, including the shoulder, elbow, and wrist/hand, is the most commonly injured anatomic area in all Para athletes,[19,26,29,37–39] unlike able-bodied athletes, for whom lower extremity injuries

Table 1
Study characteristics

Author (First), Publication Year	Title	Country (First Author)	Study Design	Study Population	Defined Injury? (Y/N)	Definition of Injury	Conclusion(s)
Akbar et al,[68] 2015	Do overhead sports increase risk for rotator cuff tears in wheelchair users?	Germany	Cross-sectional	296 patients with SCI requiring the full-time use of a manual wheelchair.	N	Not reported.	Overhead sports activities have been identified as an additional risk factor, along with age and duration of wheelchair dependence, for developing rotator cuff disease in patients with paraplegia.
Andrade et al,[50] 2013	Prevalence of oral trauma in Para-Pan American Games athletes.	Brazil	Cross-sectional	120 athletes representing 25 countries competing at the 2007 Para-Pan American Games.	N	Not reported.	A recommendation for enhanced educational efforts and the use of properly fitted mouthguards to prevent traumatic injuries among high-performance athletes with disabilities seems warranted.

Ashton-Shaeffer,[73] 2010	Survey of injuries sustained by Division II and Division III wheelchair basketball athletes.	USA	Cross-sectional	112 National Wheelchair Basketball Association Division II and III players.	Y	Any event that brought the player off the court during a game or practice, or brought any member of the coaching staff onto the court to check out an injury during a game or practice, or required first aid at any time during a game or practice.	This study raises the question of the need for medically trained professionals at wheelchair basketball games and practices so that immediate care can be administered to decrease the severity of the injury and the number of days lost playing owing to injuries.
Batts et al,[20] 1998	The medical demands of the special athlete.	USA	Prospective	2,326 athletes registered at the Hawaii Special Olympic Summer Games over 4 y.	N	Not reported.	Despite preexisting medical conditions and physical limitations of the Special Olympian, most of the medical demands encountered during athletic competition are acute, minor injuries.

(continued on next page)

Table 1
(continued)

Author (First), Publication Year	Title	Country (First Author)	Study Design	Study Population	Defined Injury? (Y/N)	Definition of Injury	Conclusion(s)
Bernardi et al,[63] 2003	Muscle pain in athletes with locomotor disability	Italy	Cross-sectional	227 athletes with locomotor disability competing at 11 national-level competitions over 2 y.	Y	Any muscle pain experienced during the past 12 mo that either occurred during sport activity (training or competition) and/or was reported as a consequence of physical exercise, causing discomfort for ≥1 d and not related to systemic disease.	Prospective studies could be devised to assess the role of anthropometric characteristics and training volume as risk factors of sports-related muscle pain.
Blauwet et al,[58] 2016	Risk of Injuries in Paralympic Track and Field Differs by Impairment and Event Discipline: A Prospective Cohort Study at the London 2012 Paralympic Games.	USA	Prospective	977 athletes competing in athletics followed over a 10-d competition period of the 2012 Paralympic Games.	Y	Any newly acquired injury as well as exacerbations of preexisting injury that occurred during training and/ or competition of the 14 d precompetition and competition period of the London 2012 Paralympic Games.	Injury patterns were specific to the event discipline and athlete impairment. The majority of injuries occurred to the thigh (ambulant athletes) or shoulder/clavicle (wheelchair or seated athletes) and did not result in time loss.

Boninger et al,[55] 1996	Upper limb nerve entrapments in elite wheelchair racers.	USA	Prospective	12 wheelchair racers participating in the United States Olympic Committee 1994 Wheelchair Sports USA training camp at California State University.	Y	Clinical signs of median or ulnar neuropathy on physical examination and orthodromic and/or antidromic responses consistent with median or ulnar neuropathy on nerve conduction study.	Despite the amount of time spent training, these wheelchair athletes have a similar or lower prevalence of median mononeuropathy than reported in the general wheelchair-using population.
Burnham,[35] 1991	Sports medicine for the physically disabled: The Canadian team experience at the 1988 Seoul Paralympic Games.	Canada	Retrospective	124 athletes with impairment representing Canada at the 1988 Seoul Paralympic Games.	N	Not reported.	Sports medicine services are important for this group of athletes and care providers should be prepared to deal with musculoskeletal injuries, general medical illnesses and disorders specific to each disability. Both type of sport and type of disability seem to be factors in injury location.

(continued on next page)

Table 1
(continued)

Author (First), Publication Year	Title	Country (First Author)	Study Design	Study Population	Defined Injury? (Y/N)	Definition of Injury	Conclusion(s)
Burnham et al,[40] 1993	Shoulder pain in wheelchair athletes. The role of muscle imbalance.	Canada	Cross-sectional	19 volunteer wheelchair athletes with paraplegia.	Y	Shoulder pain and ≥ 2 of 5 clinical signs on physical examination: (1) painful arc of abduction, (2) pain in the impingement positions, (3) pain with resisted shoulder abduction, external rotation, or forward flexion, (4) tenderness to palpation over the greater tuberosity, lesser tuberosity, or bicipital groove, and (5) wasting of the supraspinous or infraspinous fossae.	Shoulder muscle imbalance, with comparative weakness of the humeral head depressors (rotators and adductors), may be a factor in the development and perpetuation of rotator cuff impingement syndrome in wheelchair athletes.

Chung et al,[66] 2012	Musculoskeletal injuries in elite able-bodied and wheelchair foil fencers: A pilot study.	Hong Kong	Prospective	14 wheelchair and 10 able-bodied elite fencers over 3 y.	Y	Trauma that occurred during a training/competition and prohibited the athlete from continuing fencing activity for ≥1 d.	This pilot study highlighted the distinct injury incidence between the 2 different fencer groups. Large-scale epidemiologic and biomechanical studies are warranted to improve the understanding of fencing injuries to develop injury prevention/rehabilitation programs.
Curtis & Dillon,[52] 1985	Survey of wheelchair athletic injuries: Common patterns and prevention.	USA	Cross-sectional	128 wheelchair athletes with varying disabilities.	N	Not reported.	Soft tissue trauma, blisters, lacerations, decubiti and joint disorders were the most commonly reported injuries. More than 70% of all reported injuries occurred during wheelchair track, road racing, and basketball.

(continued on next page)

Table 1
(continued)

Author (First), Publication Year	Title	Country (First Author)	Study Design	Study Population	Defined Injury? (Y/N)	Definition of Injury	Conclusion(s)
Curtis & Black,[70] 1999	Shoulder pain in female wheelchair basketball players.	USA	Cross-sectional	46 female wheelchair basketball players competing at the 1997 National Women's Wheelchair Basketball tournament.	Y	Shoulder pain, as measured by the Wheelchair User's Shoulder Pain Index.	Shoulder and upper extremity pain was a very common problem reported by >90% of the subjects in this study. Prevention of pain and chronic disability in athletes who use wheelchairs should be addressed by coaches, players, and health care professionals.
Derman et al,[37] 2013	Illness and injury in athletes during the competition period at the London 2012 Paralympic Games: Development and implementation of a Web-Based Surveillance System for team medical staff.	South Africa	Prospective	2,347 male athletes and 1,218 female athletes competing at the 2012 summer Paralympic Games over 14 d.	Y	Any newly acquired injury as well as exacerbations of preexisting injury that occurred during training and/or competition of the 14 d precompetition and competition period of the London 2012 Paralympic Games.	During the competition period, the IR and IP of illness and injury at the Games were similar and comparable to the observed rates in other elite competitions. In Paralympic athletes, the IP of upper limb injuries is higher than that of lower limb injuries and nonrespiratory illnesses are more common.

| Derman et al,[45] 2016 | High incidence of injury at the Sochi 2014 Winter Paralympic Games: A prospective cohort study of 6,564 athlete days. | South Africa | Prospective | 547 athletes from 45 countries monitored daily for 12 d during the Sochi 2014 Winter Paralympic Games. | Y | Any newly acquired injury as well as exacerbations of preexisting injury that occurred during training and/or competition of the 14 d precompetition and competition period of the London 2012 Paralympic Games. | In a Winter Paralympic Games setting, athletes report higher injury incidence than do Olympic athletes or athletes in a Summer Paralympic Games setting…Our data can inform injury prevention programs and policy considerations regarding athlete safety in future Winter Paralympic Games. |
| Ferrara et al,[85] 1992 | The injury experience of the competitive athlete with a disability: Prevention implications. | USA | Cross-sectional | 426 athletes who participated at the 1989 national competition of the National Wheelchair Athletic Association, US Association for Blind Athletes, and the US Cerebral Palsy Athletic Association. | Y | Any trauma to the participant that occurred during any practice, training, or competition session that caused the athlete to stop, limit, or modify participation for ≥ 1 d. | The athlete with a disability demonstrated approximately the same percentage of injury as the athlete without a disability in similar sport activities. Biomechanical considerations of locomotion and specific sport skills shoulder be analyzed by experts to reduce the percentage of injuries. |

(continued on next page)

Table 1
(continued)

Author (First), Publication Year	Title	Country (First Author)	Study Design	Study Population	Defined Injury? (Y/N)	Definition of Injury	Conclusion(s)
Ferrara et al,[85] 1992	The injury experience and training history of the competitive skier with a disability.	USA	Cross-sectional	68 athletes who participated in the 1989 National Handicapped Sports and the US Association for Blind Athletes Winter National Games.	Y	Any trauma to the participant that occurred during any practice, training, or competitive session that resulted in the cessation, limitation, or modification of the athlete's participation for $\geq$24 h.	The skier with a disability incurred approximately the same proportion of injuries as the skier without a disability. Conditioning programs should be developed to emphasize both the aerobic and anaerobic energy systems to reduce the number of injuries.
Ferrara & Davis,[98] 1990	Injuries to elite wheelchair athletes.	USA	Cross-sectional	19 athletes at an elite wheelchair training camp.	Y	Anything the athlete expressed concern about and (a) caused a loss of participation owing to an injury or illness or (b) an injury in which a fracture, dislocation, or subluxation occurred and the athlete was able to continue participation.	The wheelchair athlete seems to have the same type and frequency of injury as the athlete without a disability. The time loss factor seems to be higher for major injuries as compared with the athlete without a disability.

Ferrara et al,[46] 2000	A longitudinal study of injuries to athletes with disabilities.	USA	Prospective	1,360 US athletes who participated in the 1990 World Games and Championships, 1991 US Paralympic Trials, 1992 Paralympic Games, the 1994 World Athletics Championship, and the 1996 Paralympic Games.	Y	An injury/illness that was evaluated by the US medical staff during these competitions.	Attention should be paid to the musculature of the thorax/spine, shoulder and hip/thigh to help reduce the number of the injuries in this region.
Galena et al,[21] 1998	Connecticut State Special Olympics: Observations and recommendations.	USA	Retrospective	674 intellectually impaired athletes who participated in the 1994, 1995, and 1996 Connecticut State Special Olympics (summer games event). Mean age of 30 y.	N	Not reported.	Minor trauma made up the largest percentage of encounters. The more serious injuries included dislocations and fractures. The incidence of seizure remained stable over these years. The highest incidence of sunburn occurred in the 1995 despite the availability of sunblock.

(continued on next page)

Table 1
(continued)

Author (First), Publication Year	Title	Country (First Author)	Study Design	Study Population	Defined Injury? (Y/N)	Definition of Injury	Conclusion(s)
Gawronski et al,[44] 2013	Fit and healthy Paralympians: Medical care guidelines for disabled athletes: A study of the injuries and illnesses incurred by the Polish Paralympic team in Beijing 2008 and London 2012.	Poland	Prospective and cross-sectional	191 athletes with impairment who competed as part of the Polish national team at the Beijing 2008 and London 2012 summer Paralympic Games.	Y	A newly acquired musculoskeletal symptom or an exacerbation of a preexisting (chronic) injury that occurred during training and/or competition.	Some groups of disabled athletes are at an increased risk of injury/illness. The more stringent medical care guidelines before London may have caused staggeringly better results.
Hawkeswood et al,[87] 2011	A pilot survey on injury and safety concerns in international sledge hockey.	Canada	Cross-sectional	10 respondents participated: 2 from each of the top 5 international sledge hockey teams, including trainers, physiotherapists, physicians, coaches, and/or general managers.	Y	Any injury that caused an athlete to stop, limit or modify participation for ≥ 1 d.	This information provides opportunity to consider implementing and evaluating safety strategies, which could include improved hand protection, cut-resistant materials in high-risk areas, increased vigilance to reduce intentional head contact, lowered rink boards, and modified bathroom floor surfacing.

Hoeberigs et al,[51] 1990	Sports medical experiences from the International Flower Marathon for disabled wheelers.	The Netherlands	Prospective and retrospective	60 participants in the 1984, 1985, and/or 1986 IFM; and 40 participants in the 1986 IFM.	N	Not reported.	The number and seriousness of injuries and other medical problems in disabled wheelers is related to environmental conditions as well as to the nature of disabilities involved. The study also shows, without doubt, that long distance events for wheelers need the support of adequate medical escorts.
Hoeberigs & Verstappen,[71] 1984	Muscle soreness in wheelchair basketballers.	The Netherlands	Cross-sectional	89 athletes representing 10 (of 21) national wheelchair basketball teams, who competed at the 1980 summer Paralympic Games.	Y	Muscle soreness.	The complaints of the athletes concerning the softness of the floor should be of interest to future organizers of wheelchair basketball tournaments.

(continued on next page)

Table 1
(continued)

Author (First), Publication Year	Title	Country (First Author)	Study Design	Study Population	Defined Injury? (Y/N)	Definition of Injury	Conclusion(s)
Laskowski & Murtaugh,[81] 1992	Snow skiing injuries in physically disabled skiers.	USA	Retrospective	4-y injury data were reviewed from 4 (of 13) US ski areas with the largest disabled skiing instructional programs.	N	Not reported.	There is a need for further prospective studies in the general able-bodied and disabled skiing populations with direct comparisons of rate, location, and severity of injury; type of disability; and experience level of the skier. We hope that this study will stimulate more ski areas to allow disabled skiers on their slopes, even if limited to participation in supervised, instructional programs.

Study	Title	Country	Design	Population		Injury definition	Findings
Magno e Silva,[62] 2013	Sport injuries in elite Paralympic swimmers with visual impairment.	Brazil	Prospective	28 elite, visually impaired swimmers (19 males, 9 females) from the Brazilian Paralympic Team surveyed over the course of 5 international competitions between 2004 and 2008.	Y	Any injury that caused an athlete to stop, limit, or modify participation for ≥ 1 more days.	Visually impaired swimmers had a relatively high proportion of overuse injuries, predominantly associated with muscle spasm in the spine, and tendinopathy in the shoulders. No differences were apparent in injury prevalence and clinical incidence among visual classes or between sexes.
Magno e Silva et al,[59] 2013	Sports injuries in Brazilian blind footballers.	Brazil	Prospective	13 male visually impaired athletes (B1 visual class - blind) who were part of the Brazilian 5-a-side football team, surveyed over the course of 5 international competitions between 2004 and 2008.	Y	Any injury that caused an athlete to stop, limit, or modify participation for ≥ 1 days.	The results are important in guiding strategies to inform the implementation of preventive pathways and provide a strong rationale for the compulsory use of additional protective equipment.

(continued on next page)

Table 1
(continued)

Author (First), Publication Year	Title	Country (First Author)	Study Design	Study Population	Defined Injury? (Y/N)	Definition of Injury	Conclusion(s)
Magno e Silva et al,[57] 2013	Sports injuries in Paralympic track and field athletes with visual impairment.	Brazil	Prospective	40 visually impaired elite Paralympic athletes who competed in 5 international competitions between 2004 and 2008.	Y	Any injury that caused an athlete to stop, limit, or modify participation for ≥1 days.	Visually impaired track and field Paralympic athletes present a pattern of overuse injuries predominantly affecting the lower limbs, particularly the thighs, lower legs, and knees.
Martinez,[27] 1989	Medical concerns among wheelchair road racers.	USA	Cross-sectional	43 wheelchair athletes participating in the 1987 Peachtree Road Race.	N		It is important that the medical community become more knowledgeable about and involved with disabled athletes and that barriers limiting wheelchair athletes be removed. All sports medicine professionals have something to contribute to the wheelchair athlete.

Study	Title	Country	Study design	Sample		Definition	Conclusions
McCormick,[83] 1985	Injuries in handicapped alpine ski racers.	USA	Cross-sectional	60 athletes competing at the 1983 Northeast Regional Handicapped Skier's Championships.	N	Not reported.	Strengthening the legs, learning to displace the outriggers to a safe position while falling and holding the ski pole correctly to avoid skier's thumb will help to reduce the injury rate among disabled skiers.
McCormick et al,[56] 1990	Injury and illness surveillance at local Special Olympic Games.	USA	Prospective	27 (of 777) athletes competing at 2 local Special Olympics Games competitions held 2 mo apart in Texas.	Y	An injury resulting directly from participation in a sports event.	Special Olympic games at the local level are safe and planners should prepare to treat more illnesses than injuries at such competitions.
Mutsuzaki et al,[75] 2017	Factors associated with deep tissue injury in male wheelchair basketball players of a Japanese national team.	Japan	Cross-sectional	20 male Japanese wheelchair basketball players on the Japanese national team at the 2012 London Paralympic Games.	Y	Low-echoic lesions on ultrasound imaging indicative of deep tissue injuries.	Players with spinal cord injury and players who used a wheelchair in daily life were more likely to have deep tissue injuries, particularly in the sacral region. The lesions were small, but a periodic medical check should be performed to maintain athletes' sporting life.

(continued on next page)

Table 1
(continued)

Author (First), Publication Year	Title	Country (First Author)	Study Design	Study Population	Defined Injury? (Y/N)	Definition of Injury	Conclusion(s)
Nyland et al,[18] 2000	Soft tissue injuries to USA Paralympians at the 1996 summer games.	USA	Prospective	304 members of the USA Paralympic Team with various physical disabilities, competing at the 1996 Paralympic Games.	Y	Soft tissue injuries were operationally defined as strain, sprain, tendonitis, bursitis, or contusion.	Differences in soft tissue injury frequency among athletes of differing impairments suggest that the competitive use of adaptive or assistive devices, in combination with sport-specific stressors and the athletes' disabilities, is related to the development of predictable soft tissue injury patterns.

Study	Focus	Country	Design	Population		Injury definition	Findings
Patatoukas et al,[19] 2011	Disability-related injuries in athletes with disabilities.	Greece	Cross-sectional	139 elite athletes with various physical disabilities.	Y	Any injury that caused an athlete to stop, limit, or modify participation for ≥1 d.	Athletes with CP sustained soft tissue injuries and lacerations more than other disability groups did because moving and walking patterns of this population add risk factors for such injuries. Fractures and blisters occur more frequently to SCI athletes because they participate in higher percentage in wheelchair basketball which is a high-risk sport.
Ramirez et al,[61] 2009	Sports injuries to high school athletes with disabilities.	USA	Prospective	210 athletes from 8 special education high schools that are part of an interscholastic sports league.	Y	"Injury episodes" were defined as events resulting in immediate removal of the athlete from the session and medical treatment by school staff or transport to a hospital. "Injury diagnoses" were defined as the physical trauma sustained to the body region of an athlete during the injury event.	The preparticipation medical examination may be an excellent opportunity to create special guidelines, particularly for athletes with autism and seizure history.

(continued on next page)

Table 1
(*continued*)

Author (First), Publication Year	Title	Country (First Author)	Study Design	Study Population	Defined Injury? (Y/N)	Definition of Injury	Conclusion(s)
Reynolds et al,[39] 1994	Paralympics, Barcelona 1992	UK	Retrospective	201 members of the British Paralympic team who attended the medical center at the 1992 Barcelona summer Paralympic Games.	N	Not reported.	The injury/illness profile was similar to those in able-bodied sport.
Robson,[54] 1990	The Special Olympic Games for the mentally handicapped, United Kingdom 1989.	UK	Cross-sectional	196 athletes competing in the 1989 Leicester Special Olympic Games, over an 8-d competition period.	N	Not reported.	The medical team played their part in contributing to the success of the games and enabling each competitor to carry out the spirit of the Special Olympic oath: "Let me win, but if I cannot win, let me be brave in the attempt."

Shimizu et al,[75] 2017	A survey of deep tissue injury in elite female wheelchair basketball players.	Japan	Cross-sectional	22 female wheelchair basketball players on the 2014 Japanese national team at the 2014 Asian Para Games.	Y	An unclear layered structure, a hypoechoic lesion, a discontinuous superficial or deep fascia, and a heterogeneous hypoechoic area on ultrasound imaging.	Central nervous system disorder, wheelchair use in daily life, pelvic instability, and lower systolic blood pressure, red blood cells, and serum creatinine increased the risk of deep tissue injuries.
Magno e Silva,[36] 2011	Aspects of Sports Injuries in Athletes with Visual Impairment.	Brazil	Prospective	131 visually impaired athletes chosen to represent Brazil at international competitions between 2004 and 2008.	Y	Any injury that has occurred with the athlete during practice, training, or competition that causes interruption, limitation, or alteration in his or her participation for $\geq$1 days.	21 diagnoses were reported, being tendinopathies, contractures, and contusions the most frequent.

(continued on next page)

Table 1
(continued)

Author (First), Publication Year	Title	Country (First Author)	Study Design	Study Population	Defined Injury? (Y/N)	Definition of Injury	Conclusion(s)
Sobiecka,[22] 2005	Injuries and ailments of the Polish participants of the 2000 Paralympic games in Sydney.	Poland	Retrospective	114 Polish athletes who competed at the 2000 Paralympic Games over 23 d.	N	Not reported.	Athletes sought medical attention most frequently owing to injuries to the motor system, common colds, and slightly elevated body temperature. Moreover, medical attention was needed for headaches, insomnia, and stomachaches after meals as well as cases of hypertension, ischialgia, abrasions and bruises, sores of the buttocks, and menstruation-related complaints.

Study	Title	Country	Design	Population		Definition	Conclusion
Taylor & Williams,[47] 1995	Sports injuries in athletes with disabilities: Wheelchair racing.	UK	Cross-sectional	53 members of the British Wheelchair Racing Association.	Y	Pain in any part of the body that affected or prevented the athlete from training or competing for ≥1 d.	There seems to be a link between overuse injuries, the presence of pain during training, and the recurrence of injuries. A lack of knowledge about sports injuries, what causes them, and what to do after an injury may contribute to the high incidence of overuse injuries in this group of athletes.
Webborn et al,[43] 2016	The Epidemiology of Injuries in Football at the London 2012 Paralympic.	UK	Prospective	70 athletes from 7 countries who participated in the football 5-a-side competition and 96 athletes from 8 countries who participated in the football 7-a-side competition over 14 d.	Y	Any newly acquired injury as well as exacerbations of preexisting injury that occurred during training and/or competition of the 14-d precompetition and competition period of the London 2012 Paralympic Games.	Protective headgear may have a role in injury prevention.

(continued on next page)

Table 1
(continued)

Author (First), Publication Year	Title	Country (First Author)	Study Design	Study Population	Defined Injury? (Y/N)	Definition of Injury	Conclusion(s)
Webborn et al,[49] 2012	The injury experience at the 2010 Winter Paralympic Games	UK	Prospective	505 athletes from 44 National Paralympic Committees participating in the 2010 Vancouver winter Paralympic Games.	Y	Any sport-related musculoskeletal complaint that caused the athlete to seek medical attention during the study period, regardless of the athlete's ability to continue with training or competition.	The injury risk was significantly higher than during the 2002 (9.4%) and 2006 (8.4%) Winter Paralympic Games. This finding may reflect improved data collection systems, but also highlights the high risk of acute injury in alpine skiing and ice sledge hockey at Paralympic Games.
Webborn et al,[25] 2006	Injuries among disabled athletes during the 2002 Winter Paralympic Games.	UK	Prospective and retrospective	39 athletes from 20 different countries competing at the Salt Lake 2002 winter Paralympic Games over 20 d.	N	Not reported.	Ongoing data collection by the International Paralympic Committee should enable feasible injury prevention strategies to be designed and implemented.

Wessels et al,[74] 2012	Concussions in wheelchair basketball.	USA	Cross-sectional	263 wheelchair basketball players at wheelchair basketball tournaments during the 2009–2010 season, in collegiate, national, women's, championship, and division III wheelchair basketball divisions.	Y	A blow to the head that causes a variety of symptoms that may last a short period, such as a few plays or minutes of a game, or a longer period.	Further work is needed in concussion assessment in persons with disability as well as greater education concerning concussion in disability sports.
Willick et al,[65] 2016	The epidemiology of injuries in powerlifting at the London 2012 Paralympic Games: An analysis of 1,411 athlete-days.	USA	Prospective	163 powerlifters representing 56 countries at the London 2012 Paralympic Games, over the 7-d competition period.	Y	Any newly acquired injury as well as exacerbations of preexisting injury that occurred during training and/or competition of the 7-d competition period of the London 2012 Paralympic Games.	The information obtained in this study opens the door for future study into the mechanisms and details of injuries into powerlifters with physical impairments.

(continued on next page)

Table 1
(continued)

Author (First), Publication Year	Title	Country (First Author)	Study Design	Study Population	Defined Injury? (Y/N)	Definition of Injury	Conclusion(s)
Willick et al,[41] 2013	The epidemiology of injuries at the London 2012 Paralympic Games.	USA	Prospective	3,565 athletes from 160 delegations who competed at the London 2012 summer Paralympic Games.	Y	Any sport-related musculoskeletal or neurologic complaint prompting an athlete to seek medical attention, regardless of whether or not the complaint resulted in lost time from training or competition.	The knowledge gained from this study will inform future injury surveillance studies and the development of prevention strategies in Paralympic sport.
Wilson & Washington,[53] 1993	Pediatric wheelchair athletics: Sports injuries and prevention.	USA	Cross-sectional	83 competitors at the 1990 Junior National Wheelchair Games.	Y	Soft tissue injuries were defined as sprains, strains and tendinitis.	Many of these injuries can be minimized by educating competitors, coaching staff, and alerting medical personnel to the unique problems encountered by junior wheelchair athletes of varying disability and age.

Abbreviations: CP, cerebral palsy; IFM, International Flower Marathon; IP, injury proportion, IR, injury rate.

Table 2
International Paralympic Committee eligible impairment categories

Impairment Category	Description
Physical impairment	
Impaired muscle power	Reduced force generated by muscles or muscle groups, such as muscles of one limb or the lower half of the body, as caused, for example, by spinal cord injuries, spina bifida, or polio.
Impaired passive ROM	ROM in ≥ 1 joints is reduced permanently, for example, owing to arthrogryposis. Hypermobility of joints, joint instability, and acute conditions, such as arthritis, are not considered eligible impairments.
Limb deficiency	Total or partial absence of bones or joints as a consequence of trauma (eg, car accident), illness (eg, bone cancer) or congenital limb deficiency (eg, dysmelia).
Leg length difference	Bone shortening in one leg owing to congenital deficiency or trauma.
Short stature	Reduced standing height owing to abnormal dimensions of bones of upper and lower limbs or trunk, for example, owing to achondroplasia or growth hormone dysfunction.
Hypertonia	Abnormal increase in muscle tension and a reduced ability of a muscle to stretch, owing to a neurologic condition, such as cerebral palsy, brain injury, or multiple sclerosis.
Ataxia	Lack of coordination of muscle movements owing to a neurologic condition, such as cerebral palsy, brain injury, or multiple sclerosis.
Athetosis	Generally characterized by unbalanced, involuntary movements and a difficulty in maintaining a symmetric posture, owing to a neurologic condition, such as cerebral palsy, brain injury, or multiple sclerosis.
Visual impairment	Vision is impacted by either an impairment of the eye structure, optical nerves or optical pathways, or the visual cortex.
Intellectual impairment	A limitation in intellectual functioning and adaptive behaviors expressed in conceptual, social and practical adaptive skills, which originates before the age of 18.

Available at: https://www.paralympic.org/classification.

predominate.[37] Advanced age and spinal cord injury may increase the risk of upper extremity injury, generally, and shoulder muscle imbalance (comparative weakness of the shoulder rotators and adductors) may contribute to seated athletes' shoulder pathology.[31,40] Male and female summer Para athletes typically have similar overall injury rates,[41] but certain sporting environments carry a higher risk. In the summer Paralympic Games setting, Football 5-a-side, Para powerlifting, Goalball, Wheelchair fencing, and Wheelchair rugby consistently have high injury rates,[41,42] with Football 5-a-side carrying the highest overall risk (**Fig. 3**).[42,43] Polish scientists have demonstrated that mandatory periodic health evaluations in the lead up to summer Paralympic Games may result in reduced overall injury rates, and improved performances.[44]

Overall injury incidence rate (IR) at the Sochi 2014 winter Paralympic Games was 2 times higher than the IR at the London 2012 summer Paralympic Games.[45] Although sprains, strains, blisters, and lacerations are the most common injuries among all Paralympians,[19] winter Paralympic sports generally carry a higher risk of head injury, fracture, and contusion, possibly owing to the high-velocity elements of competition.[45] Of note, high-velocity Para cycling (a summer sport) also poses this risk.[46–48] Para ice hockey (formerly called ice sledge hockey), Para alpine skiing, and Para snowboarding

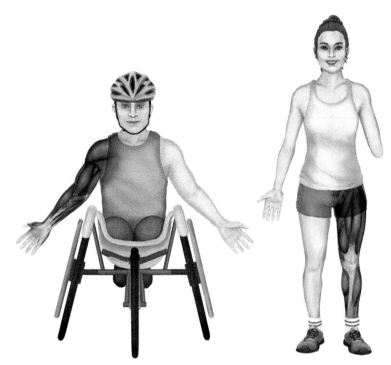

Fig. 2. Para athletes who use wheelchairs sustain upper extremity injuries in high percentages. Ambulant Para athletes sustain lower extremity injuries in high percentages. (*Courtesy of* Yetsa A. Tuakli-Wosornu, MD, MPH, New Haven, Connecticut, USA.)

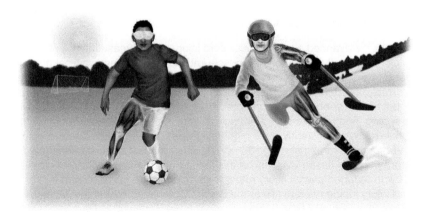

Fig. 3. During the summer Paralympic Games, the highest incidence of injury was reported in Football 5-a-side, where lower extremity injuries predominated. During the winter Paralympic Games, the highest injury incidence was reported in the Para Alpine Skiing/Snowboarding category. Among all winter sports, upper and lower extremity injuries occurred with similar frequency. (*Courtesy of* Yetsa A. Tuakli-Wosornu, MD, MPH, New Haven, Connecticut, USA.)

are particularly high-risk winter sports; Para alpine skiing/snowboarding has the highest injury risk (see **Fig. 3**).[45]

As Webborn and colleagues[49] have shown, certain injuries can be controlled by the introduction of sport-specific equipment regulations, which is discussed in greater detail elsewhere in this article.[50] Among all winter sports, upper extremity and lower extremity injury rates match, unlike summer sport injury trends.[45] Para cross-country (previously called Nordic skiing/biathlon), and wheelchair curling continue to have the lowest injury risk among winter Paralympic sports.[25,49] Certain identified sports are covered in greater detail herein.

Summer Sports

Athletics
Para athletics (track and field) is studied more than any other Para sport.[29] At all levels of competition including youth, soft tissue injuries including muscle contusions, skin abrasions, sunburn, and decubitus ulcers are more common than ominous injuries such as fractures; and chronic overuse injuries are more common than acute traumatic injuries.[47,51–54] Premature return to sport may contribute to the chronicity of certain injuries.[47] Wheelchair track athletes may develop upper extremity mononeuropathies and amputee athletes may experience residual limb pain and injury.[23,55] Intellectually impaired athletes incur more injuries in track and field than most other sports.[56] Visually impaired track athletes are at particularly high risk of chronic overuse lower extremity injury.[19,57] For example, Magno e Silva and colleagues[57] have documented a 78% overall injury prevalence and an IR of 1.93 injuries per visually impaired track athlete over a typical competitive season, within an internationally competitive track and field team.

At the London 2012 Paralympic Games, the overall injury IR was 22.1 injuries per 1000 athlete days in Para athletics.[58] There was no difference in IR between track versus field athletes, but injury patterns were specific to event and impairment type. In track events, ambulant athletes with cerebral palsy suffered a lower overall injury IR (IR, 10.2; 95% confidence interval, 4.2–16.2) compared with ambulant athletes in different impairment categories. Most injuries did not result in time loss from training or competition. Ambulant athletes experienced the greatest proportion of thigh injuries (16.4% of all injuries; IR, 4.0) predominantly on the track, and seated athletes experienced the greatest proportion of shoulder/clavicle injuries (19.3% of all injuries; IR, 3.4) predominantly in the field. Athletes in seated throwing events suffered a higher incidence of injury (IR, 23.7; 95% confidence interval, 17.5–30.0) as compared with athletes in wheelchair racing events (IR, 10.6; 95% confidence interval, 5.5–15.6).[58]

Football (5-a-side, 7-a-side, intellectual impairment, amputee)
Football for athletes with visual impairment (5-a-side), hypertonia (7-a-side), intellectual impairment, or amputation involves significant injury risk. Representative injury prevalence data is as follows: over 23 matches, the injury prevalence among a cohort of national-level Brazilian players was 84.6%.[59] In contrast, representative injury incidence data are as follows: at the London 2012 Paralympic Games, Football 5-a-side had the highest IR of all 22 sports: 22.4 injuries per 1000 athlete-days (injury incidence proportion 31.4 injuries per 100 athletes), whereas the IR for Football 7-a-side was only 10.4 per 1000 athlete-days (injury incidence proportion 14.6 injuries per 100 athletes).[43]

Collision and foul play–related acute traumatic injuries tend to predominate in elite Football 5-a-side.[41,43,59] By anatomic area, the lower limb (knee, then feet, ankle, thigh) followed by head, spine, and upper limb are affected. Common diagnoses include contusion, sprain, tendinopathy, and, more recently, head injury.[42,60] High school Para athletes also experience the highest rates of injury playing football compared with other sports, and minor, collision-related lower extremity injuries predominate.[61] Finally, injury patterns and rates among footballers with limb amputations seem to be similar to those found among able-bodied footballers.[23]

Swimming

Chronic overuse injuries are more common than acute traumatic injuries among elite Para swimmers, and there do not seem to be significant differences between injury patterns or rates based on gender or classification category.[62] The greatest proportion of injuries occur in the trunk, upper extremity (predominantly shoulder), and thoracic and lumbar spine regions. Muscle pain/spasm and tendinopathy are common diagnoses. Spinal cord injury or amputation, rather than limb deficiency, visual impairment, or other impairment, may be associated with an increased risk of muscle pain/spasm.[62,63]

Sitting volleyball

Chronic overuse injuries are more common than acute traumatic injuries in sitting volleyball players. In a large cohort of prospectively studied elite players, chronic low back pain, then acute wrist and finger sprain, and chronic rotator cuff pathology were the most common sports-related musculoskeletal injuries, in order. Older players with a longer duration of disability were disproportionately more affected by injury.[64]

Para powerlifting

At the 2016 Rio Paralympic Games, nearly 20% of Para powerlifters reported an injury, predominantly in the upper extremity/shoulder.[42] Furthermore, at the 2012 London Paralympic Games, Para powerlifters had the second highest overall IR, after Football 5-a-side: 33.3 injuries per 1000 athlete-days (injury incidence proportion, 23.3 per 100 Para powerlifters). The majority of injuries were chronic overuse, and the shoulder/clavicle was the most injured anatomic area. Most injuries occurred during the competition period, there were no significant differences in injury pattern or rate by gender, and athletes in heavier weight classes were at higher injury risk.[65]

Wheelchair fencing

Among a cohort of elite wheelchair fencers, 73.8% experienced an upper extremity injury, 32.5% of which were elbow strain and 15.8% of which were shoulder strain. Those with poor trunk control had an increased risk of injury compared with fencers with good trunk control (4.9 per 1000 hours vs 3.0 per 1000 hours; no P value reported).[66]

Para cycling

The literature on Para cycling injury epidemiology is sparse and includes a German-language cohort study.[48]

Overhead summer Para sports

Participation in overhead Para sports such as wheelchair basketball and tennis is a risk factor for upper extremity tendon, ligament, bursa, and muscle pathology, including rotator cuff disease.[19,41,51,67–70] Additional risk factors include advanced age, presence/duration of manual wheelchair dependence, and, possibly, playing surface(s).[63,68,71] Overuse upper extremity injuries are associated with repetitive motions, whereas acute injuries are due to high-force physical contact.[72,73] Comparing a large cohort of amateur wheelchair basketball players with a cohort of nonathlete wheelchair users, Akbar and colleagues[68] showed a 2.09 relative risk of rotator cuff injury (95% confidence interval, 1.68–2.59; $P<.001$).

Concussion was recently described in 6% of a large cohort of adult recreational wheelchair basketball athletes.[74] Sacral and ischial deep tissue injuries are also common in seated overhead summer Para athletes, particularly among spinally injured players as opposed to players with musculoskeletal disease.[75,76]

Para sailing and rowing
Overuse rib stress injury was reported in a single Croatian Para athlete, and authors speculate that this unique injury is potentially due to complete reliance on the upper extremity and torso in certain classes of high-level spinally injured rowers, in addition to high force transmission through certain areas of the body during rowing.[77–79]

Winter Sports

Para skiing/snowboarding
There is no significant difference in the overall injury rate between skiers with and without impairment, but patterns of injury differ.[80–83] Among able-bodied skiers, beginners are at higher risk of injury compared with advanced skiers. This association is reversed in Para skiers: elite, high-velocity skiers (either seated or standing) suffer increased injury rates and severity compared with novice, relatively low-velocity skiiers.[81,83]

Upper and lower extremity injuries seem to occur in equal proportion, and for seated Para skiers (ie, those using sit skis), upper extremity injuries seem to be most common.[25,84–86] Nordic Para skiers have a significantly lower risk of injury compared with Alpine skiers.[25,86]

Para ice hockey (formerly called IPC ice sledge hockey)
There is a similar injury incidence proportion among male and female Para Ice Hockey players at the Paralympic Games. Overuse upper extremity and spine injuries predominate, and, importantly, the frequency of relatively catastrophic injuries has been reduced over time. Between the 2002 and 2010 winter Paralympic Games, the rates of lower limb fracture in Para ice hockey decreased from 33.0% to 2.5% after the introduction of the regulation change on protective equipment and sledge height.[49] This modification illustrates the positive impact that data-driven policy changes can have on athlete health, particularly in high-risk sports like Para ice hockey. Additional safety strategies, including hand protection, and training programs to reduce intentional head contact, may be of additional benefit in this sport.[87]

DISCUSSION
The Lifetime Injury Model

To promote health through lifelong sport and physical activity, an accurate model of long-term injury risk, a so-called Lifetime Injury Model, is needed for Para athletes at various stages of their careers.[31] For reference, injury risk during and after sport has been described for able-bodied sportspeople, for example, an increased risk of lower extremity osteoarthritis in former soccer players.[88] Understanding the long-term injury risk is especially important for Para athletes, who tend to be older than able-bodied athletes, have nonmodifiable functional impairments, and among whom younger, recreational athletes are less frequently studied.[26,89]

Sports injury surveillance programs can help generate the data needed for a Lifetime Injury Model.[90] The comprehensive, Web-based Injury and Illness Surveillance Survey (WEB-IISS), for example, is currently used to prospectively capture injury and illness data at Paralympic Games (Web-based Injury and Illness Surveillance Survey data have been referenced frequently in this review).[37] Although some injury patterns can be garnered from Paralympic data, the lifetime consequences of injury remain unclear. As national and international Para sport federations create their own surveillance protocols and gather longitudinal sport- and country-specific data, a better understanding of injury patterns in both recreational and elite Para sport can be achieved.[89] Furthermore, internal and external factors such as age, skill, training intensity and volume, impairment, and secondary gain influence injury risk at the developmental, elite, and postplaying phases of a Para athletes' life.[91] As the specific components of this Lifetime Injury Model become clear, coaches, athletes, and clinicians can help to mitigate those risks.[91–95] Injury research in both recreational and elite Para sport may benefit from the use of technology, similar to Web-based Injury and Illness Surveillance Survey, longitudinal study design, focus on youth and recreational Para athletes, and the use of standardized multinational protocols.

SUMMARY

The methodology, definition of injury, population, and study size varied in the 47 studies reviewed, which made it challenging to pool data. Still, it is clear that the literature on musculoskeletal injury epidemiology in Para athletes is growing: nearly 40% of the analyses reviewed were published within the last 5 years. Although rates of musculoskeletal injury are similar for athletes with and without impairment, injury patterns differ, and injuries have magnified functional consequences for Para athletes.[80,96–98] Prevention is, therefore, paramount in this population of athletes. Fortunately, as described, injury prevention can be achieved by integrating epidemiologic data into evidence-based policy changes that protect athlete health during their competitive years.[49] Furthermore, using such data to drive lifetime injury modeling can protect Para athlete health over the life course.

REFERENCES

1. Kressler J, Cowan RE, Bigford GE, et al. Reducing cardiometabolic disease in spinal cord injury. Phys Med Rehabil Clin N Am 2014;25(3):573–604, viii.
2. Liou T-H, Pi-Sunyer FX, Laferrere B. Physical disability and obesity. Nutr Rev 2005;63(10):321–31.
3. Rimmer JH, Wang E. Obesity prevalence among a group of Chicago residents with disabilities. Arch Phys Med Rehabil 2005;86(7):1461–4.
4. Froehlich-Grobe K, Lee J, Aaronson L, et al. Exercise for everyone: a randomized controlled trial of project workout on wheels in promoting exercise among wheelchair users. Arch Phys Med Rehabil 2014;95(1):20–8.
5. Rees L, Robinson P, Shields N. Media portrayal of elite athletes with disability - a systematic review. Disabil Rehabil 2017;1–8 [Epub ahead of print].
6. Gold JR, Gold MM. Access for all: the rise of the Paralympic games. J R Soc Promot Health 2007;127(3):133–41.
7. Pedersen BK, Saltin B. Evidence for prescribing exercise as therapy in chronic disease. Scand J Med Sci Sports 2006;16:3–63.
8. Warburton DER, Nicol CW, Bredin SSD. Health benefits of physical activity: the evidence. CMAJ 2006;174(6):801–9.
9. Taylor RS, Brown A, Ebrahim S, et al. Exercise-based rehabilitation for patients with coronary heart disease: systematic review and meta-analysis of randomized controlled trials. Am J Med 2004;116(10):682–92.
10. Warburton DE, Glendhill N, Quinney A. The effects of changes in musculoskeletal fitness on health. Can J Appl Physiol 2001;26(2):161–216.
11. Dunn AL, Trivedi MH, O'Neal HA. Physical activity dose-response effects on outcomes of depression and anxiety. Med Sci Sports Exerc 2001;33(6 Suppl): S587–97 [discussion: 609–10].

12. Cragg JJ, Noonan VK, Krassioukov A, et al. Cardiovascular disease and spinal cord injury: results from a national population health survey. Neurology 2013;81(8):723–8.

13. Blauwet C, Willick SE. The Paralympic movement: using sports to promote health, disability rights, and social integration for athletes with disabilities. PM R 2012; 4(11):851–6.

14. Paulsen P, French R, Sherrill C. Comparison of wheelchair athletes and nonathletes on selected mood states. Percept Mot Skills 1990;71(3 Pt 2):1160–2.

15. Fiorilli G, Iuliano E, Aquino G, et al. Mental health and social participation skills of wheelchair basketball players: a controlled study. Res Dev Disabil 2013;34(11): 3679–85.

16. Conn JM, Annest JL, Gilchrist J. Sports and recreation related injury episodes in the US population, 1997-99. Inj Prev 2003;9(2):117–23.

17. Shephard RJ. Can we afford to exercise, given current injury rates? Inj Prev 2003; 9(2):99–100.

18. Nyland J, Snouse SL, Anderson M, et al. Soft tissue injuries to USA paralympians at the 1996 summer games. Arch Phys Med Rehabil 2000;81(3):368–73.

19. Patatoukas D, Farmakides A, Aggeli V, et al. Disability-related injuries in athletes with disabilities. Folia Med 2011;53(1):40–6.

20. Batts KB, Glorioso JE Jr, Williams MS. The medical demands of the special athlete. Clin J Sport Med 1998;8(1):22–5.

21. Galena HJ, Epstein CR, Lourie RJ. Connecticut state special Olympics: observations and recommendations. Conn Med 1998;62(1):33–7.

22. Sobiecka J. Injuries and ailments of the Polish participants of the 2000 Paralympic games in Sydney. Biology of Sport 2005;22(4):353–62.

23. Bragaru M, Dekker R, Geertzen JH, et al. Amputees and sports: a systematic review. Sports Med 2011;41(9):721–40.

24. Kocher MS, Dupre MM, Feagin JA Jr. Shoulder injuries from alpine skiing and snowboarding. Aetiology, treatment and prevention. Sports Med 1998;25(3): 201–11.

25. Webborn N, Willick S, Reeser JC. Injuries among disabled athletes during the 2002 Winter Paralympic Games. Med Sci Sports Exerc 2006;38(5):811–5.

26. Ferrara MS, Peterson CL. Injuries to athletes with disabilities: identifying injury patterns. Sports Med 2000;30(2):137–43.

27. Martinez SF. Medical concerns among wheelchair road racers. Phys Sportsmed 1989;17(2):63–8.

28. Miyahara M, Sleivert GG, Gerrard DF. The relationship of strength and muscle balance to shoulder pain and impingement syndrome in elite quadriplegic wheelchair rugby players. Int J Sports Med 1998;19(3):210–4.

29. Fagher K, Lexell J. Sports-related injuries in athletes with disabilities. Scand J Med Sci Sports 2014;24(5):e320–31.

30. Weiler R, Van Mechelen W, Fuller C, et al. Sport injuries sustained by athletes with disability: a systematic review. Sports Med 2016;46(8):1141–53.

31. Webborn N, Emery C. Descriptive epidemiology of Paralympic sports injuries. PM R 2014;6(8 Suppl):S18–22.

32. Klenck C, Gebke K. Practical management: common medical problems in disabled athletes. Clin J Sport Med 2007;17(1):55–60.

33. Miller MA, Rucker KS. Disabled athletes. Physical Medicine & Rehabilitation: state of the art reviews 1997;11(3):465–88.

34. International Paralympic Committee (IPC). Available at: https://www.paralympic. org/classification. Accessed May 15, 2017.

35. Burnham R. Sports medicine for the physically disabled: the Canadian team experience at the 1988 Seoul Paralympic Games. Clin J Sport Med 1991;1(3): 193–6.

36. Magno e Silva M. Aspects of sports injuries in athletes with visual impairment. Rev Bras Med Esporte 2011;17(5):319–23.

37. Derman W, Schwellnus M, Jordaan E, et al. Illness and injury in athletes during the competition period at the London 2012 Paralympic Games: development and implementation of a web-based surveillance system (WEB-IISS) for team medical staff. Br J Sports Med 2013;47(7):420–5.

38. Athanasopoulos S, Tsakoniti A, Athanasopoulos I, et al. The 2004 Paralympic Games: physiotherapy services in the Paralympic Village Polyclinic. Open Sports Med J 2009;3:1–9.

39. Reynolds J, Stirk A, Thomas A, et al. Paralympics–Barcelona 1992. Br J Sports Med 1994;28(1):14–7.

40. Burnham RS, May L, Nelson E, et al. Shoulder pain in wheelchair athletes. The role of muscle imbalance. Am J Sports Med 1993;21(2):238–42.

41. Willick SE, Webborn N, Emery C, et al. The epidemiology of injuries at the London 2012 Paralympic Games. Br J Sports Med 2013;47(7):426–32.

42. Derman W, Runciman P, Schwellnus M, et al. High precompetition injury rate dominates the injury profile at the Rio 2016 Summer Paralympic Games: a prospective cohort study of 51 198 athlete days. Br J Sports Med 2018;52(1):24–31.

43. Webborn N, Cushman D, Blauwet CA, et al. The epidemiology of injuries in football at the London 2012 Paralympic Games. PM R 2016;8(6):545–52.

44. Gawronski W, Sobiecka J, Malesza J. Fit and healthy Paralympians–medical care guidelines for disabled athletes: a study of the injuries and illnesses incurred by the Polish Paralympic team in Beijing 2008 and London 2012. Br J Sports Med 2013;47(13):844–9.

45. Derman W, Schwellnus MP, Jordaan E, et al. High incidence of injury at the Sochi 2014 Winter Paralympic Games: a prospective cohort study of 6564 athlete days. Br J Sports Med 2016;50(17):1069–74.

46. Ferrara MS, Palutsis GR, Snouse S, et al. A longitudinal study of injuries to athletes with disabilities. Int J Sports Med 2000;21(3):221–4.

47. Taylor D, Williams T. Sports injuries in athletes with disabilities: wheelchair racing. Paraplegia 1995;33(5):296–9.

48. Kromer P, Rocker K, Sommer A, et al. Acute and overuse injuries in elite paracycling - an epidemiological study. Sportverletz Sportschaden 2011;25(3):167–72 [in German].

49. Webborn N, Willick S, Emery CA. The injury experience at the 2010 winter Paralympic games. Clin J Sport Med 2012;22(1):3–9.

50. Andrade RA, Modesto A, Evans PL, et al. Prevalence of oral trauma in Para-Pan American Games athletes. Dent Traumatol 2013;29(4):280–4.

51. Hoeberigs JH, Debets-Eggen HB, Debets PM. Sports medical experiences from the International Flower Marathon for disabled wheelers. Am J Sports Med 1990; 18(4):418–21.

52. Curtis KA, Dillon DA. Survey of wheelchair athletic injuries: common patterns and prevention. Paraplegia 1985;23(3):170–5.

53. Wilson PE, Washington RL. Pediatric wheelchair athletics: sports injuries and prevention. Paraplegia 1993;31(5):330–7.

54. Robson HE. The Special Olympic Games for the mentally handicapped–United Kingdom 1989. Br J Sports Med 1990;24(4):225–30.

55. Boninger ML, Robertson RN, Wolff M, et al. Upper limb nerve entrapments in elite wheelchair racers. Am J Phys Med Rehabil 1996;75(3):170–6.
56. McCormick DP, Niebuhr VN, Risser WL. Injury and illness surveillance at local Special Olympic Games. Br J Sports Med 1990;24(4):221–4.
57. Magno E Silva MP, Winckler C, Costa ESAA, et al. Sports injuries in Paralympic track and field athletes with visual impairment. Med Sci Sports Exerc 2013; 45(5):908–13.
58. Blauwet CA, Cushman D, Emery C, et al. Risk of injuries in Paralympic track and field differs by impairment and event discipline: a prospective cohort study at the London 2012 Paralympic Games. Am J Sports Med 2016;44(6):1455–62.
59. Magno e Silva MP, Morato MP, Bilzon JL, et al. Sports injuries in Brazilian blind footballers. Int J Sports Med 2013;34(3):239–43.
60. Webborn N, Blauwet CA, Derman W, et al. Heads up on concussion in para sport. Br J Sports Med 2017. [Epub ahead of print].
61. Ramirez M, Yang J, Bourque L, et al. Sports injuries to high school athletes with disabilities. Pediatrics 2009;123(2):690–6.
62. Magno e Silva M, Bilzon J, Duarte E, et al. Sport injuries in elite Paralympic swimmers with visual impairment. J Athl Train 2013;48(4):493–8.
63. Bernardi M, Castellano V, Ferrara MS, et al. Muscle pain in athletes with locomotor disability. Med Sci Sports Exerc 2003;35(2):199–206.
64. Mustafins P, Vetra A, Scibrja I. The sport participation limiting injuries, musculoskeletal complains and the SF-36v2 health survey data in Paralympic volleyball players. Int J Rehabil Res 2009;32(Supplement 1):S11.
65. Willick SE, Cushman DM, Blauwet CA, et al. The epidemiology of injuries in powerlifting at the London 2012 Paralympic Games: an analysis of 1411 athlete-days. Scand J Med Sci Sports 2016;26(10):1233–8.
66. Chung WM, Yeung S, Wong AY, et al. Musculoskeletal injuries in elite able-bodied and wheelchair foil fencers–a pilot study. Clin J Sport Med 2012;22(3):278–80.
67. McCormack DAR, Reid DC, Steadward RD, et al. Injury profiles in wheelchair athletes: results of a retrospective survey. Clin J Sport Med 1991;1(1):35–40.
68. Akbar M, Brunner M, Ewerbeck V, et al. Do overhead sports increase risk for rotator cuff tears in wheelchair users? Arch Phys Med Rehabil 2015;96(3):484–8.
69. Tsunoda K, Mutsuzaki H, Hotta K, et al. Correlates of shoulder pain in wheelchair basketball players from the Japanese national team: a cross-sectional study. J Back Musculoskelet Rehabil 2016;29(4):795–800.
70. Curtis KA, Black K. Shoulder pain in female wheelchair basketball players. J Orthop Sports Phys Ther 1999;29(4):225–31.
71. Hoeberigs JH, Verstappen FTJ. Muscle soreness in wheelchair basketballers. International Journal of Sports Medicine 1984;5(Suppl):177–9.
72. Bergeron JW. Athletes with disabilities. Phys Med Rehabil Clin N Am 1999;10(1): 213–28, viii.
73. Ashton-Shaeffer C. Survey of injuries sustained by division II and division III wheelchair basketball athletes. Ann Therapeutic Rec 2010;18:87–9.
74. Wessels KK, Broglio SP, Sosnoff JJ. Concussions in wheelchair basketball. Arch Phys Med Rehabil 2012;93(2):275–8.
75. Shimizu Y, Mutsuzaki H, Tachibana K, et al. A survey of deep tissue injury in elite female wheelchair basketball players. J Back Musculoskelet Rehabil 2017;30(3): 427–34.
76. Mutsuzaki H, Tachibana K, Shimizu Y, et al. Factors associated with deep tissue injury in male wheelchair basketball players of a Japanese national team. Asia Pac J Sports Med Arthrosc Rehabil Technol 2014;1(2):72–6.

77. Smoljanovic T, Bojanic I, Pollock CL, et al. Rib stress fracture in a male adaptive rower from the arms and shoulders sport class: case report. Croat Med J 2011; 52(5):644–7.

78. Thornton JS, Vinther A, Wilson F, et al. Rowing injuries: an updated review. Sports Med 2017;47(4):641–61.

79. McDonnell LK, Hume PA, Nolte V. Rib stress fractures among rowers: definition, epidemiology, mechanisms, risk factors and effectiveness of injury prevention strategies. Sports Med 2011;41(11):883–901.

80. Pepper M, Willick S. Maximizing physical activity in athletes with amputations. Curr Sports Med Rep 2009;8(6):339–44.

81. Laskowski ER, Murtaugh PA. Snow skiing injuries in physically disabled skiers. Am J Sports Med 1992;20(5):553–7.

82. Ferrara MS, Buckley WE, Messner DG, et al. The injury experience and training history of the competitive skier with a disability. Am J Sports Med 1992;20(1):55–60.

83. McCormick DP. Injuries in handicapped alpine ski racers. Phys Sportsmed 1985; 13(12):93–7.

84. Nasuti G, Temple VA. The risks and benefits of snow sports for people with disabilities: a review of the literature. Int J Rehabil Res 2010;33(3):193–8.

85. Ferrara MS, Buckley WE, McCann BC, et al. The injury experience of the competitive athlete with a disability: prevention implications. Med Sci Sports Exerc 1992; 24(2):184–8.

86. Matthews-White JM. Training history and sports injury profiles of athletes with a disability from the VI Winter Paralympic Games [Unpublished doctoral dissertation]. Alberta (Canada): University of Alberta; 2001.

87. Hawkeswood J, Finlayson H, O'Connor R, et al. A pilot survey on injury and safety concerns in international sledge hockey. Int J Sports Phys Ther 2011;6(3): 173–85.

88. Kuijt MT, Inklaar H, Gouttebarge V, et al. Knee and ankle osteoarthritis in former elite soccer players: a systematic review of the recent literature. J Sci Med Sport 2012;15(6):480–7.

89. Ahmed OH, Hussain AW, Beasley I, et al. Enhancing performance and sport injury prevention in disability sport: moving forwards in the field of football. Br J Sports Med 2015;49(9):566–7.

90. Ekstrand J, Hagglund M, Walden M. Injury incidence and injury patterns in professional football: the UEFA injury study. Br J Sports Med 2011;45(7):553–8.

91. Webborn N. Lifetime injury prevention: the sport profile model. Br J Sports Med 2012;46(3):193–7.

92. Morrien F, Taylor MJD, Hettinga FJ. Biomechanics in Paralympics: implications for performance. Int J Sports Physiol Perform 2017;12(5):578–89.

93. Abderhalden L, Weaver FM, Bethel M, et al. Dual-energy X-ray absorptiometry and fracture prediction in patients with spinal cord injuries and disorders. Osteoporos Int 2017;28(3):925–34.

94. Giles KB. Injury resilience - let's control what can be controlled! Br J Sports Med 2011;45(9):684–5.

95. Windt J, Gabbett TJ. How do training and competition workloads relate to injury? The workload-injury aetiology model. Br J Sports Med 2017;51(5):428–35.

96. Vanlandewijck YC, Thompson WR. The Paralympic athlete. In: Vanlandewijck YC, Thompson WR, editors. Handbook of sports medicine and science. Oxford (United Kingdom): Wiley-Blackwell; 2011.

97. Ljungqvist A, Jenoure PJ, Engebretsen L, et al. The International Olympic Committee (IOC) consensus statement on periodic health evaluation of elite athletes, March 2009. Clin J Sport Med 2009;19(5):347–65.

98. Ferrara MS, Davis RW. Injuries to elite wheelchair athletes. Paraplegia 1990;28(5): 335–41.

APPENDIX 1: OVID MEDLINE SEARCH STRATEGY

1. paralympic.mp. or exp Sports for Persons with Disabilities/or adapted sport*.mp. or para sport*.mp. or athletes with impairment.mp. or adaptive sport*.mp. or para athlet*.mp. or paraathlet*.mp. para olympic*.mp. or exp Disabled Persons/ or handicapped athlet*.mp. or paralyzed athlet*.mp. or paralyzed athlet*.mp. or disabled athlet*.mp. or disabled player*.mp. or physically challenged athlet*.mp. or handicapped sport*.mp. or disabled wheeler*.mp. or (handicapped adj3 sport*).mp.
2. (wheelchair* adj2 (sport* or tennis or basketball or rugby or fencing)).mp.
3. (para adj2 (cycling or canoeing or triathalon* or rowing or tennis or archery or shooting)).mp.
4. (para adj3 (powerlift* or equestrian* or taekwondo or dance* or swim* or snowboard* or sail* or skii* or judo)).mp.
5. (exp Disabled Persons/or wheelchair*.mp. or exp wheelchairs/) and (exp Sports/or Athletes/or Sports medicine/)
6. 1 or 2 or 3 or 4 or 5
7. overuse injur*.mp. or Athletic Injuries/or exp Cumulative Trauma Disorders/or exp "Wounds and Injuries"/or sport* injur*.mp. or athletic injur*.mp.
8. 7 and 8

Autonomic Nervous System in Paralympic Athletes with Spinal Cord Injury

Matthias Walter, MD, PhD, FEBU[a],
Andrei (V.) Krassioukov, MD, PhD, FRCPC[b],*

KEYWORDS

- Autonomic nervous system • Autonomic dysfunction • Boosting
- Paralympic athletes • Spinal cord injury

KEY POINTS

- Intactness of the ANS is crucial for the performance of athletes. Following SCI, damage to critical autonomic innervation can result in changes of the response to physical activity, compromising performance.
- Athletes with SCI exhibit a lesion-dependent impairment of cardiovascular, respiratory, and thermoregulatory response to exercise that could limit endurance performance and place some athletes at a significant disadvantage during exercise training and competition.
- Individuals with SCI suffer from BP liability, either an extremely low resting BP and orthostatic hypotension or a sudden increase of BP, known as AD; both alterations in BP have a negative impact on the athletes' performance.
- If not taken care of properly, AD is a serious threat to the athletes' health and could even lead to fatal consequences.
- A combined assessment of sensorimotor and autonomic functions following SCI could help to understand the complexity of this devastating injury and to classify athletes more appropriately.

INTRODUCTION

Spinal cord injury (SCI), one of the most debilitating conditions, immediately alters an individual's life. Every year, up to half a million people worldwide sustain this

The authors have nothing to disclose. Matthias Walter is a 2017 Michael Smith Foundation for Health Research Trainee Award recipient, in partnership with the Rick Hansen Foundation.
[a] Faculty of Medicine, International Collaboration on Repair Discoveries (ICORD), University of British Columbia, 818 West 10th Avenue, Vancouver, British Columbia V5Z 1M9, Canada; [b] Division of Physical Medicine and Rehabilitation, Department of Medicine, International Collaboration on Repair Discoveries (ICORD), Blusson Spinal Cord Centre, University of British Columbia, GF Strong Rehabilitation Centre, Vancouver Coastal Health, 818 West 10th Avenue, Vancouver, British Columbia V5Z 1M9, Canada
* Corresponding author.
E-mail address: krassioukov@icord.org

devastating injury, that is, traumatic and atraumatic SCI.[1] This results in an enormous burden of disability and decreased quality of life (QoL).[2] The prevalence of traumatic SCI is high, yet differs among countries, such as Canada (1298 per million),[3] the United States (906 per million),[4] or Australia (681 per million).[1,4] Most individuals sustaining SCI are younger than 30 years of age and predominantly male.[4] Because these individuals are either planning to continue to exercise or start to compete in recreational or elite Para sport, it is important to know what potential challenges they might face following SCI.[5]

Damage to the spinal cord results in loss or impairment of sensorimotor function that presents as paralysis (ie, lost or diminished motor control) and impaired/abolished sensation. Individuals with SCI are also prone to developing secondary complications arising from damage to the autonomic nervous system (ANS). Because ANS-related impairments heavily impede QoL, recovery of ANS function is ranked among the top priorities for individuals with SCI.[2] The ANS is a control system that acts largely unconsciously and regulates multiple body functions including blood pressure (BP), heart rate (HR), breathing rate, voiding, bowel motility, and sexual arousal. Human athletic performance depends on a coordinated and fully functioning ANS.[6] According to a consensus statement from the International Olympic Committee, impairment of athletic performance "is manifested by an inability to maintain strength, power, speed, endurance, and consequently sport-specific neuromotor skill performance, prompted by premature fatigue as a result of a complex process involving multiple physiologic systems and mechanisms."[7] Therefore, loss or diminished autonomic control following SCI can have substantial negative impact on athletic performance, ranging from poor performance caused by fatigue, to life-threatening conditions.[8] For that reason, it is crucial to recognize these factors when recommending physical/exercise activities for individuals with SCI. These issues become even more obvious when individuals with SCI are involved in competitive sport. This article presents evidence that the athletic performance of individuals with SCI is affected by ANS dysfunction associated with SCI. Also discussed are factors compromising the athletic performance.

ORGANIZATION OF THE AUTONOMIC NERVOUS SYSTEM

Classically, the ANS is subdivided in two components: the sympathetic and parasympathetic nervous systems. Both sympathetic and parasympathetic ANS possess central and peripheral nervous system components. Lately, the autonomic neuronal circuits within the gastrointestinal tract have become recognized as a separate component of ANS, known as the enteric ANS.[9] The sympathetic nervous system is known to be responsible for the fast-physiologic changes in the body (eg, fight-or-flight response). Sympathoexcitatory neurons located within medulla oblongata provide tonic input via descending spinal pathways to the spinal sympathetic preganglionic neurons (SPNs).[10] The SPNs are predominately located within the lateral horn of the spinal cord from T1 to L2. Axons of these neurons leave the spinal cord through its ventral roots. Thereafter, with the exception of SPNs directly synapsing onto the adrenal glands, most SPNs conjunct with postganglionic neurons of the sympathetic chain ganglia, which are located ventrolateral to the vertebral column. The sympathetic postganglionic fibers extend to end organs (as known from animal studies), such as the heart (T1-5), gastrointestinal tract (T6-11), kidney (T10-12), lower urinary tract, and reproductive organs (T10-L2) and associated blood vessels of the upper (T1-5) and lower body (T6-L2) (**Fig. 1**).

The parasympathetic nervous system is predominantly a slower system and mostly acts while the body is at rest (eg, after eating; known as "rest and digest" responses).

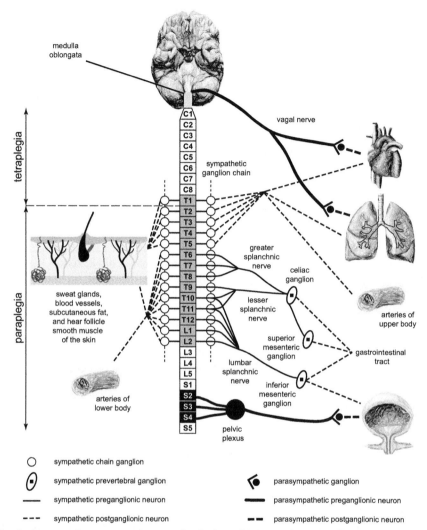

medulla
oblongata

vagal nerve

tetraplegia

sympathetic
ganglion chain

sweat glands,
blood vessels,
subcutaneous fat,
and hear follicle
smooth muscle
of the skin

paraplegia

greater
splanchnic
nerve

celiac
ganglion

lesser
splanchnic
nerve

arteries of
upper body

superior
mesenteric
ganglion

gastrointestinal
tract

lumbar
splanchnic
nerve

inferior
mesenteric
ganglion

arteries of
lower body

pelvic
plexus

○   sympathetic chain ganglion

⊘   sympathetic prevertebral ganglion   ◤●   parasympathetic ganglion

──   sympathetic preganglionic neuron   ━━   parasympathetic preganglionic neuron

---   sympathetic postganglionic neuron   ▬ ▬   parasympathetic postganglionic neuron

Fig. 1. Autonomic nervous system and spinal cord injury. Schematic diagram of the autonomic control of the cardiovascular and other systems after SCI. The brain, that is, the cerebral cortex and hypothalamus, provides excitatory and inhibitory input to the various nuclei
within the medulla oblongata, which is primarily responsible for cardiovascular control. The
vagal nerve (cranial nerve X), which provides parasympathetic control of the heart and
other organs, exits at the level of the brainstem and usually remains intact after SCI. The preganglionic fibers of the vagal nerve then synapse with postganglionic parasympathetic neurons in the ganglia on or near the target organ, such as the heart or lungs. Furthermore,
preganglionic parasympathetic neurons exit from the spinal segments S2 to S4 (*highlighted
in black*) to the pelvic plexus and synapse with postganglionic parasympathetic in proximity
of target organs, such as the urinary bladder, bowel, and reproductive organs. The neurons
within the rostroventrolateral medulla oblongata provide sympathetic tonic control to spinal SPNs involved in cardiovascular control and beyond. The SPNs are found within the
lateral horn of the spinal cord in segments T1 to L2 (*highlighted in gray*). Axons of these
neurons exit the spinal cord via the ventral root and synapse on postganglionic neurons
located in the sympathetic chain ganglia, located bilaterally to the vertebral column. Finally,

The parasympathetic preganglionic neurons, arising from the brainstem, leave the central nervous system through four different cranial nerves (CN III, VII, IX, and X). The vagal nerve (CN X) is crucial for the control of the heart, respiratory tract, and gastrointestinal tract (up to the splenic flexure). Furthermore, preganglionic parasympathetic neurons are also localized within the sacral spinal segments (S2-4) and provide control to the bladder, lower part of the bowel, and reproductive organs.[11] Postganglionic parasympathetic neurons arise either within ganglia, such as the pelvic plexus, or directly within target organs.[11] The primary neurotransmitter within the ganglia of sympathetic and parasympathetic ANS is acetylcholine. At the level of target organs within sympathetic ANS noradrenalin is the predominate neurotransmitter (with the exception of sweat glands and piloerector smooth muscles, where acetylcholine is released). Acetylcholine is also released by all postganglionic fibers at the level of target organs.

CLASSIFICATION OF SPINAL CORD INJURY
Neurologic Classification

Clinically, the severity of sensorimotor impairment following SCI is determined using the International Standards for Neurologic Classification of SCI (ISNCSCI).[12] This evaluation allows clinicians and scientists to categorize an SCI using the American Spinal Injury Association Impairment Scale (AIS).[12] This scale allows one to precisely describe the completeness and level of the injury. Furthermore, the AIS provides a standardized score that quantifies the motor function of key muscles for the upper (C5-T1) and lower (L2-S1) extremities. The AIS also assesses sensory function, such as light touch and pin prick (C2-S4/5). In addition, the AIS is used to describe a zone of partial preservation of motor and sensory function, when present. Thus, an SCI is classified as AIS A to E (**Table 1**).

Evaluation of Remaining Autonomic Functions

Unlike sensorimotor impairment, severity of autonomic dysfunction cannot be assessed by AIS. Until recently, autonomic evaluations for individuals with SCI included typical clinical tests that were previously used for the evaluation of general autonomic disorders, such as sympathetic skin response,[13,14] orthostatic challenge testing (eg, tilt table test),[15,16] sweating evaluations,[17,18] Valsalva test,[19] and peripheral catecholamine level evaluation.[20] The sympathetic skin response, for example, can quantify changes in skin conductance through a variety of stimulation that activates sweat glands.[14] The sympathetic skin response assesses the skin sweating responses within the palms and feet of individuals (sympathetic cholinergic mediated responses), which is a surrogate for evaluating the integrity of descending spinal cord autonomic pathways.[13] Many of these evaluations required sophisticated equipment, were time consuming, and mostly used in research settings.

Only recently has an international team of clinicians and scientists under the guidance of the American Spinal Injury Association and International Spinal Cord Society developed a framework for documenting autonomic dysfunction following SCI.[21,22]

---

the SPNs synapse with the target organs, such as the heart, sweat glands, and blood vessels. Afferent feedback for cardiovascular control from the central and peripheral baroreceptors is not shown. Depending on the level of SCI, consequences relating to cardiovascular control may vary significantly. This is partially explained by the number of SPNs that are independent from supraspinal control and can generate sympathetic activity below the level of injury when activated peripherally.

Table 1 Neurologic classification of SCI using the AIS according to the ISNCSCI		
Scale	Completeness	Definition
A	Motor and sensory complete	No sensory or motor function is preserved in the sacral segments S4-S5.
B	Motor complete, sensory incomplete	Sensory but not motor function is preserved below the neurologic level and includes the sacral segments S4-S5 (light touch, pin prick at S4-S5, or deep anal pressure), AND no motor function is preserved more than three levels below the motor level on either side of the body.
C	Motor and sensory incomplete	Motor function is preserved below the neurologic level and more than half of key muscle functions below the single neurologic level of injury have a muscle grade <3.
D	Motor and sensory incomplete	Motor function is preserved below the neurologic level and at least half of key muscle functions below the neurologic level of injury have a muscle grade of 3 or greater.
E	Normal	If sensation and motor function as tested with the ISNCSCI are graded as normal in all segments, and the patient had prior deficits, then the AIS grade is E. Someone without an initial SCI does not receive an AIS grade.

According to the International Standards to document remaining Autonomic Function after SCI, the Autonomic Standards Assessment Form should be used to document remaining autonomic function after SCI in a standardized manner.[22] Presently, this form has been translated into numerous languages and is implemented in clinical practice around the world.[23,24] The latest version of this form comprises two sections: assessment of general autonomic functions, such as the control of the heart, BP, sweating, bronchopulmonary system (including somatic control), and temperature regulation; and examination of lower urinary tract, bowel, and sexual function. Currently, it is recommended that clinical evaluation of individuals following SCI should include simultaneous evaluation of motor/sensory and autonomic dysfunctions using established neurologic (ISNCSCI) and autonomic (International Standards to document remaining Autonomic Function after SCI) evaluations.

Paralympic Classification

To ensure fair competition, the International Paralympic Committee (IPC) developed a classification system to determine athletes' eligibility and category assignments.[25] The IPC sport classification underwent numerous stages of development and presently includes three steps of classification: (1) eligibility impairment, (2) minimum disability criteria, and (3) sports class. According to the IPC handbook, athletes with one of the following 10 impairments are eligible to compete at IPC sanctioned events:

- Impaired muscle power
- Impaired passive range of movement
- Limb deficiency
- Leg length difference
- Short stature
- Hypertonia
- Ataxia
- Athetosis
- Visual impairment
- Intellectual impairment

Minimum disability criteria were introduced by the IPC for each sport based on which an athlete might be eligible for one sport, but not another, that is, how severe an eligible impairment must be for an athlete to be considered eligible. Once an athlete has been deemed eligible for one sport, this athlete is categorized into a sport class. Based on this classification, athletes with similar sensorimotor impairments compete against each other. Although the ANS has a crucial impact on athletic performance, little attention has been paid to the evaluation of autonomic function during sport activities among disabled athletes until recently.

CONSEQUENCES OF SPINAL CORD INJURY
Sensorimotor Dysfunction

Depending on the injury level, SCIs are classified as paraplegia or tetraplegia. Paraplegia is paralysis caused by damage to the spinal cord at the second thoracic spinal segment (T2) and below. It results in partial or total loss of motor and/or sensory function of the lower half of the body (eg, legs). Injury to T1 and above is termed tetraplegia, because it affects all four limbs and torso. According to the ISNCSCI, an SCI is classified as motor complete (AIS A and B) or incomplete (AIS C and D).[26] In individuals who sustain a motor complete SCI, the descending pathway (ie, corticospinal tract) from the motor cortex, representing the upper motor neuron within the brain, to the spinal lower motor neurons, which are located within the ventral horn or ventral root of the spinal cord, is entirely interrupted. In contrast, motor function is partially preserved in individuals with a motor incomplete SCI. Being motor complete or incomplete could be important to individuals who want to be competitive in sports, because (partial) preserved motor function (ie, of the hand and arm) is crucial to being able to maneuver a wheelchair manually. Furthermore, damage to sensory functions following SCI is categorized into sensory complete (AIS A) or incomplete lesions (AIS B to D).[26] Depending on the location and magnitude of SCI, the dorsal column and/or spinothalamic tract are affected resulting in total or partial loss of sensation of touch and vibration or pain and temperature, respectively.[27] Individuals with sensory impairments may experience numbness, paresthesia, and neuropathic pain.[28]

Autonomic Dysfunction

Impact of autonomic dysfunction on the heart

The heart is controlled by parasympathetic and sympathetic components of the ANS. The vagal nerve constitutes parasympathetic control of the heart. The sympathetic postganglionic neurons responsible for cardiovascular function receive their input from the SPNs located at the level of spinal segments T1 to T5. The impairment of sympathetic control to the heart depends on the level of injury. Thus, individuals with an autonomic complete lesion above T1 have no remaining supraspinal sympathetic control of the heart. Furthermore, there is substantial evidence that autonomic completeness of injury (ie, severity of damage to the descending autonomic pathways within the spinal cord) has an important impact on resting cardiovascular control. Individuals with an autonomic complete injury experience the most critical outage in resting cardiovascular function regardless of the level of injury.[29] The impact of the level and completeness of injury toward the resting cardiovascular control in this population has been summarized previously.[30,31] In able-bodied athletes, an appropriate cardiovascular response to physical activity is mainly facilitated by the ANS. In contrast, athletes with SCI have a compromised cardiovascular response to physical activity because of impaired supraspinal sympathetic control of the heart and blood vessels. This can limit sports performance.

Cardiovascular disease in athletes with spinal cord injury
The prevalence of cardiovascular disease in individuals with SCI ranges between 25% and 50%, which is higher compared with able-bodied adults.[32] In fact, we have demonstrated that cardiovascular dysfunction after SCI is among the primary causes of cerebrovascular decline.[33,34] Furthermore, a recent analysis of the Canadian Community Health Survey shows that individuals with SCI are at an increased risk of stroke (ie, adjusted odds ratio of 3.72) compared with the non-SCI population.[35] Physical inactivity, affecting most individuals following SCI, is associated with increased mortality,[36] prompting an expert panel to recommend physical activity to reduce risk for cardiovascular disease–related events.[37] Nevertheless, individuals with SCI participating in sports are still at an increased risk of cardiovascular abnormalities and sudden death compared with able-bodied adults.[38] Prevalence of cardiovascular abnormalities in Paralympic athletes with SCI is high (12%), and one in eight athletes demonstrates structural changes.[38] Of those, 50% of the athletes experience cardiovascular disease related to these structural changes. This evidence underpins how crucial cardiovascular function is to all individuals with SCI.

Cardiac output in athletes with spinal cord injury
Cardiac output, which is the product of stroke volume and HR, is under multifactorial control including local and central nervous (autonomic) and humoral mechanisms. In well-trained able-bodied athletes, the cardiac output can increase up to seven times during maximal exercise. Tetraplegic individuals are restricted to increase the cardiac output during maximal aerobic exercise.[39] This limitation to increase cardiac output in tetraplegics is based on a lowered HR and stroke volume. None of these limitations are evident in paraplegics.[40] However, increased cardiac output was reported from individuals with a tetraplegic SCI while under electrically induced exercise.[40] During aerobic exercise, it is well contemplated that able-bodied adults will have an increase of about half the maximal oxygen uptake. This is related to the stroke volume. Any additional rise is arranged by HR.[41] Despite the controversial literature on how the heart stroke volume reacts to exercise, an in-depth report on this matter needs a wider framework than this review.

At rest, heart stroke volume in individuals with either paraplegia or tetraplegia is similar to that of able-bodied adults.[40] During exercise (eg, submaximal using electrical stimulation), tetraplegic individuals showed an elevated, yet lower heart stroke volume than paraplegic or able-bodied adults.[40,42] However, heart stroke volume did not increase compared with the resting condition in tetraplegics in return to submaximal and maximal arm exercise.[39,43] Although nonsignificantly, the heart stroke volume response to exercise in paraplegic individuals seemed to be lower than in able-bodied adults. However, this elevation in cardiac output was based on an increase of HR.[40] Paraplegic individuals with an injury below T6 are able to increase the maximal oxygen uptake during exercise but this increase was still significantly lower compared with the age-matched able-bodied control group.[44] During submaximal exercise (20%–60% of the maximal load), oxygen uptake and the cardiac output did not significantly differ between both groups. However, HR (higher) and heart stroke volume (lower) were significantly different in paraplegics compared with able-bodied adults.[44] Recently, Currie and colleagues[45] used echocardiography to investigate structure and functional properties of the left ventricle in tetraplegic and paraplegic athletes. Besides reduced cardiac output, a reduction in global systolic function in tetraplegic compared with paraplegic athletes was found. Yet, there were no significant differences in ejection fraction or left ventricular dimensions between both groups.

Heart rate responses in athletes with spinal cord injury

There is a linear relationship between level of physical activity and HR in able-bodied adults: as physical activity increases, so does HR.[46] Individuals with an SCI are less likely to do so, because parasympathetic influence through the vagal nerve restricts the initial increase of HR related to exercise.[47] Any further increase in HR, faster than approximately 110 bpm, is facilitated through increased sympathetic activity. There are two options for the sympathetic ANS to increase the HR during exercise. One is via direct stimulation of the sinoatrial node and ventricular muscle. This is conducted through sympathetic fibers leaving the spinal cord at level T1 to T5. Second, catecholamines can stimulate β_1 adrenoceptors located within the heart, causing positive inotropic and chronotropic effects. Therefore it comes as no surprise that in tetraplegics with impaired/lost sympathetic control of the heart, the level of catecholamines at rest is significantly lower compared with paraplegics and able-bodied adults.[40] Furthermore, the exercise-related increase in noradrenaline in tetraplegic individuals is less than in paraplegics, and even less compared with able-bodied adults.[40,48] This is in line with recent data demonstrating that the increase in noradrenaline during exercise in tetraplegics is the result of a systemic release from postganglionic sympathetic nerve endings.[40,48] It has been frequently reported that during exercise the HR reaches a certain limit in tetraplegics (ie, maximum between 100 and 120 bpm), whereas paraplegics can almost reach the maximum HR of able-bodied.[48–57] With an injury level at T1 and above, tetraplegic's reduction in maximal HR is caused by a diminished or abolished positive inotropic and chronotropic effect and a reduced concentration of circulating adrenaline.[48,58] To provide more evidence on previous reports that paraplegic athletes can reach an age-predicted maximum HR,[59] West and colleagues[60] used the noninvasive sympathetic skin response technique to evaluate whether or not spinal sympathetic pathways are intact. The authors found that most athletes with a sensorimotor complete tetraplegic lesion had either partially or even entirely intact descending sympathetic pathways,[60] and the degree of preserved autonomic function was strongly associated with the maximum HR reached during exercise.[60] Tetraplegic athletes with intact descending sympathetic pathways also showed a normal age-predicted maximum HR. In contrast, individuals with a complete disruption of this pathway had a limitation in maximal HR at around 120 bpm. Preservation of autonomic spinal pathways (ie, autonomic incomplete SCI) is crucial for athletes with midthoracic and cervical lesions to increase HR during exercise. Otherwise, athletes with SCI exhibit a level-dependent limitation of HR increase during exercise compared with able-bodied adults, which is negatively correlated with athletic performance.[60]

Resting blood pressure in athletes with spinal cord injury

BP is the force exerted on the walls of arterial blood vessels when blood is circulating from the heart to periphery. Furthermore, BP depends on cardiac output, blood viscosity, and total peripheral resistance. In health, the sympathetic nervous system can increase arterial BP by elevating the force and/or the frequency of cardiac muscle activity, lowering the diameter of arteries, and reducing the kidneys' excretion of water and sodium.[61] At rest, BP is mainly under control of total peripheral resistance, which is facilitated though sympathetic activity acting on arteriolar smooth muscle. Depending on the sympathetic tone, these vessels can exhibit vasodilation or vasoconstriction, resulting in an attenuation or elevation of the BP, respectively.[62] Thus, the influence of the cardiac output on BP gradually increases with the intensity of exercise.

The relationship between cardiac output and peripheral resistance is mediated by autonomic and hormonal influences. This is facilitated through the release of vasodilatory substances from exercising muscle and vasoconstriction induced by the sympathetic nervous system.[63] Sympathetic innervation is compromised following an SCI. Depending on the extent of damage to the descending sympathetic pathways and the level of lesion, individuals with SCI exhibit impaired BP control. It is well known that an SCI above T6 is associated with life-long irregularities in systemic arterial pressure control.[64] The resting arterial pressure (ie, seated and supine) is significantly lower compared with individuals with an SCI at T7 and below or able-bodied control subjects.[45,65] Orthostatic hypotension (OH)[66,67] and autonomic dysreflexia (AD)[22] are two important examples of long-lasting cardiovascular changes. Both are often accompanied by disturbances in HR and rhythm.[68] Because of the high incidence rate and the significant health risk, OH and AD have recently become the focus of research in athletes with SCI.[69,70]

Orthostatic hypotension in athletes with spinal cord injury

OH is defined as a reduction in systolic BP of at least 20 mm Hg and/or diastolic BP of at least 10 mm Hg in response to an orthostatic challenge (eg, transfer of individuals from supine to seating or standing position).[71] During an episode of OH, the brain and heart do not receive as much blood as usual, leaving affected individuals to experience clinical symptoms including dizziness, light-headedness, fatigue, potential loss of consciousness, and cognitive impairment.[66,72]

The severity of OH is associated with increased risk of stroke and reduced cerebrovascular health,[73] and all-cause mortality.[74] Furthermore, recent compelling evidence suggests a causal relationship between low BP (ie, including episodes of OH) and cardiovascular disease and impaired cerebrovascular health and cognition.[74] Unfortunately, OH affects most of those living with SCI (~80% of tetraplegic and ~50% of paraplegic SCI).[75] Squair and colleagues[69] performed a battery of autonomic tests to evaluate whether or not autonomic control is preserved in tetraplegic athletes (AIS A to C) following SCI. Sympathetic skin response test revealed autonomic completeness of injury in 18 of 20 participants. Furthermore, using the orthostatic challenge test and cold-pressor test to the hand and foot, OH (10/20) was detected in 50% of all participants. Similar to individuals with SCI not participating in physical exercise, athletes with SCI also suffer from OH. West and Krassioukov[70] investigated tetraplegic and paraplegic athletes using the sit-up test, and found an incidence rate of 50% for OH in tetraplegic athletes, which was also equal to their self-reported incidence rate of OH. However, paraplegic athletes did not exhibit OH in this study.

It has to be acknowledged that there is substantial evidence for early onset muscle fatigue in able-bodied adults who have restricted blood perfusion (ie, applying supra-atmospheric pressure using cuffs to arrest circulation).[76] This results in reduced oxygen supply to skeletal muscles, lower force output, and increased blood lactate concentration compared with exercising subjects with normal perfusion pressure (leading to only minimal fatigue).[76–78] In individuals with SCI, a similar situation is present, when low resting BP in combination with orthostatic intolerance (ie, OH) decelerates blood flow to skeletal muscle, accelerating premature muscular fatigue.

Autonomic dysreflexia in athletes with spinal cord injury

AD is defined as an elevation in systolic BP of 20 mm Hg or more from baseline as a response to a noxious or innocuous stimuli from below the level of lesion.[68] Observed in more than half of the SCI population, that is, majority have a lesion at or above T6, AD is life-threatening because sudden elevations in systolic BP can rise up to 300 mm Hg.[79] If poorly managed, AD can result in devastating consequences including myocardial ischemia,[80] brain hemorrhage,[81,82] seizures,[83,84] and even death.[85] Squair and colleagues,[69] in the same study reporting on OH, found AD to be present during cold-pressor test (hand and foot) in 40% (8/20) of tetraplegic athletes. A high number of athletes with SCI suffer from muscular fatigue related to low BP. Therefore, athletes' desire to willingly increase BP in daily life and during physical activity to counterattack or avoid muscular fatigue is understandable. However, although it might improve performance during exercise and/or competition, this strategy to intentionally induce AD, known as boosting,[86] can be costly for athletes.

Impact of blood pressure instability on performance in athletes with spinal cord injury

In individuals with an SCI, impaired supraspinal control of the cardiovascular system (ie, heart, splanchnic blood vessels) results in reduced capacity for BP to respond during exercise.[87,88] Dela and colleagues[40] compared BP values obtained from tetraplegic and paraplegic individuals during cycling exercise with and without electrical stimulation to the leg, with data from able-bodied adults. Even though BP was elevated at the beginning of passive cycling in all individuals with SCI, tetraplegics could not maintain BP during cycling combined with electrical stimulation. In contrast, paraplegics were able to maintain BP during the latter. Because of technical difficulties, recording BP during exercise using upper extremities in SCI is difficult. However, measuring BP directly after exercise can be used as a surrogate to learn more about exercise-related BP. Claydon and colleagues[89] were able to provide evidence that paraplegic individuals with a lesion below T6 had an increased BP during exercise. On the contrary, tetraplegic individuals exhibited a decrease in exercise-induced BP.

To provide oxygen to muscles used during exercise, blood is supplied to small peripheral vessels that feed involved muscles. In able-bodied adults, this transfer of blood coming from splanchnic vessels is conveyed by the sympathetic nervous system.[87] Tetraplegic individuals lack this sympathetic input. Subsequently, reduced sympathetic tone results in the pooling of blood in the splanchnic region.[90] Thijssen and colleagues[91] used ultrasound to take a closer look at hepatic perfusion, evaluating whether portal vein flow differed during exercise executed with upper extremities only, between able-bodied adults and individuals with SCI. Those with an injury at T6 and above did not exhibit an exercise-related change in portal vein flow. In opposite to this, a change in portal vein flow was detected in those with an injury at T7 and below and in able-bodied adults. According to Thijssen and colleagues,[91] the reason for this is based on the inability of individuals with an injury at T6 and above to transfer blood to their exercising upper extremity muscles because of the pooling of blood in the splanchnic region. In another approach, Dela and colleagues[40] measured blood flow to the lower extremities to see whether or not there is an exercise-associated shift in blood volume in tetraplegics, paraplegics, and able-bodied adults. All three groups had increased blood flow to the legs in response to exercise. Yet, tetraplegics had the smallest increase in blood flow. Both studies provided evidence that the reason for this phenomenon in tetraplegic individuals is the loss of sympathetically mediated control of splanchnic vessels, hence pooling of splanchnic blood. Considering low resting BP, OH, and AD, regaining BP stability (at least partially) could have a positive impact on athletic performance by allowing athletes to establish their full athletic potential and delay the onset of muscular fatigue.

Respiratory dysfunction in athletes with spinal cord injury

It is well-known that individuals with an SCI suffer from respiratory dysfunction.[92] This complex impairment constitutes the dysfunction of respiratory muscles (reduced respiratory muscle strength resulting in lower maximal static inspiratory and expiratory pressure),[93,94] a restricted compliance (lung and chest wall),[95] and less effective expansion of the diaphragm,[96] resulting in a reduced vital capacity. West and colleagues[97] investigated whether inspiratory muscle training can improve respiratory structure and function and increase peak exercise responses in highly trained tetraplegics. They revealed that individuals who underwent 6 weeks of incremental arm-crank training had hypertrophy of the diaphragm, and increased inspiratory muscle strength and tidal volume at peak exercise (all significant) compared with baseline. Those individuals who were assigned to the sham group (ie, bronchodilator treatment) did not improve. Another study by the same group investigated the effect of abdominal binding on respiratory mechanics during exercise in tetraplegic athletes, using submaximal and maximal incremental exercise with or without abdominal binders.[98] Using abdominal binding, significant changes were already detected at rest including a reduction in residual volume and functional residual capacity and an increase in vital capacity. During exercise, the use of abdominal binders elevated Vo_2 at the final stages of exercise, whereas blood lactate level was lower compared with the unbound group. The author suggested that using abdominal binders shifts tidal breathing to lower pulmonary volumes without interfering with expiratory flow or exercise tolerability. With lower blood lactate concentration, the change in respiratory mechanics because of abdominal binding might improve blood circulation and oxygen supply, and subsequently could improve athletes' performance. Not only is inspiration affected. Haisma and colleagues[99] reported on impaired expiration in individuals with SCI. Both tetraplegic (<60%) and paraplegic (<90%) athletes were unable to reach the mean forced expiratory volume in 1 second of age- and sex-matched able-bodied adults. Respiratory dysfunction in athletes with SCI is a multidimensional challenge that limits sports performance. Tailored training and adjustments in mechanical properties (ie, abdominal binders) are two ways to successfully improve respiratory function in individuals with SCI. However, abdominal binders should be used with caution during competition to avoid an increase in arterial BP greater than 160 mm Hg, which according to the IPC would lead to the athlete's disqualification.[100]

Impairment of thermoregulation in athletes with spinal cord injury

Impairment of thermoregulation in individuals with SCI depends also on the level of lesion. The higher the level of injury, the more severe the degree of this impairment.[101] Poikilothermia,[102] defined as the inability to maintain a constant core temperature independent of ambient temperature, can influence mental state and physical well-being. Compared with paraplegic and able-bodied counterparts, tetraplegics exhibit an increased core temperature but a reduced sweating rate in response to heat exposure at rest.[101,103] The loss of afferent input to the thermoregulatory center in the hypothalamus and the loss of sympathetic vascular and sweating control below the lesion level are the main mechanisms behind the increase of core temperature.[104] Despite these potential limiting factors for thermoregulation, only little increase in core body temperature was reported in tetraplegic athletes during exercise in normothermic conditions.[105] This could have been attributed to a modest increase in metabolic rate in tetraplegics. Nevertheless, tetraplegics demonstrated a more considerable rise (higher than paraplegics and able-bodied adults) in core body temperature during prolonged training in a hot environment (ie, 60 minutes of exercise at more than 31°C).[106,107] Given these circumstances, cooling strategies to lower the core body temperature in tetraplegic athletes during exercise would be vital to avoid heat-related consequences.

Several cooling approaches (eg, hand,[108] feet,[109] ice vest,[107] or spray bottles[99]) have been shown to significantly lower core body temperature in tetraplegics during exercise in a hot environment. Only two studies have investigated various cooling techniques intended to enhance physical performance in tetraplegics. The first showed a positive effect of cooling, that is, increase in time to exhaustion during arm-crank using an ice vest before exercise (precooling) or during exercise (cooling) compared with the noncooling control group (by 31% and 45%, respectively).[110] In the second study, however, hand cooling did not improve simulated 1-km time-trial performance in wheelchair athletes (including two tetraplegics).[108] Currently, the literature on this matter is rare, but indicates that the previously mentioned cooling strategies may be beneficial to reduce core body temperature, improve performance, and delay fatigue in Para athletes.

Neurogenic lower urinary tract dysfunction in athletes with spinal cord injury

Neurogenic lower urinary tract dysfunction (NLUTD) as a result of damage to the ANS is a common consequence following SCI.[111] Depending on the lesion level, individuals experience storage and/or voiding symptoms. Athletes with an autonomic complete suprasacral SCI (at or above S1) have both. Individuals with a suprasacral SCI can suffer from involuntary loss of urine, which is caused by rapid-onset spontaneous uninhibited contractions of the detrusor muscle of the bladder, called neurogenic detrusor overactivity, and aided by the inability to voluntarily contract the external urethral sphincter.[112] Individuals with a sacral SCI only experience voiding symptoms, hence the inability to empty their bladder. This is the result of absent or reduced detrusor contraction (detrusor underactivity), caused by damage to the parasympathetic nervous system at sacral spinal segments S2 to S4.[112] Because most individuals with sacral SCI are not able to void spontaneously, another way to empty their bladder must be selected. Intermittent catheterization is the standard treatment option.[113] It mimics natural bladder emptying best (ie, complete release of urine approximately every 4 hours). In contrast, indwelling catheters establish a constant urine outflow from the bladder. Disadvantages of the latter are the increased risk of urinary tract infections (UTIs)[114] and reduced bladder volume because of continuous draining of urine. However, to perform self-intermittent catheterization, hand function must be adequate, which could be compromised in tetraplegic individuals. Otherwise, athletes must (and often do) rely on a caregiver, family member, or partner to perform intermittent catheterization.[115]

A major challenge for athletes is to coordinate their bladder management so as not to interfere with practice and/or competition. From our clinical experience, any individuals with SCI (including athletes) may not be able to empty their bladder on schedule and/or sense the state of bladder fullness, urinary incontinence, which may occur during practice and/or competition, which might leave the athlete wet, ashamed, and inconvenienced, having to change his or her sports uniform or equipment. These circumstances could potentially discourage individuals from either commencing to participate in sports in the first place or continuing to exercise in the long-term. However, some athletes delay bladder emptying or even clamp urinary catheters[116] on purpose, to boost their performance through AD.

Complications from NLUTD, such as neurogenic detrusor overactivity and UTI, are considered to be leading triggers of life-threatening episodes of AD following SCI.[31,117] Although guidelines from various urology associations on how to treat NLUTD exist, for a long time, no guidelines focusing on the prevention and management of UTI in elite athletes living with SCI were available. Finally in 2015, the Australian Institute of Sport and the Australian Paralympic committee presented a statement comprising recommendation (for physicians and health care providers) on prevention, diagnostics, treatment, and prophylaxis of UTI in this population.[118] This is crucial for athletes living with SCI, because they are predisposed to UTI,[119] which potentially can have a negative impact on athletic performance, such as fatigue.[120] Therefore, preventing UTI and activating appropriate treatment are necessary to reduce the impact on performance.

Our team revealed a significant association between the reuse of catheters and UTI within an international cohort of 61 elite Para athletes with SCI. Individuals reusing catheters (31% of all participants) had more UTIs per year (ie, four vs one) than the single user.[121] Interestingly, most athletes (83%) from developing countries were reusing catheters. In contrast, only one in four athletes (27%) from developed countries used this technique. Subsequently, the average frequency of UTIs per year in Para athletes from developing countries was significantly higher (3.5 vs 1.6) compared with their counterparts from developed countries. These findings are crucial and may demonstrate the lack of health education and resources of bladder management in developing countries.

Neurogenic bowel dysfunction in athletes with spinal cord injury
Neurogenic bowel dysfunction, a frequent complication following SCI, impedes QoL significantly.[9] Bowel evacuation for individuals with SCI is extremely time-consuming because of prolonged gastrointestinal and colorectal transit time caused by poor motility leading to chronic constipation and abdominal distention.[122] Furthermore, individuals can suffer from fecal incontinence[122] because of impaired or loss of control of the external anal sphincter. Therefore, athletes have to plan carefully in advance when to perform their bowel routine to avoid interference during practice and on competition days. Furthermore, bowel routine is physically demanding and can result in AD,[123] leaving individuals exhausted thereafter.

Enhancement of Performance During Competition

Doping was prohibited by the International Olympic Committee in 1967.[124] At the 1992 Paralympic Games in Barcelona, for the first time ever, sanctions for confirmed positive test results of doping were executed. To promote, coordinate, and observe the constant battle against the use of drugs in sports, the World Anti-Doping Agency (www.wada-ama.org) was founded in 1999. The IPC signed the World Anti-Doping code (issued from the World Anti-Doping Agency) in 2003. Similar to doping, which has been an enormous problem for decades in Olympic[125] and Paralympic athletes (including athletes with SCI),[86] boosting is a challenge within the Paralympic Movement. According to Burnham and colleagues,[125] who coined this term in 1994, boosting refers to the act of intentionally inducing AD in individuals with SCI and is used by athletes either to overcome a deficit or even to attain an advantage during competition (ie, to enhance performance).[126] Boosting is known for its performance-enhancing effect. To the present day, four studies have examined either the incidence of boosting or reported on enhancing effect of boosting on performance (**Table 2**).[116,127–129] Bhambhani and colleagues[116] found that one in six (17%) athletes performed boosting. With systolic BP reaching higher than 200 mm Hg, Wheeler and colleagues[129] and Schmid and colleagues[128] reported the highest BP values during AD boosting. The role of boosting in elite athletes with SCI has been reviewed extensively by members of our research team[130] and Mazzeo and colleagues.[131] In 2008, the IPC medical committee commenced testing BP to detect AD at any major international competition. This has been embedded in the IPC handbook (Chapter 4.3 – Position Statement on AD and Boosting).[100] In 2016, an update of this article was provided by the IPC.

Table 2
Overview on previous studies on boosting in Paralympic athletes

Study	Subject	Incidence of Boosting Increase in Performance by Boosting
Bhambhani et al,[116] 2010	Diverse sport athletes (n = 87) C5-7 (n = 70) T1-3 (n = 3) T4-6 (n = 14)	Using questionnaires, 69% (60/87) responded, of whom 17% (10/60) reported boosting.
Blauwet et al,[127] 2013	Diverse sport athletes (n = 78) Tetraplegic, C5-6 (n = 6) Tetraplegic, C7-8 (n = 47) Tetraplegic, level unknown (n = 16) Paraplegic, high thoracic lesions (n = 9)	Comprehensive testing did not reveal AD in any athlete, that is, no boosting.
Schmid et al,[128] 2001	Wheelchair athletes (n = 6) C7, complete (n = 2) C7, incomplete (n = 3) T5, unknown (n = 1)	Comprehensive testing revealed higher peak performance, peak HR, and peak oxygen consumption during boosting.
Wheeler et al,[129] 1994; Burnham et al,[125] 1994	Road race athletes (n = 8) C6-8 complete (n = 7) incomplete (n = 1)	Comprehensive testing revealed improvement in race time by 10%.

Abbreviations: C, cervical; T, thoracic.

As of now, athletes are not permitted to compete in a dysreflexic state (ie, systolic BP >160 mm Hg), and can be asked to undergo examination by a physician or para-medical staff appointed by the IPC at any given time. If an athlete fails to comply, she or he is not allowed to participate. Furthermore, any deliberate attempt to induce AD is noted and results in disqualification. Providing a base for a fair competition, athletes are tested for boosting.[127] Fortunately, there have been no documented conse-quences directly linked to boosting in athletic competition to date.

SUMMARY

Following SCI, autonomic control of bodily function is impaired. Depending on the autonomic completeness and level of injury, athletes' performance is compromised on multiple levels. There is strong evidence that exercise-related cardiovascular response depends on the integrity of descending sympathetic pathway that control the heart and blood vessels and is related to the level of SCI. Consequently, HR, stroke volume, and cardiac output are altered to varying degrees in tetraplegic versus para-plegic athletes. Furthermore, disturbances of BP, such as AD and OH, are frequent. Using autonomic tests cannot only predict cardiovascular capacity, but can also help identify individuals who are at increased risk of experiencing a life-threatening cardiovascular event during competition.

Respiratory deficits are more obvious in tetraplegic athletes than in paraplegic athletes. However, muscle training and use of abdominal binding can improve func-tioning of the respiratory system and blood circulation, respectively. However, abdominal binders must be used cautiously to avoid boosting. Cooling strategies are necessary to avoid negative heat-related events in tetraplegic athletes. Neverthe-less, significant improvements in performance in response to measures taken against poikilothermia are rare in the current literature. Appropriate bladder and bowel management is crucial for Para athletes with SCI to avoid/reduce the potential negative impact on athletic experience and performance. Boosting, the intentional induction of AD to enhance sports performance, can undermine sportsmanship. Besides enhancing athletic performance, this technique bears serious health risks, and like doping, should not be taken lightly. Taken together, the impact of autonomic dysfunction on performance in athletes with SCI is grave. Therefore, it comes as no surprise that clinicians and scientists are considering incorporating autonomic function testing into the Paralympic classification system for athletes with SCI. By creating a new categorization system for athletes with SCI, while continuing to follow the antidoping code, competition among Para athletes with SCI could become more equitable.

REFERENCES

1. Word Health Organization. International perspectives on spinal cord injury. World Health Organisation (WHO). Available at: http://apps.who.int/iris/bitstream/10665/94190/1/9789241564663_eng.pdf. Published 2013. Accessed November 1, 2017.
2. Anderson KD. Targeting recovery: priorities of the spinal cord-injured population. J Neurotrauma 2004;21(10):1371–83.
3. Noonan VK, Fingas M, Farry A, et al. Incidence and prevalence of spinal cord injury in Canada: a national perspective. Neuroepidemiology 2012;38(4):219–26.
4. Singh A, Tetreault L, Kalsi-Ryan S, et al. Global prevalence and incidence of traumatic spinal cord injury. Clin Epidemiol 2014;6:309–31.
5. Kehn M, Kroll T. Staying physically active after spinal cord injury: a qualitative exploration of barriers and facilitators to exercise participation. BMC Public Health 2009;9(1):168.
6. Fu Q, Levine BD. Exercise and the autonomic nervous system. Handb Clin Neurol 2013;117:147–60.
7. Bergeron MF, Bahr R, Bärtsch P, et al. International Olympic Committee consensus statement on thermoregulatory and altitude challenges for high-level athletes. Br J Sports Med 2012;46(11):770–9.
8. Krassioukov A, West C. The role of autonomic function on sport performance in athletes with spinal cord injury. PM R 2014;6(8):S58–65.
9. Lynch A, Antony A, Dobbs B, et al. Bowel dysfunction following spinal cord injury. Spinal Cord 2001;39:193–203.
10. Krassioukov AV, Weaver LC. Morphological changes in sympathetic preganglionic neurons after spinal cord injury in rats. Neuroscience 1996;70(1):211–25.
11. de Groat WC, Griffiths D, Yoshimura N. Neural control of the lower urinary tract. Compr Physiol 2015;5(1):327–96.
12. Kirshblum SC, Burns SP, Biering-Sorensen F, et al. International standards for neurological classification of spinal cord injury (Revised 2011). J Spinal Cord Med 2011;34(6):535–46.
13. Vetrugno R, Liguori R, Cortelli P, et al. Sympathetic skin response: basic mechanisms and clinical applications. Clin Auton Res 2003;13(4):256–70.
14. Cariga P. Organisation of the sympathetic skin response in spinal cord injury. J Neurol Neurosurg Psychiatry 2002;72(3):356–60.
15. Benditt DG, Ferguson DW, Grubb BP, et al. Tilt table testing for assessing syncope. J Am Coll Cardiol 1996;28(1):263–75.
16. Teodorovich N, Swissa M. Tilt table test today: state of the art. World J Cardiol 2016;26(83):277–82.

17. Andersen LS, Biering-Sørensen F, Müller PG, et al. The prevalence of hyperhidrosis in patients with spinal cord injuries and an evaluation of the effect of dextropropoxyphene hydrochloride in therapy. Paraplegia 1992;30(3):184–91.

18. Pritchett RC, Al-Nawaiseh AM, Pritchett KK, et al. Sweat gland density and response during high-intensity exercise in athletes with spinal cord injuries. Biol Sport 2015;32(3):249–54.

19. Berger MJ, Kimpinski K, Currie KD, et al. Multi-domain assessment of autonomic function in spinal cord injury using a modified autonomic reflex screen. J Neurotrauma 2017;34(18):2624–33.

20. Guttmann L, Munro AF, Robinson R, et al. Effect of tilting on the cardiovascular responses and plasma catecholamine levels in spinal man. Paraplegia 1963;1: 4–18.

21. Alexander MS, Biering-Sorensen F, Bodner D, et al. International standards to document remaining autonomic function after spinal cord injury. Spinal Cord 2009;47(1):36–43.

22. Krassioukov A, Biering-Sorensen F, Donovan W, et al. International standards to document remaining autonomic function after spinal cord injury. J Spinal Cord Med 2012;35(4):201–10.

23. Davidson RA, Carlson M, Fallah N, et al. Inter-rater reliability of the international standards to document remaining autonomic function after spinal cord injury. J Neurotrauma 2017;34(3):552–8.

24. Round AM, Park SE, Walden K, et al. An evaluation of the international standards to document remaining autonomic function after spinal cord injury: input from the international community. Spinal Cord 2017;55(2):198–203.

25. International Paralympic Committee. Chapter 1.3-IPC Classification code and international standards. IPC Handbook. Available at: https://www.paralympic.org/sites/default/files/document/120201084329386_2008_2_Classification_Code6.pdf. Published 2007. Accessed November 1, 2017.

26. Schuld C, Franz S, Brüggemann K, et al. International standards for neurological classification of spinal cord injury: impact of the revised worksheet (revision 02/13) on classification performance. J Spinal Cord Med 2016;39(5):504–12.

27. Haefeli J, Kramer JLK, Blum J, et al. Assessment of spinothalamic tract function beyond pinprick in spinal cord lesions: a contact heat evoked potential study. Neurorehabil Neural Repair 2013;28(5):494–503.

28. Cruz-Almeida Y, Felix ER, Martinez-Arizala A, et al. Decreased spinothalamic and dorsal column medial lemniscus-mediated function is associated with neuropathic pain after spinal cord injury. J Neurotrauma 2012;29(17):2706–15.

29. West CR, Wong SC, Krassioukov AV. Autonomic cardiovascular control in Paralympic athletes with spinal cord injury. Med Sci Sports Exerc 2014;46(1):60–8.

30. West C, Bellantoni A, Krassioukov A. Cardiovascular function in individuals with incomplete spinal cord injury: a systematic review. Top Spinal Cord Inj Rehabil 2013;19(4):267–78.

31. Teasell RW, Arnold JMO, Krassioukov A, et al. Cardiovascular consequences of loss of supraspinal control of the sympathetic nervous system after spinal cord injury. Arch Phys Med Rehabil 2000;81(4):506–16.

32. Myers J, Lee M, Kiratli J. Cardiovascular disease in spinal cord injury: an overview of prevalence, risk, evaluation, and management. Am J Phys Med Rehabil 2007;86(2):142–52.

33. Phillips AA, Krassioukov AV, Ainslie PN, et al. Perturbed and spontaneous regional cerebral blood flow responses to changes in blood pressure after

high level spinal cord injury: the effect of midodrine. J Appl Physiol (1985) 2014; 116(6):645–53.

34. Phillips AA, Warburton DE, Ainslie PN, et al. Regional neurovascular coupling and cognitive performance in those with low blood pressure secondary to high-level spinal cord injury: improved by alpha-1 agonist midodrine hydrochloride. J Cereb Blood Flow Metab 2014;34(5):794–801.

35. Cragg JJ, Noonan VK, Krassioukov A, et al. Cardiovascular disease and spinal cord injury: results from a national population health survey. Neurology 2013; 81(8):723–8.

36. Phillips AA, Krassioukov AV. Contemporary cardiovascular concerns after spinal cord injury: mechanisms, maladaptations, and management. J Neurotrauma 2015;32(24):1927–42.

37. Ginis KAM, Hicks AL, Latimer AE, et al. The development of evidence-informed physical activity guidelines for adults with spinal cord injury. Spinal Cord 2011; 49(11):1088–96.

38. Pelliccia A, Quattrini FM, Squeo MR, et al. Cardiovascular diseases in Paralympic athletes. Br J Sports Med 2016;50(17):1075–80.

39. Hostettler S, Leuthold L, Brechbühl J, et al. Maximal cardiac output during arm exercise in the sitting position after cervical spinal cord injury. J Rehabil Med 2012;44(2):131–6.

40. Dela F, Mohr T, Jensen CMR, et al. Cardiovascular control during exercise: insights from spinal cord-injured humans. Circulation 2003;107(16):2127–33.

41. Higginbotham MB, Morris KG, Williams RS, et al. Regulation of stroke volume during submaximal and maximal upright exercise in normal man. Circ Res 1986;58(2):281–91.

42. Figoni SF, Glaser RM. Acute hemodynamic responses of spinal cord injured individuals to functional neuromuscular stimulation-induced knee extension exercise. J Rehabil Res Dev 1991;28(4):9–18.

43. McLean KP, Skinner JS. Effect of body training position on outcomes of an aerobic training study on individuals with quadriplegia. Arch Phys Med Rehabil 1995;76(2):139–50.

44. Hopman MTE, Oeseburg B, Binkhorst RA. Cardiovascular responses in paraplegic subjects during arm exercise. Eur J Appl Physiol Occup Physiol 1992; 65(1):73–8.

45. Currie KD, West CR, Krassioukov AV. Differences in left ventricular global function and mechanics in Paralympic athletes with cervical and thoracic spinal cord injuries. Front Physiol 2016;7:1–8.

46. Åstrand P-O, Rodahl K. Textbook of work physiology: physiological bases of exercise. 2nd edition. New York: McGraw-Hill; 1977.

47. Fagraeus L, Linnarsson D. Autonomic origin of heart rate fluctuations at the onset of muscular exercise. J Appl Physiol 1976;40(5):679–82.

48. Schmid A, Huonker M, Barturen JM, et al. Catecholamines, heart rate, and oxygen uptake during exercise in persons with spinal cord injury subjects. J Appl Physiol 1998;85:635–41.

49. Takahashi M, Matsukawa K, Nakamoto T, et al. Control of heart rate variability by cardiac parasympathetic nerve activity during voluntary static exercise in humans with tetraplegia. J Appl Physiol 2007;103(5):1669–77.

50. Gass GC, Watson J, Camp EM, et al. The effects of physical-training on high-level spinal lesion patients. Scand J Rehabil Med 1980;12(2):61–5.

51. Lasko-McCarthey P, Davis JA. Effect of work rate increment on peak oxygen uptake during wheelchair ergometry in men with quadriplegia. Eur J Appl Physiol Occup Physiol 1991;63(5):349–53.

52. Figoni SF. Exercise responses and quadriplegia. Med Sci Sports Exerc 1993; 25(4):433–41.

53. Hopman M, Dueck C, Monroe M, et al. Limits to maximal performance in individuals with spinal cord injury. Int J Sports Med 1998;19(2):98–103.

54. Goosey-Tolfrey V. Aerobic capacity and peak power output of elite quadriplegic games players. Br J Sports Med 2006;40(8):684–7.

55. Wicks JR, Oldridge NB, Cameron BJ, et al. Arm cranking and wheelchair ergomentry.pdf. Med Sci Sports Exerc 1983;15(3):224–31.

56. Coutts KD, Rhodes EC, McKenzie DC. Maximal exercise responses of tetraplegics and paraplegics. J Appl Physiol 1983;55(2):479–82.

57. Lewis JE, Nash MS, Hamm LF, et al. The relationship between perceived exertion and physiologic indicators of stress during graded arm exercise in persons with spinal cord injuries. Arch Phys Med Rehabil 2007;88(9):1205–11.

58. Mathias C, Christensen N, Corbett J, et al. Plasma catecholamines, plasma renin activity and plasma aldosterone in tetraplegic man, horizontal and tilted. Clin Sci Mol Med 1975;49(4):291–9.

59. Lovell D, Shields D, Beck B, et al. The aerobic performance of trained and untrained handcyclists with spinal cord injury. Eur J Appl Physiol 2012;112(9): 3431–7.

60. West CR, Romer LM, Krassioukov A. Autonomic function and exercise performance in elite athletes with cervical spinal cord injury. Med Sci Sports Exerc 2013;45(2):261–7.

61. Fink GD. Sympathetic activity, vascular capacitance, and long-term regulation of arterial pressure. Hypertension 2009;53(2):307–12.

62. Thomas GD. Neural control of the circulation. Adv Physiol Educ 2011;35(1): 28–32. Available at: http://advan.physiology.org/content/35/1/28. Accessed November 1, 2017.

63. Rowell LB. Human circulation: regulation during physical stress. 6th edition. London: Oxford University Press; 1986. p. 1986.

64. Krassioukov A, Claydon VE. The clinical problems in cardiovascular control following spinal cord injury: an overview. Prog Brain Res 2006;152:223–9.

65. West CR, Mills P, Krassioukov AV. Influence of the neurological level of spinal cord injury on cardiovascular outcomes in humans: a meta-analysis. Spinal Cord 2012;50(7):484–92.

66. Claydon VE, Krassioukov AV. Orthostatic hypotension and autonomic pathways after spinal cord injury. J Neurotrauma 2006;23(12):1713–25.

67. Wecht JM, Rosado-Rivera D, Handrakis JP, et al. Effects of midodrine hydrochloride on blood pressure and cerebral blood flow during orthostasis in persons with chronic tetraplegia. Arch Phys Med Rehabil 2010;91(9):1429–35.

68. Krassioukov A, Warburton DE, Teasell R, et al. A systematic review of the management of autonomic dysreflexia after spinal cord injury. Arch Phys Med Rehabil 2009;90(4):682–95.

69. Squair JW, Phillips AA, Currie KD, et al. Autonomic testing for prediction of competition performance in Paralympic athletes. Scand J Med Sci Sports 2018;28(1):311–8.

70. West CR, Krassioukov AV. Autonomic cardiovascular control and sports classification in Paralympic athletes with spinal cord injury. Disabil Rehabil 2017; 39(2):127–34.

71. Kaufmann H. Consensus statement on the definition of orthostatic hypotension, pure autonomic failure and multiple system atrophy. Clin Auton Res 1996;6(2): 125–6.
72. Krassioukov A, Eng JJ, Warburton DE, et al. Spinal cord injury rehabilitation evidence research team. A systematic review of the management of orthostatic hypotension after spinal cord injury. Arch Phys Med Rehabil 2009;90(5):876–85.
73. Eigenbrodt ML, Rose KM, Couper DJ, et al. Orthostatic hypotension as a risk factor for stroke. Stroke 2000;10:2307–13.
74. Velilla-Zancada SM, Escobar-Cervantes C, Manzano-Espinosa L, et al. Impact of variations in blood pressure with orthostatism on mortality: the HOMO study. Blood Press Monit 2017;22(4):184–90.
75. Illman A, Stiller K, Williams M. The prevalence of orthostatic hypotension during physiotherapy treatment in patients with an acute spinal cord injury. Spinal Cord 2000;38(12):741–7.
76. Eiken O, Bjurstedt H. Dynamic exercise in man as influenced by experimental restriction of blood flow in the working muscles (L' exercice dynamique chez l' homme et l' influence de la restriction experimentale de la circulation sanguine dans les musclesactifs). Acta Physiol Scand 1987;131(3):339–45.
77. Villar R, Hughson RL. Vascular conductance and muscle blood flow during exercise are altered by inspired oxygen fraction and arterial perfusion pressure. Physiol Rep 2017;5(5):e13144.
78. Wright JR, McCloskey DI, Fitzpatrick RC. Effects of muscle perfusion pressure on fatigue and systemic arterial pressure in human subjects. J Appl Physiol 1999;86(3):845–51.
79. Krassioukov A. Autonomic dysreflexia: current evidence related to unstable arterial blood pressure control among athletes with spinal cord injury. Clin J Sport Med 2012;22(1):39–45.
80. Ho CP, Krassioukov AV. Autonomic dysreflexia and myocardial ischemia. Spinal Cord 2010;48(9):714–5.
81. Pan SL, Wang YH, Lin HL, et al. Intracerebral hemorrhage secondary to autonomic dysreflexia in a young person with incomplete C8 tetraplegia: a case report. Arch Phys Med Rehabil 2005;86(3):591–3.
82. Eltorai I, Kim R, Vulpe M, et al. Fatal cerebral hemorrhage due to autonomic dysreflexia in a tetraplegic patient: case report and review. Paraplegia 1992;30(5): 355–60.
83. Yarkony GM, Katz RT, Wu YC. Seizures secondary to autonomic dysreflexia. Arch Phys Med Rehabil 1986;67(11):834–5.
84. Fausel RA, Paski SC. Autonomic dysreflexia resulting in seizure after colonoscopy in a patient with spinal cord injury. ACG Case Rep J 2014;1(4):187–8.
85. Wan D, Krassioukov AV. Life-threatening outcomes associated with autonomic dysreflexia: a clinical review. J Spinal Cord Med 2014;37(1):2–10.
86. Webborn N, Van De Vliet P. Paralympic medicine. Lancet 2012;380(9836): 65–71.
87. Rowell LB. Regulation of splanchnic blood flow in man. Physiologist 1973;16(2): 127–42.
88. Rowell LB, Masoro EJ, Spencer MJ. Splanchnic metabolism in exercising man. J Appl Physiol 1965;20(5):1032–7.
89. Claydon VE, Hol AT, Eng JJ, et al. Cardiovascular responses and postexercise hypotension after arm cycling exercise in subjects with spinal cord injury. Arch Phys Med Rehabil 2006;87(8):1106–14.

90. Goldman JM, Rose LS, Morgan MD, et al. Measurement of abdominal wall compliance in normal subjects and tetraplegic patients. Thorax 1986;41(7): 513–8.

91. Thijssen DHJ, Steendijk S, Hopman MTE. Blood redistribution during exercise in subjects with spinal cord injury and controls. Med Sci Sports Exerc 2009;41(6): 1249–54.

92. Schilero GJ, Spungen AM, Bauman WA, et al. Pulmonary function and spinal cord injury. Respir Physiol Neurobiol 2009;166(3):129–41.

93. Hopman MT, van der Woude LH, Dallmeijer AJ, et al. Respiratory muscle strength and endurance in individuals with tetraplegia. Spinal Cord 1997; 35(2):104–8.

94. Mateus SRM, Beraldo PSS, Horan TA. Maximal static mouth respiratory pressure in spinal cord injured patients: correlation with motor level. Spinal Cord 2007; 45(8):569–75.

95. Scanlon PD, Loring SH, Pichurko BM, et al. Respiratory mechanics in acute quadriplegia. Lung and chest wall compliance and dimensional changes during respiratory maneuvers. Am Rev Respir Dis 1989;139(3):615–20.

96. Urmey W, Loring S, Mead J, et al. Upper and lower rib cage deformation during breathing in quadriplegics. J Appl Physiol (1985) 1986;60(2):618–22.

97. West CR, Taylor BJ, Campbell IG, et al. Effects of inspiratory muscle training on exercise responses in Paralympic athletes with cervical spinal cord injury. Scand J Med Sci Sport 2014;24(5):764–72.

98. West CR, Goosey-Tolfrey VL, Campbell IG, et al. Effect of abdominal binding on respiratory mechanics during exercise in athletes with cervical spinal cord injury. J Appl Physiol 2014;117(1):36–45.

99. Haisma JA, Bussmann JB, Stam HJ, et al. Changes in physical capacity during and after inpatient rehabilitation in subjects with a spinal cord injury. Arch Phys Med Rehabil 2006;87(6):741–8.

100. International Paralympic Committee. Chapter 4.3-Position Statement on Autonomic Dysreflexia and Boosting. IPC Handbook. Available at: http://www.paralympic.org/TheIPC/HWA/Handbook. Published 2016. Accessed November 1, 2017.

101. Guttmann L, Silver J, Wyndham CH. Thermoregulation in spinal man. J Physiol 1958;142(3):406–19.

102. MacKenzie MA, Hermus AR, Wollersheim HC, et al. Poikilothermia in man: pathophysiology and clinical implications. Medicine (Baltimore) 1991;70(4):257–68.

103. Petrofsky JS. Thermoregulatory stress during rest and exercise in heat in patients with a spinal cord injury. Eur J Appl Physiol 1992;64:503–7.

104. Price MJ. Thermoregulation during exercise in individuals with spinal cord injuries. Sport Med 2006;36(10):863–79.

105. Gass EM, Gass GC, Gwinn TH. Sweat rate and rectal and skin temperatures in tetraplegic men during exercise. Sport Med Train Rehabil 1992;3(4):243–9.

106. Price MJ, Campbell IG. Effects of spinal cord lesion level upon thermoregulation during exercise in the heat. Med Sci Sport Exerc 2003;35(7):1100–7.

107. Webborn N. Effects of two cooling strategies on thermoregulatory responses of tetraplegic athletes during repeated intermittent exercise in the heat. J Appl Physiol 2005;98(6):2101–7.

108. Goosey-Tolfrey V, Swainson M, Boyd C, et al. The effectiveness of hand cooling at reducing exercise-induced hyperthermia and improving distance-race performance in wheelchair and able-bodied athletes. J Appl Physiol 2008;105(1): 37–43.

109. Hagobian TA, Jacobs KA, Kiratli BJ, et al. Foot cooling reduces exercise-induced hyperthermia in men with spinal cord injury. Med Sci Sports Exerc 2004;36(3):411–7.

110. Webborn N, Price MJ, Castle P, et al. Cooling strategies improve intermittent sprint performance in the heat of athletes with tetraplegia. Br J Sports Med 2010;44(6):455–60.

111. Ruffion A, Castro-Diaz D, Patel H, et al. Systematic review of the epidemiology of urinary incontinence and detrusor overactivity among patients with neurogenic overactive bladder. Neuroepidemiology 2013;41(3–4):146–55.

112. Panicker JN, Fowler CJ, Kessler TM. Lower urinary tract dysfunction in the neurological patient: clinical assessment and management. Lancet Neurol 2015;14(7):720–32.

113. Blok B, Pannek J, Castro-Diaz D, et al. EAU Guidelines on Neuro-Urology. European Association of Urology (EAU). http://uroweb.org/guideline/neuro-urology/. Published 2017. Accessed November 1, 2017.

114. Krebs J, Wollner J, Pannek J. Risk factors for symptomatic urinary tract infections in individuals with chronic neurogenic lower urinary tract dysfunction. Spinal Cord 2016;54(9):682–6.

115. Afsar SI, Yemisci OU, Cosar SNS, et al. Compliance with clean intermittent catheterization in spinal cord injury patients: a long-term follow-up study. Spinal Cord 2013;51(8):645–9.

116. Bhambhani Y, Mactavish J, Warren S, et al. Boosting in athletes with high-level spinal cord injury: knowledge, incidence and attitudes of athletes in Paralympic sport. Disabil Rehabil 2010;32(26):2172–90.

117. Walter M, Knüpfer SC, Leitner L, et al. Autonomic dysreflexia and repeatability of cardiovascular changes during same session repeat urodynamic investigation in women with spinal cord injury. World J Urol 2016;34(3):391–7.

118. Compton S, Trease L, Cunningham C, et al. Australian Institute of Sport and the Australian Paralympic Committee position statement: urinary tract infection in spinal cord injured athletes. Br J Sports Med 2015;49(19):1236–40.

119. Balsara ZR, Ross SS, Dolber PC, et al. Enhanced susceptibility to urinary tract infection in the spinal cord-injured host with neurogenic bladder. Infect Immun 2013;81(8):3018–26.

120. Derman W, Schwellnus M, Jordaan E. Clinical characteristics of 385 illnesses of athletes with impairment reported on the web-iiss system during the london 2012 Paralympic games. PM R 2014;6(8 Suppl):S23–30.

121. Krassioukov A, Cragg JJ, West C, et al. The good, the bad and the ugly of catheterization practices among elite athletes with spinal cord injury: a global perspective. Spinal Cord 2014;53(1):78–82.

122. Krogh K, Mosdal C, Laurberg S. Gastrointestinal and segmental colonic transit times in patients with acute and chronic spinal cord lesions. Spinal Cord 2000;38(10):615–21.

123. Faaborg PM, Christensen P, Krassioukov A, et al. Autonomic dysreflexia during bowel evacuation procedures and bladder filling in subjects with spinal cord injury. Spinal Cord 2014;52(6):494–8.

124. Mottram DR. Banned drugs in sport. Sport Med 1999;27(1):1–10.

125. Burnham R, Wheeler G, Bhambhani Y, et al. Intentional induction of autonomic dysreflexia among quadriplegic athletes for performance enhancement: efficacy, safety, and mechanism of action. Clin J Sport Med 1994;4(1):1–10.

126. Harris P. Self-induced autonomic dysreflexia practised by some tetraplegic athletes to enhance their athletic performance. Spinal Cord 1994;32:289–91.

127. Blauwet CA, Benjamin-Laing H, Stomphorst J, et al. Testing for boosting at the Paralympic games: policies, results and future directions. Br J Sports Med 2013; 47(13):832–7.

128. Schmid A, Schmidt-Trucksäss A, Huonker M, et al. Catecholamines response of high performance wheelchair athletes at rest and during exercise with autonomic dysreflexia. Int J Sports Med 2001;22(1):2–7.

129. Wheeler G, Cumming D, Burnham R, et al. Testosterone, cortisol and catecholamine responses to exercise stress and autonomic dysreflexia in elite quadriplegic athletes. Paraplegia 1994;32(5):292–9.

130. Gee CM, West CR, Krassioukov AV. Boosting in elite athletes with spinal cord injury: a critical review of physiology and testing procedures. Sport Med 2015;45(8):1133–42.

131. Mazzeo F, Santamaria S, Iavarone A. "Boosting" in Paralympic athletes with spinal cord injury: doping without drugs. Funct Neurol 2015;30(2):91–8.

Athletes with Brain Injury
Pathophysiologic and Medical Challenges

Phoebe Runciman, PhD[a,b,*], Wayne Derman, MBChB, MSc (Med) (Hons), PhD, FFIMS[a,b]

KEYWORDS

- Cerebral palsy • Athlete • Elite • Paralympic • Neuromuscular • Performance
- Medical • Injury

KEY POINTS

- Movement dysfunction resulting from brain injury is typically attributed to damage to either the pyramidal (hypertonic type) or extrapyramidal tracts (dyskinetic and mixed types).
- One of the key features of brain injury is altered central efferent output, which has direct effects on neuromuscular function and exercise performance.
- Hypertonia (spasticity), athetosis, ataxia, incoordination, incorrect control of smooth movement, and coactivation are commonly observed in athletes with brain injury.
- Exercise-related medical challenges include ankle and foot deformities, pain, fatigue, musculoskeletal injury, maximal exertion and muscle spasms, and degenerative arthritis.
- Non–exercise-related medical challenges include oral health, vision and hearing impairments, higher-than-average comorbidity rates, depression, athletes with severe impairment, and psychological resilience.

INTRODUCTION

Historically, physical activity was not considered an integral component of rehabilitation or general clinical standard care for individuals with brain injury. Early studies investigating optimal rehabilitation programs have been successfully implemented in individuals with brain injury; however, these studies almost exclusively investigated function and quality of life in severely affected, sedentary children.[1–4]

However, the growth of the Paralympic movement has resulted in a concomitant increase in published scientific studies relating to athletes with brain injury. In recent years, several studies have investigated the athletic performance capacity, and associated physiologic parameters, of this group of athletes.[5–10] There is now

Disclosure: The authors have nothing to disclose.
[a] Institute of Sport and Exercise Medicine, Division of Orthopaedic Surgery, Department of Surgical Sciences, Faculty of Medicine and Health Sciences, Stellenbosch University, Francie van Zijl Drive, Tygerberg 7505, Stellenbosch, South Africa; [b] International Olympic Committee Research Centre, Francie van Zijl Drive, Tygerberg 7505, Stellenbosch, South Africa
* Corresponding author. Institute of Sport and Exercise Medicine, Tygerberg Medical Campus, Stellenbosch University, Room 4019, 4th Floor, Clinical Building, Cape Town 7505, South Africa.
E-mail address: phoebe.runciman@gmail.com

Phys Med Rehabil Clin N Am 29 (2018) 267–281
https://doi.org/10.1016/j.pmr.2018.01.004
1047-9651/18/© 2018 Elsevier Inc. All rights reserved.

an improved understanding of how these factors interact with the well-established evidence base of medical challenges associated with brain injury.[11] Therefore, the current article presents the most important pathophysiologic and medical challenges facing athletically inclined individuals with brain injury and their managing physicians and highlights the potential benefit of sport for the general brain-injured population.

DEFINITION AND CAUSES OF BRAIN INJURY
Congenital Brain Injury

Congenital brain injury (CBI), often termed cerebral palsy, is a group of permanent nonprogressive movement disorders resulting from static lesions to the immature brain.[12] With an incidence of 2.5 cases per 1000 live births, these brain lesions typically occur during pregnancy, birth, or within the first 3 years of life.[11,13–16]

Acquired Brain Injury

Acquired brain injury is an alteration in brain function that occurs later in life through either nontraumatic or traumatic origins and is not related to congenital impairment or degenerative disease.[17] In the United States, traumatic brain injury has an estimated hospitalization rate of 500,000 cases per year.[11] Traumatic brain injury is most common in men and has the highest incidence in the 15-year to 25-year age group.[11]

Recently, there has been increased interest in the study of concussion, a type of acquired brain injury, within the Para sports arena, including the long-term risk of repeated concussions.[18,19] Although concussion, mild traumatic brain injury (which is evident on computed tomography or MRI) and their sequelae are outside the scope of this article, it is important that this area of research be highlighted.

PATHOPHYSIOLOGIC CHALLENGES OF ATHLETES WITH BRAIN INJURY
Neuromuscular Control of Movement

Typical central nervous system control of movement and posture occurs at 3 levels.[20,21] First, the excitatory impulse from the brain moves from the supplementary motor cortex through the sensorimotor cortex. Second, it moves through the cerebellum, basal ganglia, and brainstem. Third, it is translated into movement patterns by the spinal cord and peripheral motor units. This last level of motor planning is regulated by stretch reflexes within skeletal muscle. Primary neurologic impairment or disturbance of this system results in several distinguishing features, which are addressed later in this article.[22]

Decreased central output
One of the key features of brain injury is altered central efferent output,[23,24] which has a direct effect on neuromuscular function and exercise performance. Research has shown that voluntary muscle activation is up to 49% lower in children with CBI, compared with able-bodied controls[25,26]; that is, the number of motor units available for activation in children with CBI is the same as for able-bodied controls, but the motor units remain inactivated unless maximally stimulated at the level of the muscle.[23,24] This finding indicates that skeletal muscle is under-recruited because of central inhibition.[25] Central inhibition also results in muscle atrophy and weakness, as well as loss of coherent movement in affected anatomic areas associated with the location of the brain injury.[27]

Movement dysfunction associated with brain injury
Movement dysfunction as a result of brain injury is typically attributed to damage to either the pyramidal or extrapyramidal tracts.[21]

Hypertonia

Hypertonia (spasticity), and resultant muscle contractures, are prominent features of brain injury. Hypertonia presents as an increase in both resting and exercise muscle tone, decreased range of movement, and rigidity.[11] For example, in running athletes, pelvic tilting and rotation may occur because of hamstring muscle spasticity. Alternatively, there may be compromised accuracy of foot strike caused by gastrocnemius muscle contracture. The transition from walking to sprint running often benefits this group of athletes. The spasticity that curtails their ability to perform a heel strike during the walking gait cycle is not a significant limitation when they are required to adopt a running gait, because the heel of the foot does not touch the ground during sprint running; the athlete first touches the ground with the forefoot.[28]

Incoordination

Incoordination is the result of the brain's inability to correctly use motor unit pathways required for synchronized, fluid movement.[29] This inability can present in awkward and ungainly walking and running biomechanics. Most incoordination is associated with damage to the cerebellum, which has been discussed previously as being an integral step in the skeletal muscle motor control pathway.[14]

Coactivation

Muscle coactivation is the simultaneous contraction of agonist and antagonist muscles during contraction of the agonist muscle group.[30] This muscle recruitment strategy is nonharmful in able-bodied individuals when there is a need for increased joint stability. For example, the anterior and posterior muscles of the lower leg may coactivate when walking over highly unstable surfaces.[31] However, in individuals with brain injury, muscle coactivation is almost always a negative component of movement and is recognized as a key functional impairment in this group of individuals, also holding an increased risk for musculoskeletal injury.[30,32,33]

Measurement of Muscle Irregularities in a Clinical Setting

Developments in technology have created a method whereby central output can be measured via the indirect measurement of voluntary muscle activation (electromyography).[34] **Fig. 1** presents electromyographic representation of 3 different examples of muscle recruitment in athletes with and without brain injury (with permission from the author).[8] **Fig. 1A** displays the typical agonist-antagonist activation pattern of the vastus lateralis (quadriceps) and biceps femoris (hamstrings) muscles of an able-bodied athlete during maximal cycling (30-second Wingate cycle test).[8] **Fig. 1B** shows the recruitment pattern of the same muscles of an athlete with brain injury and shows the complete lack of activation on the nonaffected side's pedal stroke (inhibition) and coactivation of both agonist and antagonist muscles during the pedal stroke on the affected side.[8,35–37] **Fig. 1C** shows continuous atypical muscle activation of both agonist and antagonist muscles (spasticity) throughout the pedal stroke.[23] The study presenting these data was conducted using elite Paralympic track and field athletes, indicating that these irregularities cannot be eradicated through training.

Gravitation Toward the Affected Side

It is well understood that nonathletic individuals with brain injury have movement limitation most prominently in the anatomic areas affected by the brain injury. It has been hypothesized that there is an impaired and less impaired side in individuals with hemiplegic brain injury.[38] This difference is caused by the brain's adaptation of the less impaired side's physiology toward that of the more impaired side, as a secondary response to the initial central trauma. This neuroplastic response often results in

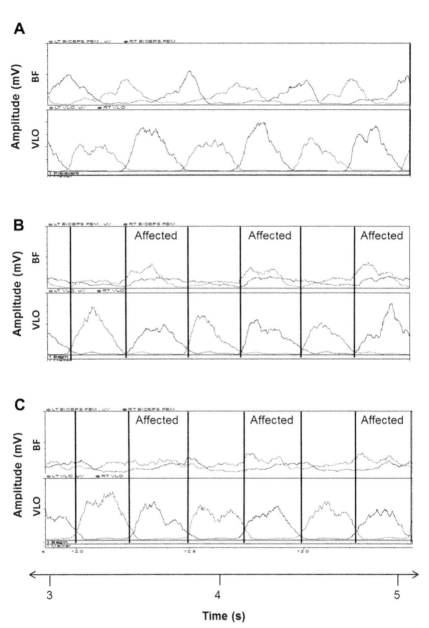

Fig. 1. A comparison of recruitment patterns of vastus lateralis (VLO) and biceps femoris (BF) muscles during maximal cycling in (A) an able-bodied athlete; (B) an athlete with brain injury, showing coactivation; and (C) an athlete with brain injury, showing spasticity during movement.

decreased muscle strength on the less impaired side, which can distort clinicians' appraisals of the individual's true functional capacity.[39] However, it has been shown that children with CBI are able to overcome significant asymmetries with the use of constraint-induced movement therapy, whereby the use of the affected side is increased by the restraint of the nonaffected side.[39,40]

Athletes May Gravitate Toward Improved Function

Athletes with brain injury, however, may be spared from developing functional limitations on the nonaffected side. A study examining power and sprinting capacity in elite Paralympic athletes with hemiplegic CBI found that there was a 33% strength deficit on the affected side during vertical jump tests. Jumping performance on the nonaffected side, in contrast, was matched to the performance of elite Olympic field hockey players.[7] The investigators postulated that this finding may indicate that athletes with brain injury may positively adapt toward the nonaffected side, rather than the affected side, because of high-load exercise training from a young age.[7] Another study conducted using the same group of elite Paralympic athletes showed that, despite the previous finding of similar performance in isolation, the same was not true for exercise performed using both legs.[7] The investigators reported that athletes with CBI used conservative pacing strategies when performing short-duration, high-intensity exercise on both legs.[6] Therefore, the athletes did perform exercise toward the capacity of the affected leg, but only when doing whole-body exercise movements (such as running or cycling).[6–8] The investigators postulated that this was a protective strategy used by the central nervous system to avoid catastrophic failure of the brain, which can result in athlete collapse, severe injury, or even death. It was further proposed that this catastrophic failure point in individuals with CBI may be lowered as a protective measure.[6]

Residual Effect of Brain Injury

In all instances, it must be kept in mind that brain injury is not reversible. That is, there is a ceiling of adaptation toward which the athlete can progress, but no further.[7] In all the studies conducted on individuals and athletes with brain injury, there were none that could rehabilitate the patients/athletes out of the spectrum of physical impairment.[9,25–27,41–43] In these referenced studies, there was significant trainability in this group of individuals, and there is now evidence that long-term exercise participation might help these individuals maintain optimal neuromuscular function over their lifespans if exercise is continued.[8,22] However, there were negative findings (discussed previously) related to the brain injury that remained static in all published studies to date. These findings represent the weakest link in the performance chain of elite athletes. Thus, if these areas are improved, the exercise capacity of the athlete's body, as a whole, will improve.

Rehabilitation of Individuals with Hemiplegic Brain Injury

There is a standard rehabilitative approach for athletes, and more prominently nonathletic individuals, with hemiplegic brain injury. It involves the rehabilitation of both sides of an individual, at the intensity and pace of the affected side.[44] However, as shown in the studies discussed earlier, if progress is made at the capacity and speed of the affected side, maximal adaptation of the nonaffected side is not facilitated.[39] A movement away from this training technique may then allow for optimized adaptation of both the nonaffected and affected sides of athletes with brain injury.[7] However, it must be kept in mind that asymmetries in such athletes would ultimately increase, as a result of training sides separately. In order to avoid incorrect compensatory muscle activation in these athletes, specific attention must be paid to this area of athletic training.

PARTICIPATION IN SPORT

Participation in sport and exercise for individuals with brain injury has grown steadily, both in the rehabilitation and sporting sectors, as shown by the growth of the

Paralympic movement.[45] There are some aspects of athletic development that are similar to those used with able-bodied athletes. However, special consideration must be paid to the athlete's individual impairment, pathophysiology, and medical challenges.

Sports for Athletes with Brain Injury

Athletes with brain injury participate in many Para sports, both within the Paralympic Games setting and independently. There are many able-bodied sports in which athletes with brain injury can compete. These sports have been adapted to make it possible for athletes with this type of impairment to participate.[46]

There are also specifically designed events included in certain Para sports that have been included for the more severely affected individuals involved in the competition. For example, the club throw is a unique event in Para athletics at the Paralympic Games, which is equivalent to the Olympic event of the hammer throw. It is scored according to the grading of the relative influence of the athlete's impairment on performance, in a group of differently classed athletes competing together (Raza points system).[46,47]

Furthermore, there are certain sports that have been designed specifically for, and performed by, athletes with brain injury. The sport of football 7-a-side was designed for athletes with neurologic impairment. The sport is played in a similar manner to the able-bodied version of the sport; however, only 7 athletes compete per side, using a maximum pitch size of 30 m by 50 m.[46] Boccia, a precision ball sport designed for severely affected athletes with neurologic impairment, was originally adapted from lawn bowls.[46] In the scant literature regarding athlete performance during Boccia, athletes who compete in this sport undergo significant physiologic demands as a result of participation.[48] The in-game average heart rate of an athlete with hypertonic quadriplegia has been reported to be 150 beats/min, over a period of 3 hours of competition (Mr Nik Diaper, English Institute of Sport, personal communication, 2017). This heart rate indicates a significant exercise load during a sport in which more severely affected individuals participate, further indicating that more research is required with regard to the physiologic demands of sports participation in severely affected athletes.

Paralympic Classification

The International Paralympic Committee (IPC) has designed the current athlete classification system in order to provide a safe and fair sporting platform for athletes with varying degrees of impairment.[49–51] Sport-specific classification is required for all Para athletes in order to compete at the national or international level, and at the Paralympic Games. All sports adhere to the classification of athletes under 10 eligible impairment categories. These categories include hypertonia, ataxia, athetosis, impaired muscle power, impaired passive range of movement, limb deficiency, leg length difference, short stature, visual impairment, and intellectual impairment. Athletes with brain injury are primarily classified into the categories of hypertonia, ataxia, or athetosis.[50]

Sport Classification

Each sport has its own classification code, which adheres to its own system of testing impairment and class allotment. The classification process for athletes with brain injury includes assessment of neuromuscular function both in the clinical and sporting setting (where the effect of the athlete's impairment on exercise capacity is investigated). This process ensures that functional deficits are observed during performance of the sport, not just in a controlled clinical setting.[50]

Performance of Athletes with Brain Injury at the Paralympic Games

To provide the clearest profile of in-competition performance deficits of athletes with brain injury, comparisons must be made within sports that do not use the Raza system of scoring. The 100 m world record for the T38 class (least impaired class for athletes competing in Para athletics with brain injury) is 10.74 seconds, compared with the able-bodied world record of 9.58 seconds. This represents a 10.9% difference in performance. In contrast, the 100 m world record for the T35 class (most impaired class for ambulant athletes with brain injury competing in Para athletics) is 12.22 seconds, indicating a 21.6% difference in performance.[52]

The wide range of deficits observed in a diverse group of athletes shows the need for more comprehensive studies to be completed in all main sports participated in by athletes with brain injury.

MEDICAL CHALLENGES OF ATHLETES WITH BRAIN INJURY

There are several medical challenges, both exercise related and non–exercise related, that face individuals with brain injury.

Exercise-Related Medical Challenges

The following are some of the most important exercise-related challenges to be cognizant of when treating this group of athletes. However, it is important to keep in mind that all athletes with brain injury require their own patient-centered management strategies, within integrated multidisciplinary teams.

Ankle and foot deformities

Ankle and foot deformities are common in individuals with CBI.[53] Athletes with deformities of the lower limb are at an increased risk of metatarsalgia, ankle instability, and increased number of overloaded areas within the foot complex. **Table 1** presents a brief description of the types and associated clinical signs of common foot deformities in this group of athletes.[53]

The inclusion of a podiatrist in the multidisciplinary team of elite athletes with brain injury is important. Orthotic and bracing considerations for these athletes are nearly always necessary, and providing services to address these needs forms an important

Table 1
Types and associated clinical signs of foot deformities associated with congenital brain injury

Type	Clinical Signs
Ankle equinus	• Limited ankle dorsiflexion (<10°) • Limited ability to clear the floor during the gait cycle
Foot equinus	• Permanent plantar flexion • Only the balls of the feet able to bear weight
Ankle equinovarus (club foot)	• Internal rotation of the foot at the ankle joint • If not treated, results in athletes walking on the lateral border of the foot
Valgus deformities	• Combination of equinus deformity of the hindfoot, pronation deformity of the midfoot and forefoot • Presents as athletes who walk on the medial border of the foot • Instability during the push-off phase of the walking gait cycle

part of patient-centered management. In more severe cases in which surgery is indicated, timely referral to an orthopedic surgeon is required.[53]

Pain

Pain occurs in up to 80% of individuals with brain injury, and most commonly affects the anatomic areas of the lower limb, hip, and lower back. The pain is thought to be related to hypertonia, dystonia, and spasticity.[54,55] Often, pain is erroneously considered to be part of the neurologic diagnosis. This error often results in the pain going unmanaged for long periods of time, particularly if the athlete has communication impairments or dysarthria. If the athlete has cognitive impairment, pain management may be required despite the lack of initiative from the athlete. Research has shown that pain is not well managed by individuals with CBI, and does not change in intensity over a 2-year observation period. Although the therapies of whirlpool, ultrasound, and transcutaneous electrical nerve stimulation were seen as successful in reducing pain during the study period, these interventions were rarely offered to the participants over the 2 years.[55] Medications used in the management of pain in these athletes include paracetamol, codeine, nonsteroidal antiinflammatory drugs, and other opiates (for more severe pain, therapeutic use exemption from the IPC is required). A spinal cord stimulator or implantable morphine pump can be used in athletes with severe refractory pain. Pain associated with muscle spasms can be managed by diazepam or baclofen. Muscle spasms can also be locally managed by nerve block, phenol, or Botox injection. Other forms of pain management include physical therapy (stretching, massage, splinting, ice, ultrasound, transcutaneous electrical nerve stimulation, and biofeedback), and, rarely, operative interventions. These interventions include tendon release, selective dorsal rhizotomy, or other surgical procedures that may be required.[11,56,57]

Fatigue

Fatigue, in association with pain, is a common complaint of athletes with brain injury.[54] A general definition of fatigue is "a reduced capacity to sustain power output over time, and experienced by the athlete as feeling tired, weak, or lacking energy."[54,58] However, a distinction between physiologic and pathologic fatigue needs to be made. Physiologic fatigue is regarded as an expected response to an exercise stimulus (including training or over-reaching). It is also rapidly reversed on the withdrawal of the stimulus (stopping exercise).[59] In contrast, pathologic fatigue can be the result of disease or disorders of the various physiologic systems affected by the brain injury. This type of fatigue should be managed according to the specific diagnosis.[30,54,60,61]

Musculoskeletal injury

Athletes with brain injury are more susceptible to injury in both upper and lower limb distributions. Athletes with brain injury constituted 16.1% of all injured athletes at the Rio 2016 Summer Paralympic Games.[62]

Hypertonia is often a causative factor regarding pain and injuries in this population.[63,64] As discussed previously, a spastic muscle has increased tone during movement and rest but has restriction in its ability to stretch, resulting in a decrease in range of motion of the affected joints.[65] As a result of this dysfunctional muscle activity, abnormally high loads are then placed on load-bearing sites in the body, which further predisposes the specific anatomic areas involved to injury. This injury risk is additive to the inherent injury risk of spasticity.

For example, a spastic gastrocnemius muscle contributes to abnormal loads on the knee, ankle, and foot directly. In response to this, the muscles that are not affected by spasticity compensate for the dysfunctional gastrocnemius. This abnormal load relationship is also present in the lower back and hip complex, as a secondary effect of the athlete having to adopt an abnormal gait cycle because of the gastrocnemius spasticity.[64]

Patellofemoral pain syndrome is another condition noted in older athletes with brain injury, caused by quadriceps muscle spasticity.[66] As discussed earlier, an abnormally high load is placed on a load-bearing aspect of the knee, the patella, by quadriceps muscle spasticity. This abnormally high load results in maltracking patterns of the patella in the trochlear groove, with resultant retropatellar cartilaginous damage.[66] The muscle spasticity also restricts knee movement with regard to the execution of well-planned movement strategies. This restriction is caused by the constant forces (and incorrect muscle activity patterns) exerted on the joint by the muscles.

Maximal exertion and muscle spasms

Clinicians working with athletes with brain injury have reported witnessing athletes experiencing acute spastic reaction following high-intensity competition. This reaction typically occurs toward the end of an event, when the athlete can develop severe spasmodic muscle contractions in all affected areas. This reaction can require medical attention, either as the result of a fall at the finish line or because of diffuse spasms if they do not spontaneously abate. However, this reaction is typically self-limiting and the spasms recede over time. If the muscle spasms are prolonged, severe, and diffuse, pharmacologic antispasmodic agents or muscle relaxants may be required, and these include baclofen, diazepam, and tizanidine.

Degenerative arthritis

Athletes with brain injury, particularly CBI, often develop osteoarthritis at an earlier age than their able-bodied counterparts.[67] This early development is caused by the inherent predisposition to injury from muscle spasticity and contracture. This condition may be caused by decreased central output[25] (less muscle activation), which reduces the protective action of surrounding muscles to susceptible joints.[68] These joints are at higher risk for injury and resultant degeneration and include the lower back, hip, knee, and ankle/foot complex. This load is compounded by the athletic training undertaken by athletes with brain injury for elite participation, which inherently increases these risks through the generation of high mechanical loads placed on joints during training and competition.[69] Sports clinicians and rehabilitation specialists should also be aware of the phenomenon of overloading of the sound (nonaffected) side in these athletes, because movement is often compensated for by the more functional side with resultant increased loads, and associated negative disturbances.

Non–exercise-related Medical Challenges

There are several medical challenges that are not exercise related but still need to be considered when managing athletes with brain injury. **Table 2** describes the types, and special considerations, of medical conditions most commonly associated with brain injury.

Postimpairment Syndrome and the Effect of Sedentary Behavior

Individuals with CBI often present with disorders additional to that of the brain injury. As discussed previously, it has been shown that these pathologic features are most probably the effect of physical inactivity and result in adaptation of the individual's physiology to the affected (weaker) side of the body.

Postimpairment syndrome is the combination of fatigue, pain, and weakness associated with joint dysfunction in individuals with CBI and, when these features are combined with physical inactivity, adaptation toward the most impaired side occurs (as discussed previously).[7,39] Contrary to the findings regarding athletic individuals, this

Table 2
Types of non–exercise-related medical challenges of athletes with brain injury, causes, and associated special considerations

Challenge	Special Considerations
Oral health	• Common problem in CBI, caused by chronic neuromuscular dysfunction • Resultant bone and oral-motor malformation and dysfunction • Increased risk for cavities and gum diseases • Drooling is common, and seen more in children and severely affected individuals • Drooling is seen when there is damage to areas of the brain that control mouth movements (masseter muscle) • Drooling is also associated with speech impediments • Despite the common misunderstanding that speech impediments are associated with intellectual impairment, no relationship has been found[70]
Vision and hearing impairments	• Vision impairment: 25%–39% • Hearing impairment: 8%–18% • Additional impairments increase the load of impairment, which is seen regularly in Paralympic athletes and has a negative effect on the quality of life and psyche of the athlete
Higher-than-average comorbidity rates	• Higher incidence of chronic diseases than the general population • Caused by/because of developmental dysfunction including malformation and specific deficiencies to the internal organs • Higher incidence of hypertension and genitourinary dysfunction • Increased risk for bone fractures as a result of low bone mineral density is also thought to be a problem in sedentary individuals with brain injury • The only study investigating bone mineral density in elite athletes with CBI showed no difference in bone mineral density to the values published by a normative database[5]
Depression	• The psychological load of physical impairment on well-being has been well established • Athletes are often required to cope with their primary impairment, secondary degenerative changes, and additional impairments • Social anxiety and negative experiences are common in the physically impaired population[71] • All athletes are equipped with their own coping mechanisms; it is the clinician's responsibility to ensure that each athlete is being managed in all aspects of well-being and health
Specific challenges in athletes with severe impairment (high needs)	• Athletes who have severe brain injury and require wheelchairs to ambulate • The use of a wheelchair automatically results in the athlete adopting a lifestyle characterized by extended periods of sitting • Medical challenges include pressure sores, neural entrapments, skin degeneration, infection • Lower back pain is also associated with sitting for long periods of time • These athletes often require full-time care and constant medical management

maladaptation usually presents in individuals who have not been given the opportunity to create healthy, exercise-based movement patterns.[22] Children or adults with CBI who wish to start high-level exercise training (either recreational or elite) may present with these combinations of factors. Therefore, sports clinicians and rehabilitation specialists should be aware of the detrimental effects of physical inactivity, and the effect it has on function. It is recommended that all patients with any form of brain injury should be referred to a physical therapist or physical medicine specialist as soon as possible to avoid these changes later in life.

Psychological Resilience

Psychological resilience is the ability to successfully adapt to life tasks in the face of social disadvantage or other highly adverse conditions. It has been noted that there is a resilience toward adversity in the impaired athletic population. Clinicians have reported that Para athletes are characterized by their ability to overcome pain and movement impairment, and even acute injury.[72] These reports show that this resilience may be a protecting factor in Para athletes' physiologic response to pain, compared with able-bodied athletes.[72] However, because of this ability to somewhat override afferent feedback, and because of the high levels of chronic pain in this population, these athletes may be able to suppress issues that require attention. If an athlete is showing signs of psychological distress, further help may be indicated.

SUMMARY

Participation in sporting activities is becoming increasingly popular for individuals with brain injury, with the associated benefits of regular physical activity. These positive effects of sport participation include an improvement in physical, mental, and emotional health as well as increased involvement in social activities. This article outlines the types of brain injury and the associated movement dysfunctions that impair the functional capacity of individuals with brain injury. In addition, specific pathophysiologic and medical challenges facing athletes with brain injury are discussed. Further research conducted using athletes with brain injury will add to the existing literature indicating the benefits of athletic training in this population. Increased scientific study within this area stands to further improve the understanding of the complex interaction between neuromuscular impairment and athletic performance.

REFERENCES

1. Damiano DL, DeJong SL. A systematic review of the effectiveness of treadmill training and body weight support in pediatric rehabilitation. J Neurol Phys Ther 2009;33(1):27–44.
2. Bar-Or O. Role of exercise in the assessment and management of neuromuscular disease in children. Med Sci Sports Exerc 1996;28(4):421–7.
3. Maanum G, Jahnsen R, Froslie KF, et al. Walking ability and predictors of performance on the 6-minute walk test in adults with spastic cerebral palsy. Dev Med Child Neurol 2010;52(6):e126–32.
4. Moreau NG, Li L, Geaghan JP, et al. Fatigue resistance during a voluntary performance task is associated with lower levels of mobility in cerebral palsy. Arch Phys Med Rehabil 2008;89(10):2011–6.
5. Runciman P, Tucker R, Ferreira S, et al. Site-specific bone mineral density is unaltered despite differences in fat-free soft tissue mass between affected and non-affected sides in hemiplegic Paralympic athletes with cerebral palsy: preliminary findings. Am J Phys Med Rehabil 2016;95(10):771–8.

6. Runciman P, Tucker R, Ferreira S, et al. Paralympic athletes with cerebral palsy display altered pacing strategies in distance-deceived shuttle running trials. Scand J Med Sci Sports 2016;26(10):1239–48.

7. Runciman P, Tucker R, Ferreira S, et al. The effects of induced volitional fatigue on sprint and jump performance in Paralympic athletes with cerebral palsy. Am J Phys Med Rehabil 2016;95(4):277–90.

8. Runciman P, Derman W, Ferreira S, et al. A descriptive comparison of sprint cycling performance and neuromuscular characteristics in able-bodied athletes and Paralympic athletes with cerebral palsy. Am J Phys Med Rehabil 2015; 94(1):28–37.

9. De Groot S, Dallmeijer AJ, Bessems PJ, et al. Comparison of muscle strength, sprint power and aerobic capacity in adults with and without cerebral palsy. J Rehabil Med 2012;44(11):932–8.

10. Kloyiam S, Breen S, Jakeman P, et al. Soccer-specific endurance and running economy in soccer players with cerebral palsy. Adapt Phys Activ Q 2011;28(4): 354–67.

11. Cuccurullo SJ. Physical medicine and rehabilitation board review. 2nd edition. New York: Demos Medical Publishing; 2010.

12. Bax MC. Terminology and classification of cerebral palsy. Dev Med Child Neurol 1964;6:295–7.

13. Rosen MG, Dickinson JC. The incidence of cerebral palsy. Am J Obstet Gynecol 1992;167(2):417–23.

14. Bialik GM, Givon U. Cerebral palsy: classification and etiology. Acta Orthop Traumatol Turc 2009;43(2):77–80 [in Turkish].

15. Reddihough DS, Collins KJ. The epidemiology and causes of cerebral palsy. Aust J Physiother 2003;49(1):7–12.

16. Johnston MV, Hoon AH Jr. Cerebral palsy. Neuromolecular Med 2006;8(4): 435–50.

17. Menon DK, Schwab K, Wright DW, et al. Position statement: definition of traumatic brain injury. Arch Phys Med Rehabil 2010;91(11):1637–40.

18. McCrory P, Meeuwisse W, Dvorak J, et al. Consensus statement on concussion in sport–the 5th International Conference on Concussion in Sport held in Berlin, October 2016. Br J Sports Med 2017;51(11):838–47.

19. Webborn N, Blauwet CA, Derman W, et al. Heads up on concussion in para sport. Br J Sports Med 2017 [pii:bjsports-2016-097236].

20. Iqbal K. Mechanisms and models of postural stability and control. Conf Proc IEEE Eng Med Biol Soc 2011;2011:7837–40.

21. Brooks VB. The neural basis of motor control. New York: Oxford University Press; 1986.

22. Runciman P, Tucker R, Ferreira S, et al. Effects of exercise training on performance and function in individuals with cerebral palsy: a critical review. South African Journal for Research in Sport, Physical Education and Recreation (SAJRSPER) 2016;38(3):177–93.

23. Rose J, McGill KC. Neuromuscular activation and motor-unit firing characteristics in cerebral palsy. Dev Med Child Neurol 2005;47(5):329–36.

24. Frontera WR, Grimby L, Larsson L. Firing rate of the lower motoneuron and contractile properties of its muscle fibers after upper motoneuron lesion in man. Muscle Nerve 1997;20(8):938–47.

25. Stackhouse SK, Binder-Macleod SA, Lee SC. Voluntary muscle activation, contractile properties, and fatigability in children with and without cerebral palsy. Muscle Nerve 2005;31(5):594–601.

26. Elder GC, Kirk J, Stewart G, et al. Contributing factors to muscle weakness in children with cerebral palsy. Dev Med Child Neurol 2003;45(8):542–50.

27. Reid S, Hamer P, Alderson J, et al. Neuromuscular adaptations to eccentric strength training in children and adolescents with cerebral palsy. Dev Med Child Neurol 2010;52(4):358–63.

28. Novacheck TF. The biomechanics of running. Gait Posture 1998;7(1):77–95.

29. Neptune RR, Kautz SA. Muscle activation and deactivation dynamics: the governing properties in fast cyclical human movement performance? Exerc Sport Sci Rev 2001;29(2):76–80.

30. Damiano DL, Martellotta TL, Sullivan DJ, et al. Muscle force production and functional performance in spastic cerebral palsy: relationship of cocontraction. Arch Phys Med Rehabil 2000;81(7):895–900.

31. Osternig LR, Hamill J, Corcos DM, et al. Electromyographic patterns accompanying isokinetic exercise under varying speed and sequencing conditions. Am J Phys Med 1984;63(6):289–97.

32. Myklebust BM, Gottlieb GL, Penn RD, et al. Reciprocal excitation of antagonistic muscles as a differentiating feature in spasticity. Ann Neurol 1982;12(4):367–74.

33. Damiano DL, Dodd K, Taylor NF. Should we be testing and training muscle strength in cerebral palsy? Dev Med Child Neurol 2002;44(1):68–72.

34. Stegeman DF, Blok JH, Hermens HJ, et al. Surface EMG models: properties and applications. J Electromyogr Kinesiol 2000;10(5):313–26.

35. Hug F, Dorel S. Electromyographic analysis of pedaling: a review. J Electromyogr Kinesiol 2009;19(2):182–98.

36. Hirokawa S. Three-dimensional mathematical model analysis of the patellofemoral joint. J Biomech 1991;24(8):659–71.

37. Solomonow M, Baratta R, Zhou BH, et al. Electromyogram coactivation patterns of the elbow antagonist muscles during slow isokinetic movement. Exp Neurol 1988;100(3):470–7.

38. Friel KM, Chakrabarty S, Martin JH. Pathophysiological mechanisms of impaired limb use and repair strategies for motor systems after unilateral injury of the developing brain. Dev Med Child Neurol 2013;55(Suppl 4):27–31.

39. Uswatte G, Taub E. Constraint-induced movement therapy: a method for harnessing neuroplasticity to treat motor disorders. Prog Brain Res 2013;207:379–401.

40. Wang TN, Wu CY, Chen CL, et al. Logistic regression analyses for predicting clinically important differences in motor capacity, motor performance, and functional independence after constraint-induced therapy in children with cerebral palsy. Res Dev Disabil 2013;34(3):1044–51.

41. Damiano DL, Abel MF. Functional outcomes of strength training in spastic cerebral palsy. Arch Phys Med Rehabil 1998;79(2):119–25.

42. van Meeteren J, van Rijn RM, Selles RW, et al. Grip strength parameters and functional activities in young adults with unilateral cerebral palsy compared with healthy subjects. J Rehabil Med 2007;39(8):598–604.

43. Hussain AW, Onambele GL, Williams AG, et al. Muscle size, activation, and co-activation in adults with cerebral palsy. Muscle Nerve 2014;49(1):76–83.

44. Brukner P, Khan K. Clinical sports medicine. 3rd edition. Sydney (Australia): McGraw-Hill; 2006.

45. Blauwet C, Willick SE. The Paralympic Movement: using sports to promote health, disability rights, and social integration for athletes with disabilities. PM R 2012;4(11):851–6.

46. International Paralympic Committee Paralympic Sports. 2017. Available at: https://www.paralympic.org/sports. Accessed March 13, 2017.
47. Picolin A. Explanatory report. Bonn (Germany): IPC Athletics Raza Point Score System. 2014.
48. Fong DT, Yam KY, Chu VW, et al. Upper limb muscle fatigue during prolonged Boccia games with underarm throwing technique. Sports Biomech 2012;11(4):441–51.
49. International Paralympic Committee Medical Code. IPC Handbook 2[1.4]. 2016. 12-15-2015.
50. Tweedy SM. International Paralympic Committee Athletics Classification Project for Physical Impairments: final report- stage 1. 2010. 1.2(2010/07/16). Available at: http://www.paralympic.org/Athletics/RulesandRegulations/Classification. Accessed November 15, 2012.
51. Tweedy SM, Vanlandewijck YC. International Paralympic Committee position stand–background and scientific principles of classification in Paralympic sport. Br J Sports Med 2011;45(4):259–69.
52. Rio 2016 Summer Paralympic Games Schedule and Results: para athletics. 2017. Available at: https://www.paralympic.org/rio-2016/schedule-results/info-live-results/rio-2016/eng/zz/engzz_athletics-daily-competition-schedule.htm. Accessed April 1, 2017.
53. Kedem P, Scher DM. Foot deformities in children with cerebral palsy. Curr Opin Pediatr 2015;27(1):67–74.
54. Brunton LK, Rice CL. Fatigue in cerebral palsy: a critical review. Dev Neurorehabil 2012;15(1):54–62.
55. Jensen MP, Engel JM, Hoffman AJ, et al. Natural history of chronic pain and pain treatment in adults with cerebral palsy. Am J Phys Med Rehabil 2004;83(6):439–45.
56. Langerak NG, Vaughan CL, Peter JC, et al. Long-term outcomes of dorsal rhizotomy. J Neurosurg Pediatr 2013;12(6):664–5.
57. Langerak NG, Hillier SL, Verkoeijen PP, et al. Level of activity and participation in adults with spastic diplegia 17-26 years after selective dorsal rhizotomy. J Rehabil Med 2011;43(4):330–7.
58. Davis MP, Walsh D. Mechanisms of fatigue. J Support Oncol 2010;8(4):164–74.
59. Weir JP, Beck TW, Cramer JT, et al. Is fatigue all in your head? A critical review of the central governor model. Br J Sports Med 2006;40(7):573–86.
60. Lundberg A. Maximal aerobic capacity of young people with spastic cerebral palsy. Dev Med Child Neurol 1978;20(2):205–10.
61. Lundberg A. Longitudinal study of physical working capacity of young people with spastic cerebral palsy. Dev Med Child Neurol 1984;26(3):328–34.
62. Derman W, Runciman P, Schwellnus M, et al. High precompetition injury rate dominates the injury profile at the Rio 2016 Summer Paralympic Games: a prospective cohort study of 51 198 athlete days. Br J Sports Med 2018;52(1):24–31.
63. Graham HK, Rosenbaum P, Paneth N, et al. Cerebral palsy. Nat Rev Dis Primers 2016;2:15082.
64. Sengupta DK, Fan H. The basis of mechanical instability in degenerative disc disease: a cadaveric study of abnormal motion versus load distribution. Spine (Phila Pa 1976) 2014;39(13):1032–43.
65. Ranatunga KW. Skeletal muscle stiffness and contracture in children with spastic cerebral palsy. J Physiol 2011;589(Pt 11):2665.
66. Choi Y, Lee SH, Chung CY, et al. Anterior knee pain in patients with cerebral palsy. Clin Orthop Surg 2014;6(4):426–31.
67. Carter DR, Tse B. The pathogenesis of osteoarthritis in cerebral palsy. Dev Med Child Neurol 2009;51(Suppl 4):79–83.

68. Tanaka M, Shigihara Y, Watanabe Y. Central inhibition regulates motor output during physical fatigue. Brain Res 2011;1412:37–43.
69. Gouttebarge V, Inklaar H, Backx F, et al. Prevalence of osteoarthritis in former elite athletes: a systematic overview of the recent literature. Rheumatol Int 2015;35(3): 405–18.
70. Tahmassebi JF, Curzon ME. Prevalence of drooling in children with cerebral palsy attending special schools. Dev Med Child Neurol 2003;45(9):613–7.
71. Vergunst R, Swartz L, Mji G, et al. 'You must carry your wheelchair'–barriers to accessing healthcare in a South African rural area. Glob Health Action 2015;8: 29003.
72. Derman W, Ferreira S, Subban K, et al. Transcendence of musculoskeletal injury in athletes with disability during major competition. South African Journal of Sports Medicine 2011;23(3):95–7.

Key Nutritional Strategies to Optimize Performance in Para Athletes

Jacque Scaramella, MS, RD, CSSD[a],
Nuwanee Kirihennedige, MS, RD, CSSD[b],
Elizabeth Broad, PhD, BSc, DipNutrDiet, MAppSc[a],*

KEYWORDS

- Bone mineral density • Carbohydrate • Protein • Vitamin D • Iron
- Spinal cord injury • Amputee • Dietary intake

KEY POINTS

- Dietary intakes of Para athletes are often insufficient to meet needs and lead to macronutrient and micronutrient deficiencies.
- Carbohydrate, protein, vitamin D, and iron are 4 key nutrients that have a great impact on athletic performance.
- When working with Para athletes, it is important to understand that there are a variety of factors related to their impairment that can impact their dietary intakes of carbohydrate, protein, vitamin D, and iron to support athletic performance.
- Depending of the nature of an athlete's impairment, a Para athlete may be at greater risk for suboptimal nutrient status, decreased bone mineral density, increased susceptibility to illness and injury, weakened oxygen utilization and transport, and a reduced ability to sustain high-intensity training.
- There is an increased need for sport nutrition education to support Para athletes by improving dietary knowledge and awareness of risk factors that may lead to decreased health and performance.

INTRODUCTION

Dietary recommendations for optimal sports performance at all competitive levels are well documented in the literature. However, there are limited studies on dietary

Disclosures: The authors have no financial or commercial conflicts of interest, or sources of income, other than the US Olympic Committee.
[a] Sport Performance, United States Olympic Committee (US Paralympics), 2800 Olympic Parkway, Chula Vista, CA 91915, USA; [b] Sport Performance, United States Olympic Committee (US Paralympics), 1 Olympic Plaza, Colorado Springs, CO 80909, USA
* Corresponding author.
E-mail address: Elizabeth.Broad@usoc.org

intake patterns in Para athletes, and those that are available are mostly focused on athletes with a spinal cord injury. Para athletes of all impairment types are at risk for inadequate dietary intakes to support athletic performance.[1–6] For example, Para athletes competing in wheelchair sports have been reported to consume inadequate total energy and specifically, inadequate carbohydrate, fat, and fiber.[1–5] These inadequate energy intakes often result in micronutrient insufficiencies, namely B vitamins, iron, vitamin D, vitamin C, calcium, and magnesium, all of which have an impact on athletic performance.[1–6] Second to inadequate intakes, the nature of an athlete's impairment may also put the athlete at greater risk for micronutrient deficiencies.

These shortfalls can lead to suboptimal nutrient status, poor bone health, and subsequently higher risk for future fractures, weakened oxygen utilization and transport, and impaired training capability.[7–9] Athletic performance aside, insufficient macronutrient and micronutrient intake weakens the immune system and increases the risk of illness, leading to time off the field of play during training and competition.[6] Limited nutrition education and lack of knowledge regarding how to balance dietary intake to meet recommended daily allowances (RDA) is likely responsible for these nutrient deficiencies in Para athletes.[5] Fewer than 50% of elite wheelchair basketball athletes surveyed on nutrition topics answered basic nutrition questions correctly.[1] Most did not have adequate general or sport-related nutrition education and support.[1,5,6] In fact, only 18% of wheelchair basketball athletes studied identified a dietitian as their source of nutrition knowledge.[1]

Provision of nutrition education and feedback significantly improved Para athletes' dietary intake and food choices. For example, 24% more Para athletes surveyed met the RDA for calcium intake after nutrition education.[5,6] Athletes' interest in further nutrition education increased 36.2% and overall attitudes about nutrition increased by 27.8% following nutrition education.[5] This highlights the need for more sports nutrition interventions and education to support the performance needs of Para athletes, and to minimize nutrient deficiencies that may impact performance, illness, and injury. An individual approach is recommended to identify risk factors associated with nutrient deficiencies unique to each Para athlete and ensure sports nutrition recommendations are individualized to the athlete's specific needs, from level of nutrition education to attitudes toward nutrition information, preferred style of learning, and impairment type.

The aim of this article was to review the current literature on nutrition recommendations for athletes, specifically nutrients that impact performance, training adaptations, and overall health, and to propose potential reasons why Para athletes may not always meet these recommendations. This article focuses on the following impairment types: spinal cord injury (SCI), amputees, cerebral palsy (CP), acquired brain injury (ABI), visual impairment (VI), and intellectual impairments. An overview of factors affecting nutrition status and performance for Para athletes is outlined and 4 key nutrients are explored: carbohydrate, protein, iron, and vitamin D.

NUTRITION CONSIDERATIONS IN PARA ATHLETES

When working with Para athletes, it is important to understand impairment-related factors that impact athletes' dietary intakes or needs. **Table 1** outlines such factors and the associated impairment types.

Table 1
Factors affecting nutrition status and performance

Factors	Cause(s)	Impact on Performance
Reduced metabolic rate and energy expenditure	• SCI • Lower-functioning CP • Double leg amputees	• At risk for macro/micronutrient deficiencies due to reduced caloric intake and needs (may negatively affect bone health, iron status, oxygen utilization, power, endurance capacity, immunity, injury risk)
Reduced muscle mass	• SCI • Lower limb amputees • CP	• Glycogen storage capacity may be smaller than in large muscle groups/where no atrophy is present
Drug nutrient interactions of medications commonly used by Para athletes	• Pain medications → constipation • Steroids → suppress immune system, weight gain, bone loss (osteoblast suppression, increased bone resorption) • Antidepressants → increased appetite, weight gain, dry mouth, dizziness • Anticonvulsant → decreased vitamin D and calcium metabolism, increased appetite • Antibiotics	• Discomfort that disrupts training and competition (nausea, diarrhea, constipation, dizziness) • Increased illness risk • Poor bone health and increased fracture risk • Negative impacts on body composition from uncontrolled hunger and weight gain • Increased illness risk due to decreases in gut bacteria → compromising gut health and immunity
Sleep disturbances	• Poor pain management • Medications • Posttraumatic stress disorder • ABI • VI • SCI	• Impaired recovery • Impaired hormone regulation (increases in ghrelin and decreases in leptin leading to poor hunger cues → indirectly affecting body composition)
Insufficient guidance at meal times and buffets (especially in unfamiliar areas and locations)	• Poor guidance from support staff during meal times for VI athletes and athletes with intellectual impairments to meet nutrient needs	• Inadequate energy intake to sustain multiple training sessions • Inadequate energy intake to maintain intensity and power • Micronutrient deficiencies → compromised immunity, suboptimal iron and vitamin D status • Excess energy intake and weight gain due to disproportionately large serving sizes

(continued on next page)

Table 1
(continued)

Factors	Cause(s)	Impact on Performance
Insufficient rest time between training sessions or hard training days for Para athletes	• Improper scheduling • Inadequate time between sessions or recovery days, especially in training camp environments (note: very few Para athletes are professional athletes, hence short-duration training camps are common)	• Limits the ability to maximize recovery, restore glycogen (refuel), and rehydrate • Increased risk for injury and illness
Swallowing difficulty and trouble preparing foods	• Improper cooking equipment and kitchen environment • CP • SCI • VI	• Inadequate energy and fluid intake to sustain training loads and recovery • Choosing highly processed, energy-dense food items • Longer circadian rhythm with complete VI → impairs strength and reaction time
Abnormal sweat rates and poor thermoregulation	• Increased sweat rates (CP) • Inadequate fluid and electrolyte replenishment to meet increased needs (CP) • Poor thermoregulation → reduced sweat rate and ability to dissipate heat (SCI and amputees) • Insufficient heat acclimation (SCI, amputees)	• Dehydration • Overheating • Spasms • Inability to finish training and competition • Increased injury and cramping risk • Heat exhaustion and stroke
Concomitant medical issues (diabetes, gastrointestinal issues, autonomic dysreflexia, autoimmune diseases, chronic inflammation)	• Side effect(s) of impairment	• Uncontrolled hypertension • Overheating/poor thermoregulation • Spasms • Inability to complete training • Limited food options • Limited ability to metabolize carbohydrates • Deficiency of key nutrients related to impaired absorption

Abbreviations: ABI, acquired brain injury; CP, cerebral palsy; SCI, spinal cord injury; VI, visual impairment; →, is connected to.

NUTRIENTS THAT IMPACT ATHLETIC PERFORMANCE
Energy

Sound nutrition recommendations for sports performance rely on the sensitive estimation of absolute energy needs, which can be challenging to achieve for Para athletes. Existing equations that estimate resting energy expenditure are based on a nonathletic population of able-bodied individuals. Exercise energy expenditure has not been assessed for many Para sports.[10] A more detailed overview of how to estimate energy requirements for Para athletes is beyond the scope of this article, but it has been recently summarized by Broad and Juzwiak.[10]

Energy expenditure

Special consideration always should be taken with each athlete's impairment and how it affects muscle mass, energy expenditure, and energy intake to maintain energy balance (see **Table 1**). For athletes with an SCI, impairments in motor function as well as the sympathetic nervous system can result in muscle atrophy below the level of lesion, and consequently reduced resting metabolic rate, lower daily and exercise energy expenditure, and reduced Vo_{2max} and power output, in comparison with preinjury values.[11] Depending on the level and completeness of injury, aerobic capacity and heart rate also may be reduced compared with able-bodied athletes.[11] Decreased energy expenditure results in lower caloric requirements. Therefore, nutrient-dense foods and small, frequent feedings to limit micronutrient deficiencies are recommended. Of note, in the setting of healing from pressure wounds and infections, common among athletes using wheelchairs or ambulating with prosthetics, total energy intakes and protein needs are higher.[11]

Athletes with lower limb amputations or CP may have lower resting energy expenditure due to reduced muscle mass. Those who ambulate by walking may counter this during activities of daily living and during exercise due to inefficient biomechanical movements, and for those with CP potentially also athetosis (ie, involuntary, writhing movements).[12] The relative change in absolute energy expenditure needs to be assessed on an individual basis,[10] and nutrition strategies, such as food quality and portion control, should be promoted to help optimize performance and achieve body composition goals.

Feeding concerns

Athletes with significant motor impairment due to CP may present with feeding difficulties, which may lead to decreased energy intake. Additionally, the prevalence of illness may be higher in these athletes, resulting in higher energy and protein requirements to avoid losses in muscle strength and immune function.[12] Depending on the area of the brain affected, picky eating behaviors may ensue, causing food aversions, which may lead to nutrient deficiencies.[12] Individualized fueling and recovery strategies should be used to promote well-tolerated foods rich in carbohydrate and protein to adequately meet needs, especially during hard training phases and while traveling for training and competition. Food-based supplements may be warranted to help meet an athlete's needs when issues with food aversions arise, particularly during times of limited access to common foods, such as during travel.

Inadequate energy intake

Insufficient energy intake, especially during high-volume training, decreases the body's ability to sustain exercise capacity and maintain power output. In addition, it reduces the ability to refuel and recover properly between sessions, ultimately increasing illness and injury risk. Para athletes are often reported to have inadequate energy intakes, which commonly result in performance-related micronutrient insufficiencies, such as low iron and vitamin D.[1–6] The recent International Olympic Committee consensus statement on Relative Energy Deficiency in Sport (RED-S) highlights the negative effects of chronic energy insufficiency on athletic performance, including decreases in bone health, skeletal muscle function, immunity, metabolism, and cardiovascular and endocrine function.[13] The prevalence of RED-S has not yet been reported in Para athletes, but is an area of concern.[14] All individuals working with Para athletes, including the sports physician, should remain mindful of energy needs and the need to fuel athletes sufficiently.

Carbohydrate

Sufficient carbohydrate intake is necessary to maintain training intensity, combat fatigue, protect immune function, and sustain training adaptations.[15] Therefore, optimizing carbohydrate stores in the muscle and liver is key for ensuring athletic success.

Carbohydrate intakes of athletes should be varied from day-to-day according to the total volume and intensity of training. The ranges of recommended carbohydrate intakes are presented in **Table 2**. These estimates are based on trained able-bodied athletes of average body weight and body-fat levels. It is therefore more appropriate to use the lower end of the range for smaller athletes, and for those Para athletes with substantially less active muscle mass proportional to their body weight (ie, SCI, spina bifida, double leg amputees). Increased energy needs due to inefficiency of movement of ambulant athletes with lower limb amputations may increase glycogen utilization and therefore carbohydrate needs.[16] Adequate stores of muscle glycogen are reported to sustain approximately 90 to 120 minutes of continuous moderate to high-intensity exercise in an able-bodied athlete.[17] In contrast, although no evidence has been published on the muscle glycogen storage capacities of Para athletes, experience suggests those using smaller muscle groups (eg, SCI, double leg amputees) are able to sustain approximately 75 to 90 minutes of continuous moderate to high-intensity exercise.

Table 2
Daily carbohydrate guidelines for athletes by g/kg body mass

	Training Load	Carbohydrate Intake Targets, g/kg body mass/day
Light	Low-intensity or skill-based activities	3–5
Moderate	Moderate exercise program (ie, ~1 h/d)	5–7
High	Endurance program (ie, 1–3 h/d of moderate to high-intensity exercise)	6–10
Very High	Extreme commitment (ie, at least 4–5 h/d of moderate to high-intensity exercise)	8–12

Data from Burke L. Nutrition for recovery after training and competition. In: Burke L, Deakin V, editors. Clinical sports nutrition. 5th edition. Sydney (Australia): McGraw-Hill Education; 2015. p. 420–62.

Fueling recommendations

Ensuring the athlete is adequately fueled and hydrated before starting physical activity is key to supporting sustained muscle function and power throughout the session. As **Table 3** outlines, carbohydrate intake during exercise is not always necessary. However, in practice, there can be benefits to consuming carbohydrate during training to contribute to total daily carbohydrate needs. For example,

a. If the athlete has not eaten before a training session, and the session involves skill or high-intensity work
b. If the athlete is undertaking a hard training block, resulting in limited time available to eat, potentially reduced appetite, and less time to recover muscle glycogen stores between training sessions
c. If the athlete needs to practice the intake of carbohydrate for competition and train the gut to tolerate carbohydrate during intense exercise

Muscle glycogen resynthesis post exercise

After exercise, co-ingestion of carbohydrate with a high-protein recovery snack is recommended to help restore muscle glycogen effectively (see **Table 3**), especially if recovery times are short.[18] The highest rates of muscle glycogen resynthesis occur during the first 2 hours after exercise, when insulin sensitivity is elevated and glycogen synthesis enzymes are activated.[19] Some athletes may experience a decrease in appetite after intense exercise, reducing the desire to consume food. If this is the case, a liquid carbohydrate and protein snack (such as chocolate milk) can help combat restrained hunger cues and allow recovery processes to get under way.

Gastrointestinal concerns

The same guidelines for able-bodied athletes should be used in athletes with intellectual and visual impairments and high-functioning ABI and CP, as there is no indication for a need to modify macronutrient guidelines. For wheelchair-dependent athletes, positioning in the wheelchair can contribute to gastrointestinal disturbances such as nausea and vomiting.[11] Some may experience early satiety resulting in a reduced amount of food tolerated per feeding, especially before and during exercise. Slower gastric emptying rates, affected by the sympathetic

Table 3
Carbohydrate guidelines during and after exercise

During Exercise		
During brief exercise	<45 min	Not needed
During sustained high-intensity exercise	45–75 min	Small amounts including a carbohydrate mouth rinse
During endurance exercise, including "stop and start" sports	1–2.5 h	30–60 g/h
During ultra-endurance exercise	>2.5–3 h	Up to 90 g/h[a] 1 g/kg per h for 4 h
After exercise (for rapid refueling of energy stores)		1 g/kg per h for 4 h

[a] With a ratio of glucose:fructose = 2:1.
Adapted from Burke L. Nutrition for recovery after training and competition. In: Burke L, Deakin V, editors. Clinical sports nutrition. 5th edition. Sydney (Australia): McGraw-Hill Education; 2015. p. 433; with permission.

Table 4
Protein recommendations for athletes

Recommendations	Dosing	Example Based on 68-kg Athlete
Protein intake per dose	0.3 g/kg per meal/snack	20 g per meal/snack
Protein intake per day	1.2–1.7 g/kg/d (or up to 2.3 g/kg per day if energy restricted)	82–116 g throughout the day or 156 g throughout the day
Protein intake per dose when energy restricted	0.3–0.4 g/kg per meal/snack	20–27 g per meal/snack

Adapted from Moore D, Phillips S, Slater G. Protein. In: Burke L, Deakin V, editors. Clinical sports nutrition. 5th edition. Sydney (Australia): McGraw-Hill Education; 2015. p. 94–113; with permission.

nervous system, are reported in people with SCI; thus, timing of meals (eg, before exercise and before competition) may have to be adjusted.[11] Small frequent feedings of energy-dense food, or liquid calorie sources, such as meal replacements, smoothies, and fruit juice may be beneficial to provide adequate carbohydrate to meet exercise needs. Customization of guidelines is needed to ensure the athlete's actual needs are well understood and practical measures to achieve these needs are taken.

Protein

Protein intake distributed throughout the day, and especially after training, improves muscle protein synthesis and net protein balance, and may enhance training adaptations.[20] Protein recommendations for athletes are presented in **Table 4**. Adequate protein intake as part of a recovery nutrition plan should be consumed shortly after training sessions, especially from high biological value sources, like beef, fish, poultry, eggs, and dairy products.[20] Furthermore, this recovery strategy should be repeated throughout the week, as recovery processes are ongoing 24 to 48 hours after exercise.[20] During calorie-restricted phases of training, such as athletes competing in weight making sports, protein intake should be increased to preserve muscle mass (see **Table 4**).

Meal plan example for a moderate training day

The following meal plan is based on a female Para triathlete with an SCI. She typically trains twice a day. An example of a training day may include a morning low to moderate-intensity pool swim and a moderate to high-intensity interval hand cycle in the afternoon. Assuming a body mass (BM) of 48 kg (105 lb), approximate carbohydrate (CHO) requirements for this day are 5 g/kg BM (240 g). Adequate carbohydrate intake during and between sessions ensures energy stores are replenished to support repeated training sessions. This is particularly critical for Para triathletes with SCI, as they use the same muscle groups for each session. Although able-bodied recommendations might be closer to 6 to 8 g CHO/kg BM for this training day, the proportional muscle mass of an athlete with an SCI is less, as is total energy expenditure for the day. Aiming for 5 g CHO/kg BM allows for adequate intake of other nutrients within this athlete's smaller calorie budget.

Pretraining snack (6:00 AM)	1 cup whole grain cereal with ½ cup chocolate soy milk	30 g CHO	6 g PRO
Training (6:30 AM)	2500-m pool swim water during session		
Breakfast (8:00 AM)	2 slices whole wheat toast with 1 tablespoon peanut butter 4 oz strawberry Greek yogurt	50 g CHO	20 g PRO
Work (9:30 AM–1:30 PM)	Fruit smoothie: 4 oz orange juice, 4 oz water, 6 oz Greek yogurt, spinach, frozen pineapple, ½ banana	50 g CHO	15 g PRO
Lunch (1:30 PM)	2 oz sliced turkey on whole wheat bread with avocado, sliced tomato Baby carrots with 1 tablespoon hummus	30 g CHO	12 g PRO
Pretraining snack (4:15 PM)	12 oz sports drink	20 g CHO	0 g PRO
Afternoon training (4:30 PM)	75-min hand cycle ride with high-intensity intervals 8 oz sports drink with water	15 g CHO	0 g PRO
Post-training recovery (6:00 PM)	Protein shake (provides ~15 g protein and ~20 g carbohydrate)	20 g CHO	15 g PRO
Dinner (7:30 PM)	3 oz lean beef and vegetable stir-fry Brown rice (1/2 cup)	25 g CHO	30 g PRO
TOTALS		240 g CHO (5 g/kg)	98 g PRO (2 g/kg)

Abbreviation: PRO, protein.

Iron

Iron is an important nutrient for athletes to ensure optimal delivery of oxygen to working muscles. Athletes have greater iron requirements due to increased red blood cell production and higher turnover due to hemolysis, sweating, gastrointestinal bleeding, and other factors.[7] Inadequate matching of iron intake to requirements leads to early fatigue, decreased time to exhaustion, increased rate of perceived exertion, decreased aerobic capacity, and inhibited adaptations to training, especially at altitude.[7] Inadequate iron intake may result from poor quality and quantity of food intake, inadequate protein intake, or increased requirements from training adaptations (ie, erythropoiesis).[7] Assessing iron status of Para athletes should be prioritized, as research indicates a high prevalence of low iron intakes.[1-4]

Iron testing in athletes

It is recommended to perform blood testing of iron status for all athletes at least annually. If status is suboptimal to meet performance needs, more frequent follow-ups are encouraged to check on the effectiveness of treatment. **Table 5** outlines different stages of iron depletion and deficiency, highlighting the importance of assessing ferritin, total iron-binding capacity, and transferrin saturation in athletes. Athletic performance can be negatively impacted even at subclinically low iron levels, hence iron supplementation of athletes should occur earlier than the diagnosis of clinical anemia.[7]

Collaboration between the sports medicine physician and sport dietitian is critical to ensure the athlete's care is comprehensive and includes improvement in iron-rich foods in addition to supplementation if insufficiency is present. Iron-rich heme food sources (animal-based), such as beef, fish, poultry, and whole eggs, should be encouraged for all Para athletes. Non-heme iron-rich foods, such as fortified cereal, tofu, oatmeal, raisins, and cooked spinach, are best absorbed when combined with

Table 5
Reference ranges for hematological iron status markers

Stage 1 Iron depletion (ID)	<35 µg/L ferritin >115 g/L hemoglobin (Hb) >16% transferrin saturation
Stage 2 Iron-deficient non-anemia (IDNA)	<20 µg/L ferritin >115 g/L Hb <16% transferrin saturation > TIBC >500 µg/dL
Stage 3 Iron-deficient anemia (IDA)	<12 µg/L ferritin <115 g/L Hb <16% transferrin saturation

Physicians need to take into account that the same reference standards for hemoglobin, hematocrit, and mean corpuscular volume do not apply to all ethnic groups.[21] Note that ferritin is an acute-phase reactant so may be abnormally elevated in periods of inflammation.

TIBC, total iron-binding capacity.

Adapted from Deakin V, Peeling P. Prevention, detection and treatment of iron depletion and deficiency in athletes. In: Burke L, Deakin V, editors. Clinical sports nutrition. 5th edition. Sydney (Australia): McGraw-Hill Education; 2015. p. 267; with permission.

vitamin C–rich foods. If iron status values are too low or do not improve with the increased consumption of iron-rich foods, supplementation is recommended. **Table 6** outlines iron supplementation recommendations for athletes.

Treatment considerations

Ingestion of oral iron (typically in the form of ferrous sulfate) is recommended to be taken with food to avoid gastrointestinal discomfort. Although the treatment goal is to use the best dose to improve iron status, side effects, such as constipation and diarrhea, may occur. If an athlete continues to experience these symptoms, alternating days on/off, recommending a smaller dose or alternative forms of iron, such as iron bisglycinate, may be necessary. Athletes training, competing, or living at altitude are at increased risk for iron insufficiency and are recommended to increase intake of iron-rich foods or take a low-dose supplement (9–18 mg alone or via multivitamin) as a prophylactic measure. Iron supplements greater than 45 mg/d should not be undertaken by athletes for long periods of time and should be implemented only in those athletes with a proven depletion or deficiency.

Inhibition and enhancement of iron

After exercise and during times of high stress or infection, the liver releases a hormone called hepcidin that inhibits intestinal iron absorption and directs iron away from hemoglobin and red blood cell synthesis.[7] Other inhibitors of non-heme iron absorption include the following:

- Phytates, commonly found in fiber-rich foods, such as cereal grains, legumes, nuts, and seeds

Table 6
Iron supplementation protocol[a]

	>35	<35	<20
Serum ferritin, ng/mL			
Elemental iron recommendation, mg/d	0	25–65	65–100

[a] US Olympic Committee, (Shawn Hueglin, personal communication, 2014)

- Polyphenols from coffee, tea, cocoa, and red wine
- Calcium-rich foods

Vitamin C–rich foods and meats strongly enhance iron absorption and can even neutralize the inhibitory effects of phytates, polyphenols, and calcium.[7] For this reason, iron supplementation is best timed well after exercise, either in the evening with a meal containing meat or before bed combined with a source of vitamin C to enhance absorption.

Vitamin D and Bone Health

Vitamin D has become an emerging area of interest and research in athletic populations far beyond calcium homeostasis and bone health. Para athletes are at high risk of being deficient in vitamin D for many reasons, including, but not limited to, the nature of their impairment, inadequate energy intakes, and micronutrient deficiencies, as outlined in **Table 7**. Low bone mineral density (BMD) and risk of bone injury are higher in athletes with SCI and lower limb amputations due to less gravitational forces and muscular loads. High risk of fractures and low BMD are documented in patients with spina bifida, especially those who are nonambulatory.[22] Amputation level has been seen to influence bone characteristics, with above-knee amputees having greater bone atrophy than below-knee amputees, leading to greater risk of osteoporosis and fractures in the hip.[23] Athletes with amputations may be at higher risk for sustaining osteoporotic fractures at a younger age compared with nonamputees. Furthermore, greater reductions in BMD may occur after traumatic amputations, as compared with nontraumatic amputations.[24]

Table 7
Risk factors by Para population of suboptimal vitamin D status and low BMD

Para Population	Risk Factors
SCI	• Limited weight-bearing activity • Less gravitational and muscular loads to lower extremities • Decreased energy expenditure and energy intake → vitamin D deficiency • Anticonvulsant use • Limited sun exposure (covering up the skin with clothing, keeping in the shade due to thermoregulation challenges)
Amputees	• Level of amputation (greater risk in above knee than below knee) • Prosthesis fit • Insufficient weight bearing on residual limb • <6 h/d spent on prosthesis • Compensatory loading on intact limb
CP and ABI	• Insufficient energy and micronutrient intake • Poor growth rates • Delayed puberty • Disrupted hormone production • Anticonvulsant use • Swallowing difficulties and the need for food/fluid texture modification → decreased dietary intake
Intellectual impairments	• Suboptimal micronutrient intake • Difficulty coping with unfamiliar foods • Anticonvulsant use
VI	• Limited sun exposure in prevention of sunburn and skin cancer (albinism)

Abbreviations: ABI, acquired brain injury; CP, cerebral palsy; SCI, spinal cord injury; VI, visual impairment.

Benefits of optimal vitamin D status in athletes

Vitamin D can impact morphology and functionality of human skeletal muscles, substrate utilization, including long-chain fatty acid oxidation and glycogen metabolism, aerobic fitness, and maximal oxygen uptake.[8,9] Optimal levels of vitamin D also help enhance the ability of muscle to make quick, explosive movements as supported by the positive effect of vitamin D on velocity, jump height, power, and force.[9] According to Allison and colleagues,[25] athletes with lower vitamin D status (<25 nmol/L) had smaller atrial and ventricular structures compared with those who had vitamin D status of more than 50 nmol/L. Innate and adaptive immunity is closely related to vitamin D status, and some studies support the possibility of the capacity of vitamin D to reduce upper respiratory infections, commonly reported by highly trained athletes due to high training volume and intensities.[9]

Causes of vitamin D insufficiency

Vitamin D deficiencies and insufficiencies in athletes with SCI are well documented. A recent meta-analysis reported a 32% to 93% prevalence of suboptimal vitamin D status in athletes with SCI from a range of indoor and outdoor sports, higher than able-bodied counterparts.[26] Risk of low vitamin D status seems to increase after ABI. Jamall and colleagues[27] found 46.5% of 353 patients tested 0.3 to 56.5 months post injury were vitamin D deficient, with a total of 80.2% being insufficient. Importantly, those deficient in vitamin D were found to have lower scores on a cognitive examination.[27] Inadequate vitamin D levels may be due to poor dietary intake, living/training location (northern latitudes), type of sport (indoor vs outdoor), insufficient skin exposure to sun due to the nature of the impairment and/or thermoregulatory challenges, low or high body-fat levels, darker skin pigmentation, sunscreen use, and time spent outdoors.[28] Symptoms of vitamin D deficiency in athletes include low BMD, stress fractures, fatigue, unexplained muscle and joint pain, and frequent illness.[28]

Anticonvulsants are often prescribed to populations with ABI, CP, SCI, and intellectual impairments to manage seizures, but these may decrease serum vitamin D by increasing catabolism of 25(OH)D and 1,25(OH)2D,[29] and impair calcium metabolism by reducing absorption.[30] Prophylactic intake of calcium and vitamin D is recommended for all patients on anticonvulsants to protect against altered bone health.[31]

Vitamin D testing in athletes

Due to the impact vitamin D can have on both bone health and performance, and the high prevalence of vitamin D insufficiency in Para athletes, testing vitamin D status is highly recommended. **Table 8** presents the reference ranges of vitamin D status in athletic populations. In addition, routine assessment of BMD, such as dual-energy X-ray absorptiometry, parathyroid hormone, bioavailable vitamin D,[32] and dietary calcium intake, are important to detect risk factors of suboptimal bone health.

Recommendations to optimize vitamin D status

Reported dietary intake of vitamin D in elite athletes with SCI is between 115 and 121 IU per day,[36] which is well under the current dietary reference intake for vitamin D of 600 IU per day.[35] Safe exposure to sunlight and promotion of vitamin D–rich food sources, such as salmon, tuna, sardines, and vitamin D–fortified milks and cereals should be encouraged in Para athletes, as they may consume insufficient amounts of these foods.[1,2,4–6]

Because the evidence presented suggests it is challenging for many Para athletes to meet daily vitamin D needs with dietary sources, supplementation may be warranted to restore optimal status, such as that outlined in **Table 9**. Flueck

Table 8
Reference ranges for vitamin D in athletes

Vitamin D Status	ng·mL^{-1}	nmol·mL^{-1}
Vitamin D toxicity	>150	>375
Optimal status (bone and muscle)	40–70	100–175
Normal vitamin D status	30–80	75–200
Vitamin D insufficiency	21–29	52.5–72.5
Vitamin D deficiency	≤20	≤50

Conversion factor between units is 2.5.
Data from Refs.[33–35]

and colleagues[37] reported that 12 weeks of supplementation with 6000 IU vitamin D in Swiss wheelchair athletes with insufficiency significantly improved their vitamin D status and improved their performance in an elbow isokinetic dynamometer test on their nondominant hand. Furthermore, Stark[38] show the supplementation protocol in **Table 9** was effective in restoring or maintaining adequate vitamin D status in 91% of athletes with an SCI over 12 to 16 weeks, and improved handgrip strength.[38]

Recommendations to optimize bone health

As discussed previously, many Para athletes are at higher risk of low bone density. There is also increasing evidence of low bone density due to participation in certain sports, such as swimming and cycling.[39] Therefore, it is important to optimize all nutrients and factors that support bone health. Calcium-rich foods, such as dairy products, tofu, fish with soft bones, and calcium-fortified foods, should be encouraged, as Para athletes are often found to consume insufficient calcium.[1,2,4–6] Calcium loss via sweat has been investigated as a factor contributing to athletes' low bone density. Haakonssen and colleagues[40] reported on the feeding of a calcium-rich dairy-based preexercise meal 2 hours before 90 minutes of high-intensity exercise in 32 female cyclists. This resulted in an attenuation of the exercise-induced rise of bone resorption markers, thereby protecting bone in addition to supporting adequate total daily calcium intake.[40] Other micronutrients important to bone health, such as magnesium and phosphorus, also were below the estimated average requirements in surveyed Para athletes[1,2,4–6] and should be encouraged as part of a nutrient-dense diet. Finally, strategies to increase load-bearing activity and other forms of bone stimulation should be encouraged in all Para athlete populations. For example, amputees who wore a prosthesis for more than 6 hours per day had significantly greater hip BMD than those who wore a prosthesis for less than 6 hours per day.[24]

Table 9
Proposed supplementation protocol for ages 18 years and older[a]

Vitamin D Status, ng·mL^{-1}	Supplementation	Duration, wk	Maintenance, IU/d
≤20	50,000 IU/wk or 10,000 IU 5 d/wk	8	1500–3000
21–30	35,000 IU/wk or 4000–5000 IU/d	8	1500–2000
30–40	2000–4000 IU/d		1500–2000

[a] US Olympic Committee, (Shawn Hueglin, personal communication, 2014).

SUMMARY/DISCUSSION

Analysis of Para athlete dietary intakes, specifically carbohydrate, protein, iron, and vitamin D status, are important to detect nutrient insufficiencies that greatly impact athletic performance. Negative effects on performance from suboptimal nutrient status include inadequate muscle glycogen to sustain power output, impaired recovery, diminishing bone health, delayed injury repair, decreased aerobic capacity and training adaptations, and increased susceptibility to illness and injury. Individualized dietary approaches are most effective in achieving behavior change and should be used when working with Para athletes to account for differences in impairment type, learning style, and dietary preferences. Sport nutrition support is critical to empowering Para athletes with the knowledge to understand their individual nutrition needs and risk factors for nutrient insufficiencies, to achieve optimal health and athletic performance. More research is needed on nutrition-related topics that affect performance measures in Para athletes.

REFERENCES

1. Eskici G, Ersoy G. An evaluation of wheelchair basketball players' nutritional status and nutritional knowledge levels. J Sports Med Phys Fitness 2016;56:259–68.
2. Gerrish H, Broad E, Lacroix M, et al. Nutrient intake of elite Canadian and American athletes with spinal cord injury. Int J Exerc Sci 2017;10(7):1018–28.
3. Goosey-Tolfrey VL, Crosland J. Nutritional practices of competitive British wheelchair games players. Adapt Phys Activ Q 2010;27:47–59.
4. Krempien JL, Barr SI. Risk of nutrient inadequacies in elite Canadian athletes with spinal cord injury. Int J Sport Nutr Exerc Metab 2011;21:417–25.
5. Rastmanesh R, Taleban FA, Kimiagar M, et al. Nutritional knowledge and attitudes in athletes with physical disabilities. J Athl Train 2007;42:99–105.
6. Grams L, Garrido G, Villacieros J, et al. Marginal micronutrient intake in high-performance male wheelchair basketball players: a dietary evaluation and the effects of nutritional advice. PLoS One 2016;11. https://doi.org/10.1371/journal.pone.0157931.
7. Deakin V, Peeling P. Prevention, detection and treatment of iron depletion and deficiency in athletes. In: Burke L, Deakin V, editors. Clinical sports nutrition. 5th edition. Sydney (Australia): McGraw-Hill Education; 2015. p. 266–309.
8. Cannell JJ, Hollis BW, Sorenson MB, et al. Athletic performance and Vitamin D. Med Sci Sports Exerc 2009;41:1102–10.
9. Todd JJ, Pourshahidi LK, Mcsorley EM, et al. Vitamin D: recent advances and implications for athletes. Sports Med 2014;45:213–29.
10. Broad E, Juzwiak C. Determining the energy requirements of para athletes. Aspetar Sports Med J, in press.
11. Goosey-Tolfrey V, Krempien J, Price M. Spinal cord injuries. In: Broad E, editor. Sports nutrition for paralympic athletes. Boca Raton (FL): CRC Press; 2014. p. 67–90.
12. Crosland J, Boyd C. Cerebral palsy and acquired brain injuries. In: Broad E, editor. Sports nutrition for paralympic athletes. Boca Raton (FL): CRC Press; 2014. p. 91–106.
13. Mountjoy M, Sundgot-Borgen J, Burke L, et al. The IOC consensus statement: beyond the female athlete triad—Relative energy deficiency in sport (RED-S). Br J Sports Med 2014;48:491–7.
14. Blauwet CA, Brooke EM, Tenforde AS, et al. Low energy availability, menstrual dysfunction, and low bone mineral density in individuals with a disability:

implications for the para athlete population. Sports Med 2017. https://doi.org/10.1007/s40279-017-0696-0.

15. Burke L. Preparation for competition. In: Burke L, Deakin V, editors. Clinical sports nutrition. 5th edition. Sydney (Australia): McGraw-Hill Education; 2015. p. 346–76.

16. Meyer NL, Edwards S. Amputees. In: Broad E, editor. Sports nutrition for paralympic athletes. Boca Raton (FL): CRC Press; 2014. p. 107–26.

17. Jeukendrup A, Carter J, Maughan R. Competition fluid and fuel. In: Burke L, Deakin V, editors. Clinical sports nutrition. 5th edition. Sydney (Australia): McGraw-Hill Education; 2015. p. 377–419.

18. Burke L. Nutrition for recovery after training and competition. In: Burke L, Deakin V, editors. Clinical sports nutrition. 5th edition. Sydney (Australia): McGraw-Hill Education; 2015. p. 420–62.

19. Ivy JL, Katz AL, Cutler CL, et al. Muscle glycogen synthesis after exercise: effect of time of carbohydrate ingestion. J Appl Physiol (1985) 1988;64:1480–5.

20. Moore D, Phillips S, Slater G. Protein. In: Burke L, Deakin V, editors. Clinical sports nutrition. 5th edition. Sydney (Australia): McGraw-Hill Education; 2015. p. 94–113.

21. Beutler E, West C. Hematologic differences between African-Americans and whites: the roles of iron deficiency and thalassemia on hemoglobin levels and mean corpuscular volume. Blood 2005;106:740–5.

22. Marreiros H, Loff C, Calado E. Osteoporosis in paediatric patients with spina bifida. J Spinal Cord Med 2012;35:129–30.

23. Sherk VD, Bemben MG, Bemben DA. BMD and bone geometry in transtibial and transfemoral amputees. J Bone Miner Res 2008;23:1449–57.

24. Leclercq MM, Bonidan O, Haaby E, et al. Study of bone mass with dual energy x-ray absorptiometry in a population of 99 lower limb amputees. Ann Readapt Med Phys 2003;46:24–30.

25. Allison RJ, Close GL, Farooq A, et al. Severely vitamin D-deficient athletes present smaller hearts than sufficient athletes. Eur J Prev Cardiol 2015;22:535–42.

26. Flueck JL, Perret C. Vitamin D deficiency in individuals with a spinal cord injury: a literature review. Spinal Cord 2016;55:428–34.

27. Jamall OA, Feeney C, Zaw-Linn J, et al. Prevalence and correlates of vitamin D deficiency in adults after traumatic brain injury. Clin Endocrinol (Oxf) 2016;85:636–44.

28. Larson-Meyer E, Willis KS. Vitamin D and athletes. Curr Sports Med Rep 2010;9:220–6.

29. Holick MF, Binkley NC, Bischoff-Ferrari HA, et al. Evaluation, treatment and prevention of vitamin D deficiency: an endocrine society clinical practice guideline. J Clin Endocrinol Metab 2011;96:1911–30.

30. Verrotti A, Coppola G, Parisi P, et al. Bone and calcium metabolism and antiepileptic drugs. Clin Neurol Neurosurg 2010;112:1–10.

31. Meier C, Kraenzlin ME. Antiepileptics and bone health. Ther Adv Musculoskelet Dis 2011;3:235–43.

32. Allison RJ, Farooq A, Cherif A, et al. Why don't serum vitamin D concentrations associate with BMD by DXA? A case of being 'bound' to the wrong assay? Implications for vitamin D screening. Br J Sports Med 2017. https://doi.org/10.1136/bjsports-2016-097130.

33. Holick MF. A D-Lightful health perspective. Nutr Rev 2008;66(suppl 2):S182–92.

34. Holick MF. Vitamin D status: measurement, interpretation, and clinical application. Ann Epidemiol 2009;19:73–8.

35. Institute of Medicine. Dietary reference intakes for calcium and vitamin D. Washington, DC: National Academies Press; 2010.

36. Pritchett K, Pritchett R, Ogan D, et al. 25(OH)D Status of elite athletes with spinal cord injury relative to lifestyle factors. Nutrients 2016;8:374.

37. Flueck J, Schlaepfer M, Perret C. Effect of 12-week vitamin D supplementation on 25[OH]D status and performance in athletes with a spinal cord injury. Nutrients 2016;8:586.

38. Stark L. Effect of a sliding scale vitamin D supplementation protocol on 25(OH)D status in elite athletes with spinal cord injury [masters thesis]. Ellensburg (WA): Central Washington University; 2017.

39. Scofield KL, Hecht S. Bone health in endurance athletes: runners, cyclists and swimmers. Curr Sports Med Rep 2012;11:328–34.

40. Haakonssen EC, Ross ML, Knight EJ, et al. The effects of a calcium-rich pre-exercise meal on biomarkers or calcium homeostasis in competitive female cyclists: a randomised crossover trial. PLoS One 2015;10:e0123302.

Concussion in Para Sport

James Kissick, MD, CCFP (SEM), Dip Sport Med[a],*,
Nick Webborn, MB BS, FFSEM, MSc[b]

KEYWORDS

- Concussion • Para sport • Para athlete • Athletes with a disability • Injury

KEY POINTS

- Para athletes are exposed to concussion risk, particularly in speed, collision, and contact sports.
- There are few incidence data on concussion in Para athletes.
- Current assessment guidelines and tools (eg, Sport Concussion Assessment Tool—5th Edition) are not applicable to some Para athlete populations.
- The management of concussion in the Para athletes may need to be adapted depending on the athlete impairment and sport.
- Risk reduction strategies, in particular education, must be implemented.

It is probably safe to say that there has been no sport medicine topic more newsworthy than concussion over the past decade. In addition to intense interest from athletes, parents, the media, and others, concussion has been a popular subject of research, which has grown exponentially over the years. For the Para athlete (the International Paralympic Committee [IPC] term for a sportsperson with a disability), however, concussion struggles to attract interest and attention.[1,2] For example, a search strategy developed to find articles regarding athletes and concussion retrieved more than 6000 results, whereas one developed for athletes with disabilities and concussion only returned 60 articles. Furthermore, the recent Fifth International Consensus Conference on Concussion in Sport featured 202 oral and written abstracts, but only 2 were specific to athletes with a disability. Despite this, participation in sport by Para athletes continues to grow, and these athletes are exposed to the risk of concussion in sports that involve speed, collision, and contact. This review examines what is currently known about concussion in Para sport and how assessment, management, and risk reduction in this group of athletes might differ from the general athletic

Disclosure Statement: The authors have nothing to disclose.
[a] Department of Family Medicine, University of Ottawa Carleton University Sport Medicine Clinic, Ottawa, Ontario, Canada; [b] Centre for Sport and Exercise Science and Medicine (SESAME), University of Brighton, The Welkin, Carlisle Road, Eastbourne BN20 7SN, UK
* Corresponding author.
E-mail address: jameskissick@me.com

Phys Med Rehabil Clin N Am 29 (2018) 299–311
https://doi.org/10.1016/j.pmr.2018.01.002
1047-9651/18/© 2018 Elsevier Inc. All rights reserved.

population. Current and future challenges are discussed, but, more importantly, opportunities for further study are identified.

INCIDENCE

As described by Van Mechelen and colleagues[3] in their 4-step injury prevention model, the first step in prevention is to determine the incidence and severity of any injury that is hoped to be prevented. Although there are several Para sports where a greater risk of concussion would be anticipated, there are few incidence data. **Table 1** gives an example of best estimate risk assessment by IPC Medical Committee members for Summer and Winter Paralympics sports, based on their experience and the available data of concussion risk considering the impairment type, speed, collision potential, protective wear, and risk rating. This table needs refinement as more data become available but is a useful starting point for field-of-play clinicians and event organizers to consider.

Paralympic Games Injury Surveillance

The IPC has conducted injury surveillance studies at the Winter Paralympic Games since 2002, and at the Summer Paralympic Games since 2012. A Web-based injury and illness surveillance system (WEB-IISS) was introduced at the 2012 London Paralympic Games to enter injury data and has been used at all subsequent Summer and Winter Games. Questions specifically related to concussion, however, were not added to the WEB-IISS until the 2016 Rio Summer Paralympics. In 2002, alpine skiing (now termed, Para alpine skiing) and ice sledge hockey (now termed, Para ice hockey) had the highest risk of any musculoskeletal injury of all sports contested at the Winter Paralympic Games. A higher risk of concussion might be expected in both sports due to the speed and impact involved, but no head injuries were reported.[4] The 2006 Torino Paralympic Games surveillance study was hampered by some methodological issues; still, it noted 2 head injuries (1 in alpine skiing and 1 in Nordic skiing) of 39 recorded injuries, but there is no further information on the specific type of head injury (eg, scalp laceration, contusion, facial fracture, or concussion).[5] At the 2010 Vancouver Winter Paralympics, 2 of 40 reported injuries in Para ice hockey and 3 of 42 reported injuries in Para alpine skiing (all standing skiers with visual or physical impairment) were to the head, but, again, there was no further differentiation into injury type. Data on Nordic skiers indicated 1 concussion of 26 reported injuries.[6] The most recent Winter Games study was done at the 2014 Sochi Paralympic Games. Of 174 total reported injuries, 31 injuries to the head, face, and neck were reported, accounting for 4.8% of athletes with an injury and an incidence rate (IR) of 4.7 injuries per 1000 athlete days (95% CI, 3.2–6.7). The investigators noted that, overall, there was a higher injury incidence at the Sochi Paralympic Winter Games than in the Sochi Winter Olympics or 2012 London Summer Paralympic Games.[7]

Although the incidence of concussion intuitively might be expected to be higher in a Winter Games setting, with speed sports, such as Para alpine skiing, and collision sports, such as Para ice hockey, the Summer Paralympic Games includes several contact sports, such as wheelchair basketball, wheelchair rugby, judo, and visually impaired (VI) Football 5-a-side. In addition, in some Para sports, there is a risk of concussion even though the sport's able-bodied equivalent is not traditionally associated with this injury. Although the risk of concussion in an Olympic track event is unreported, the risk of a crash in wheelchair track athletes resulting in head injury is not uncommon, with 2 documented concussions from crashes occurring at the last 2 World Para Athletics Championships (**Fig. 1**). At the 2012 London Paralympic Games,

Table 1
Summer and Winter Paralympic sports with best estimate of concussion risk based on impairment impact speed, collision potential, head protection and risk rating (1 = low to 5 = high)

Summer Sports	Impairment	Collision Potential	Impact Speed	Head Protection	Risk Rating
Archery	Multiple	Very low	Very low	No	1
Boccia	CP	Very low	Very low	No	1
Cycling road	Handcycle	Moderate	High	Yes	5
Cycling road	Trike	Moderate	Moderate–High	Yes	3
Cycling road	Bike	Moderate	High	Yes	5
Cycling track	Multiple	Moderate	Moderate	Yes	3
Equestrian	Multiple	Low	Moderate	Yes	2
Football 5-a-side	VI	High	Low	No	4
Football 7-a-side	CP	Moderate	Low–Moderate	No	2
Goalball	VI	Moderate	Moderate	No	3
Judo	VI	Moderate	Moderate	No	2
Para athletics field	Wheelchair	Low	Very low	No	1
Para athletics field	Amputee	Low	Moderate	No	2
Para athletics field	VI	Low	Moderate	No	2
Para athletics field	CP	Low	Moderate	No	2
Para athletics track	Wheelchair	Moderate	Moderate	Yes	3
Para athletics track	Amputee	Low	Moderate	No	1
Para athletics track	VI	Low	Moderate	No	1
Para athletics track	CP	Low	Moderate	No	1
Para canoe	Multiple	Low	Low	No	2
Para powerlifting	Multiple	Very low	V low	No	1
Para swimming	Multiple	Low	Low	No	2
Para triathlon—bike	Multiple	Moderate	High	Yes	4
Para triathlon—run	Multiple	Low	Low	No	2
Para triathlon—swim	Multiple	Low	Low	No	2
Rowing	Multiple	Very low	Low	No	2
Sailing	Multiple	Moderate	Moderate	No	3
Shooting Para sport	Multiple	Very low	Very low	No	1
Sitting volleyball	Multiple	Low	Low	No	2
Table tennis	Multiple	Low	Low	No	1
Wheelchair basketball	Multiple	Low	Low	No	2
Wheelchair fencing	Multiple	Low	Low	Yes	2
Wheelchair rugby	SCI	High	Low	No	3
Wheelchair tennis	Multiple	Low	Low	No	2

Winter Sports	Impairment	Collision Potential	Impact Speed	Head Protection	Risk Rating
Para alpine downhill	Sit-ski	Very high	Very high	Yes	5
Para alpine downhill	VI	Very high	Very high	Yes	5
Para alpine downhill	Standing	Very high	Very high	Yes	5
Para alpine other	Sit-ski	High	High	Yes	4

(continued on next page)

Table 1
(continued)

Winter Sports	Impairment	Collision Potential	Impact Speed	Head Protection	Risk Rating
Para alpine other	VI	High	High	Yes	4
Para alpine other	Standing	High	High	Yes	4
Para alpine slalom	Sit-ski	Moderate	High	Yes	3
Para alpine slalom	VI	Moderate	High	Yes	3
Para alpine slalom	Standing	Moderate	High	Yes	4
Para cross-country skiing/biathlon	Sit-ski	Low	Low	No	2
Para cross-country skiing/biathlon	VI	Low	Low	No	2
Para cross-country skiing/biathlon	Standing	Low	Low	No	4
Para ice hockey	Multiple	High	Moderate	Yes	1
Para snowboard	Standing	High	Moderate	Yes	2
Wheelchair curling	Multiple	Very low	Very low	No	1

Abbreviations: CP, cerebral palsy; SCI, spinal cord injury; VI, visually impaired.

2.2% of reported injuries (14/633) were to the head and face; however, there was no differentiation into injury type.[8] The 2016 Rio Paralympic Games study was the first to include specific reporting questions on concussion, with team physicians from 78 of the 81 participating countries using the WEB-IISS. If an injury to the head, face, or neck was noted, the physician then received specific questions regarding concussion: 1.6% of total injuries (7/440) were to the head and face, and 8.4% (37/440) to the neck, giving incidence rates of 0.1 (95% CI, 0.1–0.3) and 0.7 (95% CI, 0.5–1.0) per 1000

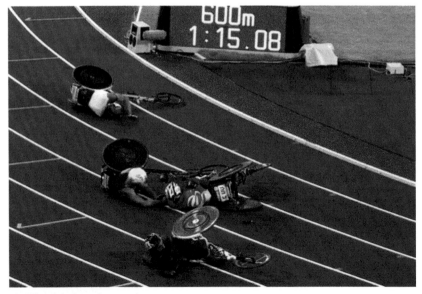

Fig. 1. Wheelchair racing crash.

athlete days, respectively. Despite these injuries, however, no concussions were reported.[9] Concussions cannot be diagnosed from the stands with certainty; however, during Football 5-a-side matches, the authors witnessed clear head-to-head contact followed by players holding their heads and exhibiting apparent balance issues. These incidents were also observed on review of video footage from the matches and were suspicious of concussion. Thus, although no concussions were reported via WEB-IISS, this may not mean that none occurred, pointing to the importance of improving concussion education for players, coaches, officials, and health care staff.

Concussions will again be specifically questioned in the injury surveillance survey at the 2018 Pyeonchang Winter Paralympic Games, and the pre-event team physician seminar will highlight this issue. The smaller nature of the Winter Games may make injury follow-up easier, potentially yielding more information.

Sport-Specific Studies

Football 5-a-side

Football 5-a-side refers to football (soccer) for players with visual impairment. Goalkeepers are sighted and call out defensive strategy to 4 VI players who wear eyeshades to ensure all have no vision. The ball has a bell within it, and players are required to call out "voy!' ("I go!" in Spanish) as they approach the player with the ball. In addition to being VI, which reduces their ability to brace for or block a blow to the head, players tend to play in more of an upright position than non-VI players, potentially exposing them to a greater risk of head to head collision[10] (**Fig. 2**). Webborn and colleagues[10] found a high incidence of head and face injuries in this sport at the 2012 London Paralympic Games (13.6% of total injuries), although this was in only 22 total injuries. Injury incidence in the total Games population, as discussed previously, was only 2.2%. The other Paralympic football type is cerebral palsy (CP) football, or Football 7-a-side played by athletes with CP. Players have full vision, and there is no heading of the ball allowed, which reduces the risk of head collision. Again, the number of total injuries was low, but only 1 of 17 total injuries was to the head and face (7.1%).

A preliminary analysis of the data from Rio (Webborn, unpublished data, 2017) showed that 5 of 17 (29%) injuries in competition were to the head and face, and, furthermore, Football 5-a-side remained the sport with the highest rate of injury of all sports at the Games. Magno e Silva and colleagues[11] reported that head injuries made up 8.6% of all injuries to VI international Brazilian footballers over 4 years (5 competitions).

Wheelchair basketball

Wheelchair basketball is played by both men and women on a standard-sized basketball court. It is fast paced, and contact certainly occurs. Wessels and colleagues[12] reported on a self-report survey of 263 athletes from ages 18 to 60 playing in tournaments during the 2009–2010 season: 6.1% of players reported having had a concussion, similar to the reported incidence in able-bodied basketball; 44% did not report their symptoms to team staff—of these, 67% said it was because they did not want to be removed from play, and 50% did not know they had a concussion at the time. Women had a 2.5-times higher concussion rate, but there were a limited number of women in the study. Although some athletes use a wheelchair regularly, some have impairments that do not necessitate regular wheelchair use. This group had a higher rate of concussions than habitual wheelchair users. Wessels and colleagues[12] speculated that this finding reflects regular users having more experience and better balance in their chairs or that some of the nonregular users were able to rise up in their chairs more, perhaps making them more unstable.

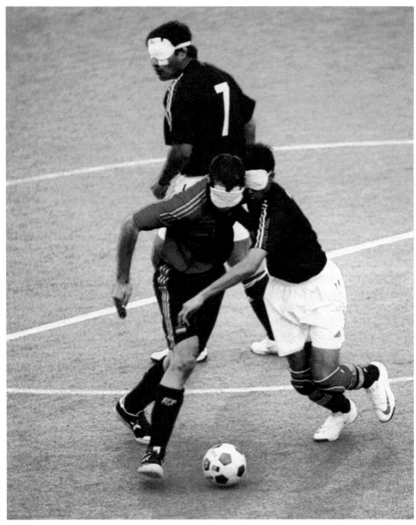

Fig. 2. Football 5-a-side action.

Para ice hockey

Like its stand-up counterpart, Para ice hockey is a fast game played on an ice surface surrounded by hard boards. Body contact is part of the game and collisions, both intentional and unintentional, occur regularly. Accordingly, the risk for concussion seems significant. There are no published studies, however, regarding concussion in this sport; the only relevant data come from the Paralympics surveillance studies, described previously. Hawkeswood and colleagues[13] surveyed team representatives (physician where the team had one, therapist, coach, and manager) of the top-ranked Para ice hockey teams at the 2010 Vancouver Paralympic Games. Concussions were a significant concern, with body checking believed the main mechanism of injury. Although this was a small anecdotal study, it may indicate that concussions are under-reported because none was recorded in the 2010 Games survey and thus more of a concern than surveillance studies have indicated thus far.

Summary

Although concussion risk in Para sports seems intuitively and anecdotally significant, there are few data. Sport-specific incidence studies, using consistent injury definition and well-designed methodology are needed; this is an excellent opportunity for researchers to provide valuable information and address this important first step in injury prevention.

ASSESSMENT

The consensus statement from the Fifth International Consensus Conference on Concussion in Sport states, "The recognition of suspected SRC (sport related concussion) is therefore best approached using multi-dimensional testing guided by expert consensus. The SCAT5 currently represents the most well-established and rigorously developed instrument for sideline assessment."[14] The Sport Concussion Assessment Tool (SCAT) 5 and its predecessors have been widely used by clinicians throughout the world to guide their sideline assessment of concussion. Because there is little published research on concussion assessment in Para athletes specifically, most clinicians working with these athletes likely look to existing assessment tools for the general sport population, like the SCAT5, for guidance. There are portions of the SCAT5, however, that are not appropriate or valid for use in the Para athlete and need to be modified. In an accompanying article to the consensus statement regarding the SCAT5, it is noted that the systematic review performed for the development of this tool found there was "scant information on the use of the SCAT in athletes with disabilities, as well as across different cultures and language groups."[15] In addition, Para athletes do not represent a homogeneous population; there are a wide range of impairments not only within Para sport as a whole but also within individual Para sports. Thus, a 1-size-fits-all approach is not possible.

Table 2 looks at potential challenges to the use of the SCAT5 in the disabled population. The challenges noted are not an exhaustive list, and some, such as learning disability or hearing impairment, may also be present in the general sporting population. Cognitive testing may be similarly difficult in some cultures and languages. It serves as reminder, however, that, as discussed by the authors of the SCAT5[15], a systematic approach is needed to adapt the SCAT5 for use among athletes with disabilities and across diverse cultures and language groups.

A growing body of normative data has been obtained over the years the SCAT has been used. Is this applicable, however, to the Para athlete population? Weiler and colleagues[16] compared baseline SCAT3 scores in football (soccer) players with a disability and those without and found significant differences. Male VI players had higher scores for total concentration and delayed recall (reflecting better scores than the group without a disability). Male players with CP scored higher on immediate memory and balance testing (which reflects a greater number of errors on balance tests). Female players with hearing impairment scored higher for total concentration and balance (again, greater number of errors) than female players without a disability.

Although the Concussion in Sport Group did not recommend baseline or postinjury neuropsychological testing as mandatory for all athletes,[14] brief computerized neuropsychological tests are frequently used, particularly in more elite sports with a higher concussion risk. Use of these tools is not possible in athletes with significant visual impairment and may be difficult to use in athletes who have difficulty using a computer mouse or those with a cognitive impairment or learning disability.

As noted in **Table 2**, balance testing may pose a significant challenge. The modified Balance Error Scoring System is not possible for athletes in a wheelchair. There are no

Table 2
Potential challenges to the use of sections of the Sport Concussion Assessment Tool—5th Edition in the Para athlete

Sport Concussion Assessment Tool—5th Edition Section	Potential Challenges
1. Immediate or on-field assessment • Red flags • Observable signs • Maddocks questions • Glasgow Coma Scale • Cervical spine assessment	Motor/sensation impairment, VI Balance/coordination impairment Balance difficulty, motor incoordination Hearing impairment, cognitive impairment, speech impairment Hearing impairment, VI, motor impairment, speech impairment Neck movement impairment
2. Symptom evaluation	More likely to have preexisting symptoms; different baseline
3. Cognitive screening	Cognitive impairment, learning disability, speech impairment
4. Neurologic screen • Reading aloud • Cervical spine movement • Looking up and down without diplopia • Finger-nose test • Tandem gait • Balance examination (modified Balance Error Scoring System)	VI, cognitive impairment, speech impairment, learning disability Neck movement impairment VI, including physical conditions, anophthalmia Amputation, coordination impairment Wheelchair user, coordination impairment, amputation Wheelchair user, amputation/prosthetic use, coordination impairment
5. Delayed recall	Hearing impairment, cognitive impairment, speech impairment, learning disability

data on its use for athletes with lower limb amputations wearing a prosthesis. As discussed previously, Weiler and colleagues[16] found increased balance errors in male CP footballers and female footballers with a hearing impairment.

Wessels described a proposed Wheelchair Error Scoring System, which consists of 6 tests to measure seated postural control: sitting on a hard surface, feet not touching the floor, hands on hips (eyes open and closed); sitting on a balance disc, feet not touching the floor (eyes open and closed); and holding a wheelie (front wheels off the ground) with eyes open and closed. Although there were a small number of participants, good intertester and intratester reliability was found, and it was possible to detect changes in postural control in each of the 5 cases of concussion during the study. The addition of a cognitive task increased postural control during the wheelie position; the authors proposed that this could be due to the participants' focus being diverted to the cognitive task, allowing balance to occur subconsciously, as it would normally.[17]

Knowledge of concussion assessment and assessment tools may be an issue in the Para sport world. West and colleagues[18] commented on their experience at the 2015 CP Football World Championships, where physicians and physiotherapists working with teams were surveyed. Although most reported some education in concussion assessment and management, as well as experience in managing players with a concussion, several reported they relied more on subjective factors like their knowledge of their players. There was a low rate of use of the SCAT3 or any other assessment tool and a high reliance on imaging. It was not identified why this might be; it may have been a lack of awareness of existing assessment tools, or perhaps the clinicians did not find them helpful, given aforementioned challenges in their use among Para athletes. If the former, although it may not be generalizable to other Para sports, it speaks to the need for education for health care providers working with Para athletes. The latter reinforces the need to develop assessment tools that are applicable to Para athletes.

MANAGEMENT

To date, there are no published guidelines or clinical consensus statements specific to the management of concussion in the Para athlete. The experience of the authors, and of other experienced clinicians, is to adhere to the recommendations of the Concussion in Sport Group, who recommend removal of an athlete from game, practice, or activity if a concussion is suspected and, where a concussion is diagnosed, a brief period of rest followed by resumption of daily activities and then a graduated return to play protocol.[14] As with assessment, however, there may be some challenges, or at least nuances, in Para athletes, depending on their disability and sport. The functional consequences of concussion to a Para athlete can be greater than to an able-bodied athlete.[4] For example, a brief initial period of rest is recommended, and many athletes with a concussion find that physical (and cognitive) exertion worsens their symptoms early on. Rest may be more difficult for wheelchair athletes who must wheel, transfer, and use other forms of physical exertion during regular activities of daily living, particularly if they live on their own.

Other questions arise: computerized neuropsychological testing is often used to assess cognitive recovery and clearance for resumption of contact activity. As discussed previously, the use of this tool may be limited in some athletes. In addition, is it valid where certain impairments exist? Does the 6-step return-to-play strategy need to be made more gradual or altered for some athletes? For example, for a Para ice hockey player who has to look down at the puck more when resuming noncontact drills than does a stand-up counterpart, this strategy could potentially cause more dizziness and neck discomfort if introduced too early.

West and colleagues'[18] CP Football World Cup study identified several clinicians who were returning concussed athletes to play faster than recommended by the Concussion in Sport Consensus recommendations (at that point, consensus statement on concussion in sport: the 4th International Conference on Concussion in Sport held in Zurich, November 2012). Several reported they were unaware of the existence of any concussion management guidelines. It is critical that clinicians providing care Para athletes are aware of existing guidelines and recommendations.

RISK REDUCTION

The Van Mechelen model is still at step 1, in "establishing the extent of the injury"[3] in relation to concussion incidence in Para sport. Risk reduction strategies, however, can and should be developed using existing principles of risk reduction but with specific consideration of a Para athlete's impairment and the specific sport. The athlete's impairment may increase collision risk; the example of a Football 5-a-side athlete with a visual impairment is previously described. Strategies must also address the specifics of the sport, including potential for collision, impact velocity, whether head protection is used and what type, and sport rules. As noted by Caroline Finch,[19] "To prevent injuries, sports injury prevention measures need to be acceptable, adopted and complied with by the athletes and sports bodies they are targeted at. If the athletes, coaches or sports administrators we are trying to work with will not use or adopt any of the prevention measures that we advocate, then all of our preventive efforts will fail."

Renowned injury epidemiologist Susan Baker described the "3 E's of Injury Prevention" in 1973: education, enforcement, and engineering (or environment). Although these originally arose from her work in motor vehicle accident prevention, they have been widely adapted for injury prevention in general, including in sport, and provide a useful framework for risk reduction strategies in Para sport.[20]

Education

Effective education, or knowledge translation, is the most critical component of injury prevention; without appropriate knowledge and understanding of the injury that is wished to be prevented, it is unlikely there will be good uptake of other strategies, such as safer play, protective equipment use, and adherence to rules. Wessels'[17] wheelchair basketball study found that 50% of those who had a concussion did not report it at the time because they did not know it was a concussion, and 42% thought it was just part of the game. The authors' experience in working with Para athletes also suggests that some Para athletes may not consider concussion a significant issue for them, given previous illness or injury, such as cancer or severe trauma: "Thanks for the information, doc, but I'm not really worried about a bump to my head when I have been through far worse." Many Para athletes may be risk takers, which for some may have been a contributing factor to a traumatic injury leading to an impairment. This behavior may not have changed afterward, making potentially higher-risk sports more attractive. Educational strategies must, therefore, emphasize that despite their past experiences, it is still critically important to protect the brain.

Educational initiatives must be directed at multiple levels—not only athletes but also health care providers, coaches, officials, sport administrators, and, in the case of younger athletes, parents. As previously discussed, there seems to be a need to educate health care providers regarding concussion recognition, assessment, and management. The most effective method for knowledge translation must be considered, and this may differ for each group. West and colleagues[18] noted that clinicians prefer to receive concussion education through courses or online materials. Athletes may prefer to receive information through social media. In addition to providing information about concussion, educational interventions can also include advice or instructions about safe play techniques, equipment use, and the importance of rules designed to reduce injury risk.

Enforcement

In sport, *enforcement* refers to the rules or laws of the game, which are put in place to ensure fair competition and to protect athletes from injury. It is, therefore, important that all involved, including athletes, coaches, and officials, understand and support these rules, not just when they are called against an opponent. Research in able-bodied ice hockey has demonstrated that hits to the head are associated with increased risk of concussion, which resulted in the no head checking rule, which is also used in Para ice hockey. Referees can enforce a more stringent penalty, including ejection from the game and possible suspension from future games, if a player hits another player on the head. This is designed to act as a deterrent, because it could have a significant impact on both a player and the team. In Football 5-a-side the voy rule requires that a player approaching another player in possession of the ball call out "voy." Strict enforcement of this rule is likely to reduce the frequency and severity of impacts, because the possessor of the ball should be more aware of a potential impact and take measures to try to avoid or protect.

Engineering

Engineering refers to the sport and athlete environment, which includes the venue, field of play, and equipment. The problem of player collisions in Football 5-a-side has been previously discussed. Players are often in an upright position as they compete for the ball, and their lack of vision makes anticipation of the collision difficult—it is difficult to try to avoid the collision or to brace by assuming a more protected position or by pretensioning muscles.[21] Players are required to wear eyeshades to ensure equal lack of vision, and, although acknowledging that no head protection in general use thus far can prevent concussion or reduce rotational forces to the brain, it was postulated that a combined eyeshade with head protection might confer a protective benefit in the head-to-head collisions seen in this sport. Examples are shown in **Fig. 3**. The majority of research into protective headgear has taken place in high-impact sports, such as National Football League football and Rugby Union, neither of which is directly comparable to Football 5-a-side. The results of the 2012 London study[10] opened up the opportunity to approach the International Blind Sports Federation Football to consider this option, which met with a favorable response. Consequently, pilot work is being undertaken using a wearable sensor system to measure linear acceleration and then through various algorithms also estimate angular acceleration. This will be attached to the mandatory eyeshade of the players. When combined with the clinical data after head collisions and their consequences, it may then be possible to design protective equipment that can defend against the measured forces.

The advent of new materials to reduce force impact has raised the possibility of more easily customizable sport specific wear. Already in use in industry and the military, products made from materials that are rate-sensitive, soft, and flexible but with high shock-absorbing properties are increasingly used in protective sports products.[22] As the cost reduces, they will become more affordable and become mandatory in sports if risk reduction benefit can be shown. As noted, however, by Finch,[19] "Sports bodies will not implement sports safety policies until they are sure that the

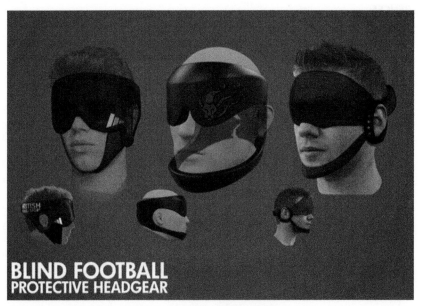

Fig. 3. Proposed Football 5-a-side eyeshade/headgear design.

safety measures actually prevent injuries, are acceptable to their participants, do not change the essential nature or appeal of the sport, and do not adversely affect participation or performance."

The high rate of injury in Para alpine skiing at the Sochi Winter Paralympics also raises the issue of the safety of the field of play. During the Games, temperatures during competition reached 18°C and did not often fall below 0°C at night. The warm climate may have substantially contributed to poor snow conditions, potentially putting athletes at higher risk of injury.[7]

"MIND THE GAP"

Passengers on the London Underground are reminded to "Mind the gap" to help ensure their safety in boarding and disembarking trains. This safety message can also be an important direction to clinicians and researchers regarding the current state of knowledge about concussion in Para athletes. Although ever-increasing study into concussion in the able-bodied population has provided information that can be applied to Para athletes, there is a significant gap in knowledge about the specifics and nuances of concussion in the latter group. Recent editorials have emphasized the importance of addressing this issue[1,23]; however, this gap presents a valuable opportunity for clinically relevant research. Incidence data, mechanisms of injury, specific assessment tools, appropriate management and return to play, and risk reduction strategies are all fertile ground for study and will play an important role in helping Para athletes compete safely. Although not the final frontier, it is hoped that concussion in Para sport will be the next frontier, including being a subject at the next International Consensus Conference on Concussion in Sport. As *Star Trek* Captain James T. Kirk said, "…there is no such thing as the unknown, only things temporarily hidden and not understood."[24] For the health and safety of Para athletes and all those with a disability, it is imperative that the concussion knowledge gap be addressed.

REFERENCES

1. Webborn N, Blauwet CA, Derman W, et al. Heads up on concussion in para sport. Br J Sports Med 2017. Available at: http://bjsm.bmj.com/content/early/2017/06/29/bjsports-2016-097236. Accessed July 24, 2017.
2. Blauwet C, Lexell J, Derman W, et al. The Road To Rio: medical and scientific perspectives on the 2016 paralympic games. PM R 2016;8(8):798–801.
3. Van Mechelen W, Hlobil H, Kemper HC. Incidence, severity, aetiology and prevention of sports injuries. A review of concepts. Sports Med 1992;14(2):82–9.
4. Webborn N, Willick S, Reeser J. Injuries among disabled athletes during the 2002 winter paralympic games. Med Sci Sports Exerc 2006;38(5):811–5.
5. Webborn AD. IPC injury survey Torino 2006. The Paralympian 2007;(2):11.
6. Webborn N, Willick S, Emery CA. The injury experience at the 2010 winter paralympic games. Clin J Sport Med 2012;22:3–9.
7. Derman W, Schwellnus M, Jordaan E, et al. High incidence of injury at the Sochi 2014 Winter Paralympic Games: a prospective cohort study of 6564 athlete days. Br J Sports Med 2016;50:1069–74.
8. Willick SE, Webborn N, Emery C, et al. The epidemiology of injuries at the London 2012 paralympic games. Br J Sports Med 2013;47:426–32.
9. Derman W, Schwellnus MP, Jordaan E, et al. Sport, sex and age increase risk of illness at the Rio 2016 Summer Paralympic Games: a prospective cohort study of 51 198 athlete days. Br J Sports Med 2018;52:17–23.

10. Webborn N, Cushman D, Blauwet C, et al. The epidemiology of injuries in football at the London 2012 paralympic games. PM R 2016;8(6):542–52.
11. Magno e Silva MP, Morato MP, Bilzon JL, et al. Sports injuries in brazilian blind footballers. Int J Sports Med 2013;34:239–43.
12. Wessels K, Broglio S, Sosnoff J. Concussions in wheelchair basketball. Arch Phys Med Rehabil 2012;93:275–8.
13. Hawkeswood J, Finlayson H, O'Connor R, et al. A pilot survey on injury and safety concerns in International Sledge Hockey. Int J Sports Phys Ther 2011;6(3): 173–85.
14. McCrory P, Meeuwisse W, Dvorak J, et al. Consensus statement on concussion in sport – the 5th international conference on concussion in sport held in Berlin, October 2016. Br J Sports Med 2017;51:838–47.
15. Echemendia R, Meeuwisse W, McCrory P, et al. The sport concussion assessment tool fifth edition (SCAT5). Br J Sports Med 2017;51:848–50.
16. Weiler R, van Mechelen W, Fuller C, et al. Do neurocognitive SCAT3 baseline test scores differ between footballers (Soccer) living with and without disability? A cross-sectional study. Clin J Sport Med 2018;28(1):43–50.
17. Wessels KK. Concussion assessment in wheelchair users: quantifying seated postural control. Ann Arbor (Michigan): University of Illinois at Urbana-Champaign, ProQuest Dissertations Publishing; 2013. p. 3632369.
18. West LR, Griffin S, Weiler R, et al. Management of concussion in disability sport: a different ball game? Br J Sports Med 2017;51:1050–1.
19. Finch C. A new injury framework for research leading to sports injury prevention. J Sci Med Sport 2006;9:3–9.
20. Baker SP. Injury control. In: Rosenau MJ, Maxcy KF, Sartwell PE, editors. Preventive medicine and public health. 10th edition. New York: Appleton-Century-Crofts; 1973.
21. Bose D, Crandall JR. Influence of active muscle contribution on the injury response of restrained car occupants. Ann Adv Automot Med 2008;52:61–72. Available at: http://www.ncbi.nlm.nih.gov/pubmed/19026223. Accessed December 4, 2017.
22. Kajta Z, Karren J, Subic A. Experimental investigation into the suitability of smart polymers as an impact-absorbing material for an improved rugby headgear. International Conference on Mechanics, Materials, Mechanical Engineering and Chemical Engineeering (MMMCE 2015). 2015. Available at: http://www.inase.org/library/2015/books/MMMCE.pdf. Accessed December 4, 2017.
23. West LR, Griffin S, Weiler R, et al. Management of concussion in disability sport: a different ball game? Br J Sports Med 2017;51(14):1050–1.
24. Knapp A. Five leadership lessons from James T. Kirk. Jersey (NJ): Forbes; 2012. Available at: https://www.forbes.com/sites/alexknapp/2012/03/05/five-leadership-lessons-from-james-t-kirk/#46d401bd2631. Accessed December 2, 2017.

Applying Scientific Principles to Enhance Paralympic Classification Now and in the Future

A Research Primer for Rehabilitation Specialists

Sean M. Tweedy, PhD*, Mark J. Connick, PhD, Emma M. Beckman, PhD

KEYWORDS

- Activity limitation • Descriptive science • Impairment • Para sport
- Para athlete taxonomy

KEY POINTS

- Para sport classification permits the realization of the Paralympic Vision by defining who is eligible to compete as a Para athlete and by providing a structure for competition that aims to control for the impact of impairment on the outcome of competition.
- Development of classification systems based on scientific evidence is required but has only recently been made possible by adoption of a clear, unambiguous statement of the purpose of classification by the International Paralympic Committee and its member organizations.
- Rigorous descriptive science with its focus on measuring, recording, analyzing, and predicting can improve extant systems of classification and lead to the development of new systems of classification. Both paths should be pursued.
- The absence of valid ratio-scaled measures of impairment is currently the most significant barrier to the development of evidence-based systems of classification and addressing this is the Paralympic Movement's most pressing scientific challenge.
- A recently published study demonstrated that development of data-driven classification structures based on ratio-scaled measures of impairment is possible and yields a valid class structure that is superior to the extant system.

The authors have nothing to disclose.
School of Human Movement and Nutrition Sciences, The University of Queensland (UQ), Blair Drive and Union Road, St Lucia QLD 4072, Australia
* Corresponding author.
E-mail address: s.tweedy@uq.edu.au

Phys Med Rehabil Clin N Am 29 (2018) 313–332
https://doi.org/10.1016/j.pmr.2018.01.010
1047-9651/18/© 2018 Elsevier Inc. All rights reserved.

INTRODUCTION
Vision of the Paralympic Movement and Evidence-Based Classification

The Vision of the Paralympic Movement is "to enable Para athletes to achieve sporting excellence and inspire and excite the World."[1] Para sport classification systems perform 2 functions that are critical for the realization of this vision. First, they define who is eligible to compete in Para sport and, therefore, who can be a Para athlete. In this way classification is fundamental to Para sport, providing a framework for determining who can and who cannot compete. Second, they group athletes into sport classes that control for the impact of impairment on the outcome of competition and ensure that, as far as possible, sporting excellence determines which athlete or team is ultimately victorious.[2,3]

In this way, Para sport classification systems provide a unique framework that permits Para athletes to demonstrate that elite athletic performance is a relative, rather than an absolute, concept, and that achieving excellence in the context of significant physical, sensory, or intellectual impairment can be particularly inspiring.

Classification systems that are invalid, or perceived to be invalid, pose a significant threat to the Vision of the Paralympic Movement. At the elite level, the legitimacy of an individual or team's competitive success can be significantly diminished by the perception that they are in the wrong class. The perception can also have potentially adverse personal and financial consequences for that athlete or team. At the grassroots level, a classification system that is perceived to be unfair will discourage participation among people with disabilities rather than achieve the goal of fostering it.[2] Therefore, the organizations governing the Paralympic Movement have a duty to ensure that systems of classification are valid, defensible, and based on the best available scientific evidence.

Governance and Terminology in Para Sport

The International Paralympic Committee (IPC) is the global governing body of the Paralympic Movement.[4] Its constitutional duties include the preparation and delivery of the Summer and Winter Paralympic Games, the flag-ship sporting events for the Paralympic Movement. The IPC is structurally and administratively independent from the International Olympic Committee but, as the prefix Para indicates, the Paralympic Games run parallel with the Olympic Games and have been held in the same year as the Olympic Games since their inception in 1948.[5]

The IPC is also the governing body for 10 of the 40 Para sports; a Para sport is a sport that is either governed directly by the IPC or by a member organization. Not all Para sports are Paralympic sports, this term being reserved for sports that are contested at the Paralympic Games. Para dance sport (governed by the IPC) and Para world sailing (governed by World Sailing), are examples of Para sports that are not currently included in the Paralympic program. Similarly, Para athlete refers to any athlete competing in a Para sport, whereas Paralympic athlete denotes someone who has competed at the Paralympic Games.

Table 1 presents the 28 sports currently on the Paralympic program, 22 of which will be contested at the 2020 Tokyo Paralympic Games, and the remaining 6 will be contested at the 2018 PyeongChang Winter Paralympic Games. As **Table 1** indicates, athletes with physical impairments are eligible for 25 Paralympic sports, those with visual impairment are eligible for 13, and those with an intellectual impairment are eligible for 3. This article focuses on the classification of Para athletes with physical impairments.

Table 1
Sports in the 2020 Tokyo Summer Paralympic Games and the 2018 PyeongChang Winter Paralympic Games

			Impairment Group		
	Paralympic Sport	Governing Organization	Physical	Visual	Intellectual
Sports for 2020 Tokyo Paralympic Games (N = 22)	Archery	World Archery	✓	✓	—
	Badminton	Badminton World Federation	✓	—	—
	Boccia	Boccia International Sports Federation	✓	—	—
	Canoe	International Canoe Federation	✓	—	—
	Cycling	International Cycling Union	✓	✓	—
	Equestrian	International Equestrian Federation	✓	✓	—
	Football 5-a-Side	International Blind Sport Association	—	✓	—
	Goalball	International Blind Sport Association	—	✓	—
	Judo	International Blind Sport Association	—	✓	—
	Para athletics	World Para Athletics (IPC)	✓	✓	✓
	Para powerlifting	World Para Powerlifting (IPC)	✓	—	—
	Para swimming	World Para Swimming (IPC)	✓	✓	✓
	Rowing	International Rowing Federation	✓	✓	—
	Shooting Para sport	World Shooting Para Sport (IPC)	✓	—	—
	Table Tennis	International Table Tennis Federation	✓	—	✓
	Taekwondo	World Taekwondo	✓	—	—
	Triathlon	International Triathlon Union	✓	✓	—
	Volleyball (Sitting)	World Para Volley	✓	—	—
	Wheelchair Basketball	International Wheelchair Basketball Federation	✓	—	—
	Wheelchair Fencing	International Wheelchair and Amputee Sports Federation	✓	—	—
	Wheelchair Rugby	International Wheelchair Rugby Federation	✓	—	—
	Wheelchair Tennis	International Tennis Federation	✓	—	—
Sports for 2018 PyeongChang Winter Games (N = 6)	Para alpine skiing	World Para Alpine Skiing (IPC)	✓	✓	—
	Para biathlon	World Para Nordic Skiing (IPC)	✓	✓	—
	Para cross-country skiing	World Para Nordic Skiing (IPC)	✓	✓	—
	Para ice hockey	World Para Ice Hockey (IPC)	✓	—	—
	Para snowboard	World Para Snowboard (IPC)	✓	—	—
	Wheelchair curling	World Curling Federation	✓	—	—

The second column presents the governing organization for each sport, 9 of which are directly administered by the IPC, whereas the others are structurally and administratively independent. The final 3 columns indicate which of the 3 impairment groups (physical, visual, or intellectual) are eligible to compete in each sport.

Implications of Para Sport Governance for Researchers

Eighteen separate organizations govern the 28 Paralympic sports (see **Table 1**). Nine sports are governed by the IPC and the remaining 19 sports are governed by 17 organizations that are members of the IPC, including the International Blind Sports Association, which governs 3 Paralympic sports, and 16 other organizations, each of which governs single Para sport (see **Table 1**).

Each of the 18 governing organizations has endorsed the IPC Classification Code[6] which includes, inter alia, a commitment to developing systems of classification for their sports based on scientific evidence. The collective commitment of all Para sports to the development of evidence-based classification systems is critical for reasons considered in the next section. However, from the perspective of performing classification research, the individual commitment of each of these 18 organizations is important because each is an autonomous entity with the right to determine whether research findings will be incorporated into their classification procedures and, if so, how they will be implemented. Researchers who engage with governing organizations in the planning stages of the research process will not only enhance the prospects of producing results that affect classification practice, they can also gain an authentic, grounded understanding of the sport, which can assist with the identification of key areas of research need. Governing organizations are also in an ideal position to assist researchers to recruit participants for classification projects and help to overcome a perennial challenge in Para sport research: obtaining an adequate sample size.

Taxonomic Evolution of Para Sport Classification

Until recently, the principal barrier to the development of evidence-based systems of classification was that there was no consensus among Para sport governing organizations regarding the purpose of classification. Furthermore, if there was agreement, the purpose was ambiguous (eg, to provide a framework for fair competition).[7] **Table 2** presents the chronologic evolution of the taxonomic principles for Para sport, together with the research required for the development of evidence-based systems of classification.

In 2002, the first paper applying the principles of taxonomy to a Para sport, or Para athletics (then referred to as disability athletics), was published. One of the key contributions of the paper was to propose that, based on a taxonomic analysis of extant systems of classification, the purpose of the Para athletics classification system should be to minimize the impact of eligible impairments on the outcome of competition.[7] This proposal gained traction within the sport of Para athletics and, with support from the sport's governing bodies, a project to develop a taxonomically valid classification framework for Para athletics was launched in 2003. The first report was submitted in 2006; however, the findings did not receive the approvals required for implementation until 2009.[8]

In the meantime, the first IPC Classification Code was published and endorsed by the General Assembly of the IPC,[9] which includes all organizations governing Para sports. The Code was significant because, for the first time, the principles and procedures required in classification for all Para sports were codified and compliance with the Code was mandatory for all IPC member organizations. Significantly, the Code included a statement about the purpose of classification in Para sports that was consistent with the 2002 proposal.[7] Another significant inclusion in the Code was the mandatory requirement for all Para sports to pursue the development of evidence-based systems of classification (Article 15.2). The code was recently revised and has retained the same statement of purpose for classification (Article 2), as well as the requirement for the development of evidence-based systems of classification (Article 10.2).[6]

Table 2
Evolution of taxonomic principles for Para sport classification

Year	Title	Advances in Taxonomic Principles for Para Sports, Including Research Required for Evidence-Based Systems
2002	"Taxonomic Theory and the ICF: Foundations for a Unified Disability Athletics Classification" (Tweedy, 2002)	• First application of taxonomic theory to classification in Para sport (the sport of Para athletics), including defining classification • Demonstrated taxonomic relationship between Para athletics and the International Classification of Functioning, Disability, and Health (ICF), and advocated aligning the language and taxonomic structure of the Para athletics classification system with the ICF (World Health Organization, 2001) • Identified primary barrier to development of evidence-based systems of classification was that organizations did not agree about the purpose of classification or, if there was agreement, the statement of purpose was ambiguous (eg, to make sport fair) • The following unambiguous statement of purpose was proposed: the purpose of classification should be to minimize the impact of eligible impairments on the outcome of competition

2007	International Paralympic Committee Classification Code and International Standards (IPC, 2007)	• Consensus about the purpose of classification was achieved when the General Assembly of the IPC formally adopted the IPC Classification Code, which specifies, inter alia:
		  ○ That the purpose of classification is to minimize the impact of eligible impairments on the outcome of competition
		  ○ That systems of classification should be based on scientific evidence

2011	"International Paralympic Committee Position Stand–Background And Scientific Principles of Classification in Paralympic Sport" (Tweedy, 2011)	• The authoritative position on the scientific principles of classification in Para sports, officially adopted by the IPC and incorporated verbatim into the governance documents for the Paralympic Movement (IPC, 2003) provides the scientific underpinnings of the Classification Code (the Code being a policy, rather than a scientific, document)
		• The taxonomic structure proposed for the sport of athletics in 2002 (Tweedy, 2002) is made a requirement for all Para sports, including the definition and purpose of classification and alignment with the language and structure of the ICF
		• Defines the term evidence-based classification system, this being a system in which:
		  ○ The purpose is stated unambiguously
		  ○ Scientific evidence indicates that the methods used for assigning class will achieve the stated purpose
		• The 10 impairment types eligible for Paralympic sport are specified
		• Describes the research required for development of evidence-based systems of classification (ie, determine the strength of association between measures of impairment and performance in sport with the aim of quantifying the extent of activity limitation resulting by impairment)

(continued on next page)

Table 2
(continued)

Year	Title	Advances in Taxonomic Principles for Para Sports, Including Research Required for Evidence-Based Systems
		• Identifies weighting and aggregation of measures of impairment as a fundamental threat to the validity of current systems of classification
		• Specifies the measurement properties required of valid measures of impairment, these being that they should be objective, reliable, precise, specific to the impairment of interest (eg, assesses strength or co-ordination but not both), parsimonious (smallest number of measures that account for the greatest variance in performance), and (as far as possible) training resistant (ie, when athletes undertake rigorous, sport-specific training, the difference between pretraining and posttraining measures of impairment should be minimal)
2014	"Paralympic Classification: Conceptual Basis, Current Methods, and Research Update" (Tweedy, 2014)	• First schematic representation of the sequence of steps required for the development of new evidence-based systems of classification with the aim of facilitating engagement of researchers in the Para sport classification research agenda
		• Development of valid measures of impairment identified as most pressing scientific challenge in development of evidence-based systems of classification
		• Posits that, in addition to the measurement features specified in the position stand, a valid measure of impairment should be ratio-scaled and that ordinal scales (eg, those currently used to assess impaired strength) (Hislop, 2007)[18] and hypertonia (Ashworth, 1964)[19] could not lead to evidence-based systems of classification
2016	"Research Needs for the Development of Evidence-based Systems of Classification for Physical, Vision and Intellectual Impairments" in *Training and Coaching the Paralympic Athlete* (Tweedy, 2016)	• Detailed operational translation of principals articulated in the 2011 position stand to athletes with vision impairment and intellectual impairment
		• Expanded format (11,000 words) permitted detailed description and examples of research design and measurement methods required for the development of evidence-based classification systems for each of those impairment groups
		• Updated schematic representation of the research required to develop new systems of classification, including issues applicable to vision impairment and intellectual impairment and incorporating the need for research to address issues, such as how to detect deliberate submaximal performance (intentional misrepresentation) and quantifying the training responsiveness of measures of impairment

	• Recognized the term measurement of impairment is a term of convenience; impairment is a loss or absence and, therefore, cannot be directly measured but must be inferred based on measurement of extant body structures or functions
2017 "Evolution and Development of Best Practice in Paralympic Classification," in *Palgrave Handbook of Paralympic Studies* (Connick, 2017)[25]	• Recognition that, although the goal of evidence-based classification systems is critical, assessment of a system should not be binary (either evidence-based or not evidence-based) but take into account the strength of the evidence on which the system is based • Expands on the statistical decision-making methods that can be used to assign new athletes a class
This article	• Identifies the central importance of the principles of descriptive science (rather than experimental science) to the development of evidence based systems of classification (ie, to describe the relationship between measures of impairment and activity limitation) • Highlights how the principles of descriptive science can not only be applied to developing new systems of classification but also can be applied to the evaluation and improvement of current systems; scientific analysis of current systems can provide research directions for the development of new systems • Underscores that at the point of system change (from current system of classification to a new system of classification) the new system should be based on the very highest level of evidence and preceded by rigorous translational research projects assessing athlete acceptability, the impact on athletes currently competing, feasibility and face-validity

In 2011, the "International Paralympic Committee Position Stand–Background and Scientific Principles of Classification in Paralympic Sport"[2] was published. This document sets forth the scientific principles of classification in Para sport and outlines the essential research agenda for the development of evidence-based classification systems. This important paper has passed through a rigorous, scientific peer-review process, has been approved by the Governing Board of the International Paralympic Committee, and has been incorporated verbatim into the IPC handbook.[10] Since its publication, 3 additional peer-reviewed papers have contributed to the taxonomic advancement of Para sport classification, including specific descriptions of the research required for the development of evidence-based classification systems. The contributions of these papers are presented in **Table 2**.

Specific Aims

This is the fourth paper published on the taxonomic principles of Para sports classification since the publication of the position stand; its aim is to provide specialists in physical medicine and rehabilitation (PM&R) with descriptions of:

- The current classification process as described in the recently revised Code,[6] with which all Para sports are required to comply
- Ways the scientific method can be applied to the development of new, evidence-based systems of classification, as well as to enhancing extant systems of classification
- A recent advance in wheelchair track racing classification that has led to the first valid, data-driven classification structure for any Para sport
- The diverse and critical roles that PM&R specialists can play in the delivery and advancement of Para sports classification.

THE CURRENT CLASSIFICATION PROCESS

All Para sports are required to have and publish classification rules and regulations for their sport (Article 1.6)[6] and the elements of central importance to this article are presented in **Fig. 1**.

Taxonomic Foundations for an Evidence-Based Classification System

Fig. 1 presents the taxonomic foundations that must be in place in order for a sport to develop an evidence-based classification system. These foundations come from Articles 2.1 and 2.2 of the Code,[6] and the former is a clear, unambiguous statement of purpose. In the interest of clear communication, it is ideal if the statement is accompanied by a description of how the classification system aims to achieve this purpose. Following is a model statement of purpose for the sport of wheelchair basketball[11]:

> The purpose of classification in wheelchair basketball is to minimize the impact of eligible impairments on the outcome of wheelchair basketball games. Conceptually, the wheelchair basketball classification system aims to achieve this purpose by placing athletes into classes according to how much their impairment affects fundamental activities required for optimal wheelchair basketball performance. If this aim is achieved, each wheelchair basketball class will comprise athletes who have impairments that cause approximately the same amount of disadvantage in wheelchair basketball, independent of skill level, training history or assistive equipment.

The other foundational element of a Code-compliant classification system is specification of the eligible impairment types. There are a 10 eligible impairment types in

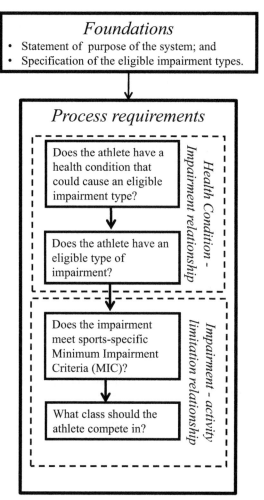

Fig. 1. Key elements required for a code-compliant, evidence-based, Para sport classification system. The taxonomic foundations of a code-compliant classification system (*top*) are derived from Article 2.1 and 2.2 of the IPC Classification Code. The key elements of a code-compliant classification process (*bottom*) are derived from Articles 2.2.2 to 2.2.4 of the IPC Classification Code. Compliance with these elements of the Code will permit the development of evidence-based systems of classification.

Para sport: vision and intellectual impairment, as well as 8 physical impairments: hypertonia, ataxia, athetosis, impaired muscle power, impaired range of movement, limb deficiency, leg-length difference, and short stature.[2,3] There is no requirement for each Para sport to have classification systems for all eligible impairment types. For example, people with short stature are eligible to compete in Para athletics and Para swimming but not Para boccia or Para canoe. Thus, Boccia and Para canoe need not account for short stature in their classification systems.

The Athlete Classification Process

Fig. 1 also summarizes the process requirements of a Code-compliant classification system, presented as 4 key questions derived from Articles 2.2.2 to 2.2.4 of the

Classification Code. The first 2 questions require assessments that are essentially medical in nature, being required to establish the health condition–impairment relationship (see **Fig. 1**). The final 2 questions require a range of assessments that permit evaluation of the extent to which impairment adversely affects sports performance.

The first key question is whether or not the athlete has a health condition that could lead to 1 or more of the 10 eligible impairment types. For example, health conditions such as spinal cord injury, cerebral palsy, traumatic brain injury, and achondroplasia all typically lead to an eligible impairment type, whereas health conditions such as fibromyalgia and complex regional pain syndrome do not.[3] Code-compliant classification systems should have processes in place for gathering and assessing an athlete's medical information. Best practice procedures include having new athletes submit medical documentation well ahead of competition, and engaging a panel of medical practitioners with relevant specializations to assess the documentation and provide authoritative input.

If it is determined that an athlete does have a health condition that could lead to an eligible impairment type, they are then required to attend a face-to-face assessment that is usually conducted immediately before an approved competition. The assessment is conducted by a classification panel comprising a minimum of 2 accredited classifiers, 1 medical (with a medical or physiotherapy qualification) and 1 sports technical (with a coaching or sports science qualification), who have both completed an accredited classification course.[6]

When the athlete presents, the next 2 questions that the panel must address are whether the athlete does, in fact, have an eligible type of impairment and, if so, whether the impairment is severe enough to meet eligibility criteria.[6] The second question must be addressed because the IPC Classification Code requires that, to be eligible to compete in a given Para sport, an athlete should have an impairment severe enough to affect sports performance.[6] Thus, each Para sport' classification system is required to set minimum impairment criteria (MIC), which are operational descriptions of the minimum severity of each eligible impairment type. It stands to reason that there is considerable variability in MIC from sport to sport. For example, although limb deficiency is an eligible impairment type for both athletics (ie, track and field) and swimming, a person with a unilateral below-wrist amputation is not eligible for athletics events, but is eligible for swimming, because such an impairment will affect swimming performance but will have minimal or no impact on performance in athletic events (eg, running, jumps or throws).

Methods of physical impairment assessment used to assess MIC commonly include anthropometric techniques for assessing limb deficiency, short stature, and leg-length difference[12]; manual muscle testing for assessing impaired strength,[12] frequently with sport-specific adaptations[13]; goniometry for range of movement; and the Ashworth scale for hypertonia.[12] Methods for assessing impaired coordination, such as that associated with hypertonia, ataxia, and athetosis, are rarely drawn from the peer-reviewed literature but some systems include the Scale for the Assessment and Rating of Ataxia.[14] In general, classification processes require very little equipment, enabling a great variety of competition locations to serve as classification sites. However, achieving acceptable precision and interrater and intrarater reliability is challenging.

The fourth and final key question addressed in the classification process is "What class should the athlete compete in?" Each sport has its own class profiles presented in sport-specific classification rules and regulations. Class profiles describe impairments and activities that are typical of athletes in each class. The classification panel must match each athlete with the most appropriate class profile.[9] Ideally, methods for classifying impairments and determining class profile are evidence-based; that is, based on scientific data that ensures the creation of homogeneous classes of athletes with impairments that cause the same amount of difficulty in a given sport.[2]

Unfortunately, such evidence does not exist[2] and current best practices require classification panels to assign a class by subjectively considering outcomes from the impairment assessment (described previously), combined with outcomes from 4 other forms of assessment: (1) Novel motor tasks are tasks that are unlikely to have been practiced by the athlete in the usual course of training for their sport. For example, in the sport of Para athletics this might include rapid hand-rubbing, alternating heel-toe tapping in a seated position, or backwards tandem walking; (2) Sport-specific activities are likely to have been frequently practiced by athletes training for the sport. For example, in the sport of athletics this might include standing broad jump, 4 bounds for distance, or speed-skipping; (3) An activity in which the athlete, as far as possible, kinematically replicates the sports activity they will compete in. For example, a runner would complete 40-m sprint and a shot putter would throw a shot put; (4) A detailed training history and other personal and environmental factors that are, together with impairment, likely to affect sports proficiency. This includes age, time since injury, and whether they have access to a qualified coach.[15]

The classification process is completed after the classification panel observes the athlete during competition, the purpose of which is to check that, as far as possible, the athlete's performance in competition is consistent with the results of preceding assessments.[6]

USING THE SCIENTIFIC METHOD TO ENHANCE CLASSIFICATION
Descriptive Versus Experimental Science

The scientific method is a way of using unbiased, objective observations to generate new knowledge and can be divided into descriptive and experimental scientific methods.[16] Rigorous descriptive science requires accurate, objective measurement of variables but, unlike experimental science, manipulation of variables is not required. As a result, descriptive science cannot be used to test causal hypotheses, although it can act as a catalyst for them.[16]

Scientific description requires 4 sequential steps[16]:

1. Scientific measurement: The first and foundational step of rigorous scientific description is scientific measurement; that is, measurement that is accurate, objective, reliable (ie, free of bias and random error), and valid (ie, measures the intended variable).
2. Scientific recording: Data should be recorded in a way that is systematic, secure, and searchable;
3. Scientific analysis to identify relationships: Well-recognized statistical procedures can be used to assess whether variables are related and the strength of the relationship.
4. Scientific evaluation of whether identified relationships can be generalized: This is done by reproducing results in large representative samples and using statistics to evaluate the extent to which the relationships observed in the sample truly reflect the relationships in the population. Results from this step determine the predictive validity of the variables measured.

Most branches of science have specialized taxonomic structures that have been developed through rigorous descriptive science. For example, it was the accurate scientific description of plants and animals that underpinned their classification into kingdom, phylum, genus, and species; and observation of chemical elements that led to the development of the periodic table. The authors posit that the development of evidence-based systems of classification for Para sports requires rigorous application of descriptive scientific methods and that these methods can be used to both improve extant systems of classification and develop new ones.

Improving Extant Systems of Classification Through Science

Fig. 2 provides a schematic summary of the ways in which descriptive science can enhance extant Para sport classification systems. Note that, consistent with the descriptive scientific method, the first step for improving each of the elements of the process is the identification or development of scientific measures (ie, measures that are objective, reliable, and valid). Specifically

- The process for assessing medical documentation to determine whether an athlete has a health condition that could lead to an eligible impairment type

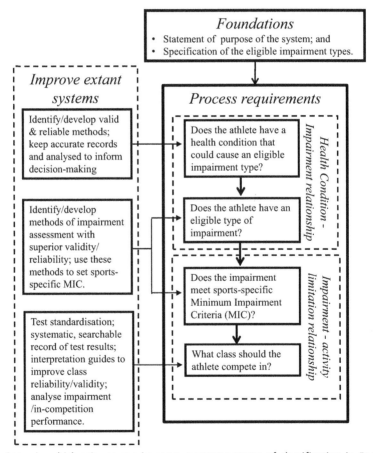

Fig. 2. Areas in which science can improve current systems of classification in Para sport. (*Top* and *center*) **Fig. 1** reproduced. (*Left*) An overview of areas in which science can improve extant Para sport classification systems by applying principles of scientific measurement and record-keeping that will enhance objectivity and permit analysis that can be used to further improve current decision-making and guide the development of new systems of classification (see **Fig. 3**).

depends on specialist medical knowledge. However, this decision is not typical of medical specialists' routine decision-making and this decision-making process is not well-developed. A scientific approach would commence with medical specialists making an inventory of the tests required for more common health conditions, then systematically broadening and updating the inventory as case diversity increases and advances in medical science occur. This should be complemented by a process for systematic, searchable recording of decisions made. These strategies can help to ensure pending decisions are consistent with previous decisions (reliability) and analysis of decision-making over time could help to differentiate more useful from less.

- Identification or development of methods for assessing impairments with improved reliability and/or validity, with particular emphasis on evaluation of very mild presentations, can help to ensure consistency of decision-making when determining whether an athlete has an eligible impairment type and could be used to revise or update MIC. Scientific recordkeeping of results from such assessments would help to improve the reliability of these decisions. Investigation of the relationship between the outcomes and in-competition performance could eventually lead to the development of MIC that is more valid or better defined. The physical impairments with greatest scope for enhancement are hypertonia, ataxia, and athetosis.
- As indicated previously, class allocation is based on the outcomes of a range of different tests, including tests of impairment, novel motor tasks, practiced motor tasks, and kinematic replication. In general, test standardization, recording of results, and interpretation guides are not well-developed in Para sport classification systems. A more scientific approach in these areas could significantly enhance the reliability of class allocation. Analysis of the relationship between measures of impairment obtained during classification and in-competition performance could help inform the development of more sports-specific MIC and help to guide the development of research projects aiming to develop new systems of classification.

Notably, such analyses (ie, the relationship between impairment data collected during athlete classification and the in-competition performance of those athletes) cannot provide the basis for new systems of classification. The development of new systems requires dedicated research projects conducted away from competition for several reasons:

- Potential underperformance on tests of impairment: Although athletes are required to give maximal effort during classification, there is an incentive to underperform on tests of impairment to be placed into a class for athletes with more severe impairments and increase chances of competitive success. The only way to eliminate this incentive is to conduct research in settings completely removed from the classification process to ensure athletes are convinced impairment test results will not affect class allocation and, therefore, will be confident to give maximal effort.
- Submaximal competition performance: Competition performance is not always maximal for a range of reasons, including injury, heavy competition schedules, or tactical reasons. Research results would be confounded if submaximal competition performance were included in the analysis.
- Variability in environmental or emotional status during competition: Environmental conditions during competition can vary markedly, particularly for outdoor sports (eg, wind, rain, extreme temperatures), as can emotional status (eg,

effects of team selection pressure, opponent tactics, media, and internal team dynamics). These confounding influences can be eliminated or controlled to some extent in a standardized research environment.

Until recently, the notion that science can improve extant systems of Para sport classification has received relatively little attention in the literature. Although there is little doubt that the long-term future of Para sport requires the development of new systems of classification, the development and implementation of these new systems is likely to take several years at least. In the meantime, improving the validity and integrity of extant systems of classification can help to ensure that athletes currently competing do so under the fairest possible circumstances. In addition, there are relatively good prospects that a more scientific approach to measurement and recording in extant systems could generate knowledge that could help optimize the design of dedicated research programs required to develop new systems of classification. These prospects are described in the next section.

Developing New Systems of Classification

The most comprehensive and up-to-date description of the research required to develop evidence-based methods of classification is presented in a recent book chapter.[17] A summary of that 5-step process is presented in **Fig. 3**.

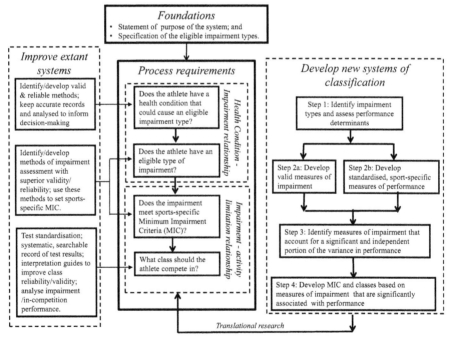

Fig. 3. Research required for developing new systems of classification. (*Top, center,* and *left*) **Fig. 2** reproduced. (*Right*) The research required for development of new systems of classification in which the structure and the number of classes are based on scientific evidence regarding the relative strength of association between valid measures of impairment and sports performance. Once developed, and before full-scale implementation, translational research is required in which the new system is implemented on a small scale and the success of the implementation is evaluated in relation to outcomes such as feasibility, data collection, storage and security processes, acceptability, influence on competition format, and a range of other areas.

Just as the methods for improving current systems of classification clearly align with the principles of descriptive science, so do the published methods for developing new systems of classification presented in **Fig. 3**.[16] Specifically, the 5-step process is sequential, moving from step 1, which requires specification of the impairment types to be classified and that the extant literature is reviewed; to steps 2a and 2b, which focus on the development of measures of the 2 key constructs: impairment (step 2a) and sports performance (step 2b); to step 3 in which measures of impairment that are significantly associated with sports performance are identified; to using appropriate statistical analyses to develop data-driven MIC and class structures. However, there are some essential differences between the approaches used for improving extant systems and those used for developing new systems. Some of the most important include

- Improvements in extant systems of classification can be made based on the methods of impairment assessment that are already in place. For example, the reliability of manual muscle testing assessment was improved in Para athletics when methods of manual muscle testing were standardized across classifiers.[13] However, the development of a new, evidence-based classification system requires measures of impairment have all of the following attributes: reliability, precision, parsimony, training resistance, and a ratio scale. Manual muscle testing is based on an ordinal, 6-point scale in which a muscle with a grade of 2 is not necessarily twice as strong as the muscle with a grade of 1 or one-half as strong as a muscle with a grade of 4. As a consequence, manual muscle testing is not a suitable method of impairment assessment for the development of an evidence-based methods of classification.[15] Methods for assessment of strength impairment that are suitable for the development of evidence-based systems of classification are described in the next section.
- To evaluate the extent of activity limitation resulting from impairment, standardized, sport-specific measures of performance that predict overall sports performance need to be developed. This is relatively straightforward in sports in which performance is measured with a single, ratio-scaled measure. Either distance or time may be used; for example, track (eg, 40-m sprint), field (eg, throw distance), or swimming (eg, 25-m sprint). However in team sports such as wheelchair basketball, wheelchair rugby, or 7-side football, the development of sports-specific measures is a considerable scientific challenge.[17]
- The structure of a new system (ie, the number of classes and the relationship between classes) will be data-driven and may result in a structure that is similar to or radically different from the extant system of classification. In contrast, methods used for improving current systems of classification will rarely lead to a change in the number of classes because such a change requires knowledge of the extent of activity limitation resulting from different impairment types and, as previously pointed out, this evidence does not currently exist.

In summary, extant systems of classification can be improved through selective application of the principles of descriptive science to address specific issues, whereas the development of new, evidence-based systems of classification requires rigorous execution of the entire descriptive science process.

It remains the case that the most pressing scientific challenge for researchers in evidence-based classification is the development of valid and reliable measures of impairment.[15] This is because of the development of such measures occurs relatively early in the sequence of steps required to develop evidence-based systems of classification and no sport will be in a position to progress the research agenda until the development of appropriate measures of impairment have been developed.[15,18,19]

THE FIRST DATA-DRIVEN PARA SPORT CLASSIFICATION STRUCTURE

The sport in which the classification research agenda has progressed the farthest is wheelchair track racing for athletes currently competing in classes T51 to T54. This is the first sport in which all 5 steps of the classification research agenda presented in **Fig. 3** have been completed. The program of research has resulted in a classification structure that has been published in a peer-reviewed journal[20] and could be transferred directly to the sport.[20]

An overview of the program of research includes the following:

- As per step 1, impairment types eligible for this sport were identified, including limb deficiency (eg, results from amputation or dysmelia), leg-length differences, impaired range of movement (eg, results from arthrogryposis or contracture), and impairments of strength (eg, results from spinal cord injury, spina bifida, or polio). Consultation with an expert panel, reference to seminal literature,[21] and some original research by our group in collaboration with others[22] resulted in identification of the following key muscle actions being identified for assessment: shoulder flexors, elbow extensors, forearm pronators, and forward trunk flexion.
- In relation to step 2a, it should be noted that, although 4 impairment types are eligible, tests for assessing impaired muscle strength were developed because athletes who are eligible based on 1 of the other 3 impairment types frequently do not have impairments that affect the key wheelchair propulsion muscle actions. More specifically
  ○ Leg-length difference only affects lower limbs by definition.
  ○ Limb deficiency is almost exclusively lower limb; very few upper limb amputees compete.
  ○ Significant impairments of upper limb range of movement are not very common among athletes and, although impairments of trunk range of movement occur relatively more frequently in people with muscle power impairment (especially scoliosis, kyphosis, or kyphosis scoliosis), it is particularly difficult to measure. The authors' research indicated that trunk impairment was not likely to have a significant influence on performance and some of the effects would be reflected in the lower muscle strength scores that we intended to measure.
- Other work conducted in relation to step 2a included
  ○ Detailed review of the literature to identify the most appropriate voluntary strength assessment method for inferring strength loss in Para athletes[23]
  ○ The development of 7 ratio-scaled isometric strength tests and reporting sex-specific normal performance ranges in 118 nondisabled participants (63 men and 55 women) aged 23.2 plus or minus 3.7 years, test–retest reliability, and evaluation of the relationship between the measures and body mass.[23]
- Three preliminary studies helped to identify the best protocols for sports-specific assessment, refine impairment testing protocols, and gain insight into the influence of trunk flexion strength on start and top speeds.[2,22,24]

The capstone study that comprehensively covered both steps 3 and 4, "Cluster Analysis of Novel Isometric Strength Measures Produces a Valid and Evidence-Based Classification Structure for Wheelchair Track Racing,"[20] used a sample of 32 international-level wheelchair track racers and demonstrated that

- Six novel isometric strength tests were significantly correlated with measures of wheelchair racing performance, including right and left isometric arm extension strength, isometric trunk flexion strength, a combined measure of isometric arm extension plus trunk flexion strength, and a combined measure of pronation and grip strength.
- Cluster analysis of the strength tests produced 4 clusters and there were significant between-cluster differences in strength: cluster 4 was stronger than 3, which was stronger than 2, which was stronger than 1. Nineteen percent of athletes were in a cluster that did not align with their current class; for example, some athletes in cluster 3 were in current class T54.
- In relation to sports performance, the mean speeds achieved by the clusters was hierarchical, such that cluster 4 was faster than 3, which was faster than 2, which was faster than 1. In contrast, current classes were not hierarchical: there was no difference between speeds achieved by T53 and T54.

Based on these findings, the strength tests reported can be used as the basis for developing a new classification system for those wheelchair track racers currently competing in T51 to T54, pending replication of the findings in a sufficiently large, representative sample. The positive findings should encourage other Para sports specialists to use scientific methods to develop evidence-based systems of classification, and this article can provide valuable conceptual and methodological guidance.

Translational Research: Getting Evidence-Based Systems of Classification into Practice

The results of the wheelchair racing classification study provide a reason to be optimistic that other researchers will be able to produce data-driven systems for allocating athletes to classes based on the extent of activity limitation resulting from their impairment in a wide range of sports and in other impairment types. The goal of creating Para sport classification systems that are valid, transparent, and relatively free of contested decisions seems attainable. However, as indicated in **Fig. 3**, the authors contend that the final step, implementing the system in practice, should not take place until results from relevant translational studies indicate that implementation is appropriate. Translational research would include analyses of areas such as stakeholder acceptability (eg, athletes, coaches, classifiers, administrators, and sports fans); advanced indication of the impact on current athletes, including medal winners and record holders at the national and international level; development of suitable data recording, reduction, storage, retrieval, and protection; and any influence on athlete access to classification opportunities.

Relatively sophisticated change management strategies will also be required because a change from a system of classification to another, including a possible increase or decrease in the number of classes, is likely to have far-reaching effects. For example, under new systems of classification, several previously successful athletes may be less successful, possibly substantially so, and this is unlikely to occur without reaction from athletes, their coaches, and their national sports organizations. In addition, historical records may have to be retired and new records started. One transitional strategy with merit is having a period of time during which athletes continue competing in the old system but are also classified according to the new system. This would provide a valid basis on which to evaluate many of the effects of transitioning to a new system. The ultimate determinant of whether the change will be worthwhile is a balanced consideration of whether the benefits that will be accrued (ie, more transparent, defensible scientifically based classification systems) justify the inevitable human and/or financial costs previously outlined.

ROLES FOR PHYSICAL MEDICINE AND REHABILITATION SPECIALISTS IN PARA SPORT CLASSIFICATION

PM&R specialists can play a wide range of highly valuable roles in Para sport classification, including

- Encouraging patients in acute settings to consider becoming involved in Para sports once they have been discharged. PM&R specialists can help streamline this process by endeavoring to establish working relationships between rehabilitation centers in which they work and community sports organizations for people with disabilities.
- Training to become a classifier for 1 of the 25 sports that provide competitive opportunities to athletes with physical impairments. Clinicians with particular interest in physical assessment and medical reasoning are likely to find this work interesting and challenging, particularly if they also have a working knowledge of the sport they are classifying. Pathways into classification vary from sport to sport and direct contact with the governing organization offers the most efficient path.
- For those with a particular interest in diagnostics and assessing medical reports, an ideal way to contribute would be through medical panels that assess whether an athlete has a health condition that could lead to an eligible impairment type. This would have minimal or no travel requirement and would suit those who are time poor.
- Finally, for those who are trained in research, engagement with a governing organization to begin the conversation about ways in which the scientific method can be used to improve current methods of classification and develop new evidence-based methods is a way to make a lasting contribution to the ongoing success of the Paralympic Movement.

SUMMARY

Para sport classification permits the realization of the Paralympic Vision by defining who is eligible to compete as a Para athlete and by providing a structure for competition that aims to control for the impact of impairment on the outcome of competition. Development of classification systems based on scientific evidence is required but has only recently been made possible by adoption of a clear, unambiguous statement of the purpose of classification by the IPC and its member organizations. Rigorous descriptive science with its focus on measuring, recording, analyzing, and predicting can improve extant systems of classification and lead to the development of new systems of classification. Both these paths should be pursued. The absence of valid ratio-scaled measures of impairment is currently the most significant barrier to the development of evidence-based systems of classification and addressing this is the Movement's most pressing scientific challenge. A recently published study demonstrated that development of data-driven classification structures based on ratio-scaled measures of impairment is possible and yields a valid class structure that is superior to the extant system. However, implementation of this and other evidence-based systems of classification should be supported by the results of translational research projects. Finally, PM&R specialists can make important contributions by encouraging their patients to participate in Para sport; training to become a classifier; assessing medical records to evaluate athlete eligibility; and, for those who are trained in research, assisting Para sport organizations to improve their classification processes using the scientific method.

REFERENCES

1. International Paralympic Committee. Paralympic vision and mission. IPC handbook. Bonn (Germany): Author; 2003.
2. Tweedy SM, Vanlandewijck YC. International Paralympic Committee position stand–background and scientific principles of classification in Paralympic sport. Br J Sports Med 2011;45(4):259–69.
3. International Paralympic Committee. International standard for eligible impairments. International Paralympic Committee athlete classification code. Bonn (Germany): Author; 2015.
4. International Paralympic Committee. Strategic plan 2015-18-strategic outlook for the International Paralympic Committee. Bonn (Germany): Author; 2015. p. 22.
5. International Paralympic Committee. IPC handbook. Bonn (Germany): Author; 2003.
6. International Paralympic Committee. International Paralympic Committee athlete classification code. Bonn (Germany): Author; 2015.
7. Tweedy SM. Taxonomic theory and the ICF: foundations for a unified disability athletics classification. Adapt Phys Activ Q 2002;19(2):220–37.
8. Tweedy SM, Bourke J. IPC athletics classification project for physical impairments: final report - stage 1. Bonn (Germany): IPC Athletics; 2009.
9. International Paralympic Committee. International Paralympic Committee classification code and international standards. Bonn (Germany): Author; 2007.
10. International Paralympic Committee. Position Statement on background and scientific principles of classification in Paralympic sport. IPC Handbook. Bonn (Germany): Author; 2003.
11. International Wheelchair Basketball Federation (IWBF) Player Classification Commission. IWBF functional player classification manual. Winnipeg (Canada): IWBF; 2014.
12. International Paralympic Committee. IPC athletics classification rules and regulations. Bonn (Germany): Author; 2017.
13. Tweedy SM, Williams G, Bourke J. Selecting and modifying methods of manual muscle testing for classification in Paralympic sport. European Journal of Adapted Physical Activity 2010;3(2):7–16.
14. Schmitz-Hübsch T, du Montcel ST, Baliko L, et al. Scale for the assessment and rating of ataxia: development of a new clinical scale. Neurology 2006;66(11):1717–20.
15. Tweedy SM, Beckman EM, Connick MJ. Paralympic classification: conceptual basis, current methods, and research update. PM R 2014;6(8):S11–7.
16. Mitchell ML, Jolley JM. Research design explained. 8th edition. Belmont (CA): Wadsworth Cengage Learning; 2013.
17. Tweedy SM, Mann DL, Vanlandewijck YC. Research needs for the development of evidence-based systems of classification for physical, vision and intellectual impairments. In: Vanlandewijck YC, Thompson WR, editors. Training and coaching the Paralympic athlete. London: John Wiley & Sons, Ltd; 2016. p. 122–49.
18. Hislop H, Montgomery J. Daniels and Worthingham's muscle testing: techniques of manual examination. St Louis (MO): Saunders Elsevier; 2007.

19. Ashworth B. Preliminary trial of carisoprodal in multiple sclerosis. Practitioner 1964;192:540–2.
20. Connick MJ, Beckman E, Vanlandewijck Y, et al. Cluster analysis of novel isometric strength measures produces a valid and evidence-based classification structure for wheelchair track racing. Br J Sports Med 2017. [Epub ahead of print].
21. Vanlandewijck Y, Theisen D, Daly D. Wheelchair propulsion biomechanics: implications for wheelchair sports. Sports Med 2001;31(5):339–67.
22. Vanlandewijck YC, Verellen J, Beckman E, et al. Trunk strength effect on track wheelchair start: implications for classification. Med Sci Sports Exerc 2011; 43(12):2344–51.
23. Beckman EM, Connick MJ, Tweedy SM. Assessing muscle strength for the purpose of classification in Paralympic sport: a review and recommendations. J Sci Med Sport 2017;20(4):391–6.
24. Vanlandewijck YC, Verellen J, Tweedy SM. Towards evidence-based classification – the impact of impaired trunk strength on wheelchair propulsion. Adv Rehabil 2010;3(1):1–5.
25. Connick MJ, Beckman EM, TSM. Evolution and development of best practice in Paralympic classification. In: Brittain I, Beacom A, editors. Palgrave Handbook of Paralympic Studies, London: Palgrave Publishing Ltd.

Performance Characteristics of Para Swimmers

How Effective Is the Swimming Classification System?

Brendan Burkett, PhD[a],*, Carl Payton, PhD[b],
Peter Van de Vliet, PhD[c], Hannah Jarvis, PhD[b], Daniel Daly, PhD[d],
Christiane Mehrkuehler, MSc[d], Marvin Kilian, MSc[e],
Luke Hogarth, PhD[f]

KEYWORDS

- Swimming classification • Paralympics • Swimming performances • Impairments

KEY POINTS

- Paralympic swimming classification began with a sports medicine–driven medical-based system.
- The current functional classification system is a swimming-specific system that assigns and integrates athletes with eligible impairments into classes.
- Based on performance characteristics of swimmers within the current classification system, the relationship between swimming class and performance is inconsistent, potentially disadvantaging some athletes.
- A new evidence-based swimming classification system is currently under development, built on the knowledge from the sport medicine assessment.

INTRODUCTION

The sport of swimming has been part of every Paralympic program since the games began in 1960 and is one of the most popular sports for Para athletes

[a] High Performance Sport, Faculty of Science, Health, Education and Engineering, School of Health and Sport Sciences, University of the Sunshine Coast, Sippy Downs, Queensland 4558, Australia; [b] HEAL Research Centre, Manchester Metropolitan University, Crewe Green Road, Crewe CW1 5DU, United Kingdom; [c] Medical and Scientific Department, International Paralympic Committee, Adenauerallee 212-214, Bonn 53113, Germany; [d] Faculty of Kinesiology and Rehabilitation Sciences, KU Leuven, Tervuursevest 101, Heverlee 3001, Belgium; [e] Institute of Training Science and Sport Informatics, German Sport University, Am Sportpark Müngersdorf 6, Cologne 50933, Germany; [f] School of Health and Sport Sciences, University of the Sunshine Coast, Sippy Downs, Queensland 4558, Australia
* Corresponding author.
E-mail address: bburkett@usc.edu.au

Phys Med Rehabil Clin N Am 29 (2018) 333–346
https://doi.org/10.1016/j.pmr.2018.01.011
1047-9651/18/© 2018 Elsevier Inc. All rights reserved.
pmr.theclinics.com

with a physical, visual, or intellectual impairment. For all Paralympic sports, an international classification system determines athlete eligibility and the subsequent 'grouping' of athletes for competition. The aim of classification is to achieve fair competition by minimizing the impact of an individual's impairment on the outcome of the competition so that sporting ability, skill level, and training alone determine success and the final result.[1] Despite this long history of inclusion within the Paralympic Games, questions have often been raised on the effectiveness of the classification system. Indeed, the International Paralympic Committee (IPC) has mandated the development of evidence-based classification systems of classification,[1] which highlights the need for a review of the current classification system for swimming.

As Paralympic sport evolved from an initial medical rehabilitation program, sports medicine formed the original swimming classification system. This inaugural classification system was based purely on a medical model with athletes 'grouped' within 5 classes of impairment: (i) athletes with an amputation, (ii) athletes with cerebral palsy, (iii) athletes with a spinal cord injury, (iv) Athletes with a visual impairment, and (v) athletes with les autres.

IPC swimming introduced the Functional Classification System in 1990, which involved 2 forms of assessment, a sports medicine bench test that screens the musculoskeletal function of the athlete. The philosophy of this system was to combine the previous medical assessment with sport-specific measures. This assessment involved a modified format of the traditional medical range of movement and strength assessment. The functional classification system is a sport-specific system of classification that assigns and integrates athletes with eligible impairments, predominately physical impairments, into classes to maintain equitable and fair competition among these athletes.[2] The cumulative score from these equally weighted dry land measures would determine into which classification the athlete would be placed, because each classification was represented by a specific range of bench test scores. This test was followed by an in-water assessment, which required the registered IPC swimming classifier to observe the athlete swim in the water, and based on this observation, if necessary, adjust the bench test score and ultimately the final classification. This combination of medical and sport-specific assessment currently forms the activity limitation tests for Para swimming. The system has been in place for 7 consecutive Paralympic Games from 1992 to 2016, with some modifications over time.

The separate classes distinguish between the distinct arm-dominant freestyle, backstroke, and butterfly strokes; the leg-dominated breaststroke; and the individual medley, which includes all 4 strokes and, therefore, warrants its own unique classification system. Athletes rated as a 10 on the classification scale (eg, S10, SB10, SM10) have the greatest function. Function gradually decreases (the scope of the impairment increases) as one moves closer to a 1 rating (S1, SB1, SM1).

Although the requirement for fairness and equity has been stipulated,[3] there has been no quantitative research that has examined if the current classification system results in discrete categories of swimming performance for all events and genders for each class. To date, analysis of Paralympic swimming performance has focused on the factors that contribute to the final outcome, swimming time.[4–6] Therefore, the aim of this study was to investigate how effective the current classification system creates clearly differentiated Paralympic competition classes, based on performance time for all swimming strokes and events. This new knowledge provides the required evidence for the effectiveness of this important Para sport.

METHODOLOGY

The swim time performances for male and female medalist swimmers since the inception of the current functional classification system were obtained from 6 major competitions, the

- 1992 (Barcelona),
- 1996 (Atlanta),
- 2000 (Sydney),
- 2004 (Athens),
- 2008 (Beijing), and
- 2012 (London) Paralympic and Olympic games.

The swim time performance for the male and female Olympic swimmers in corresponding events provided a benchmark comparison. In total, 2370 race performance times were investigated, with all data downloaded from official, publicly accessible swimming and sporting websites (www.ipc-swimming.org, www.databaseolympics.com).

The swim times for male and female medalists in the Paralympic classes and the corresponding swim times for the 3 Olympic medalists in the following events were recorded:

- The 50-m, 100-m, and 400-m freestyle,
- The 100-m backstroke,
- The 100-m breaststroke,
- The 100-m butterfly, and
- The 200-m individual medley.

These events were analyzed because they were common to both Paralympic and Olympic games. Because the data were publicly available and deidentified, human ethics approval was not required. To determine if there were clear differences between performances in each class, the mean swimming speeds (m/s) for Paralympic performances were expressed as a percentage of the corresponding Olympic performance. This percentage index allowed for a uniform comparison of race performance between classes, events, and genders.

Statistical analysis was performed with the Statistical Package for the Social Sciences (SPSS, version 17.0, SPSS, Inc, Chicago, IL). The normality of distribution of data was confirmed using a Shapiro-Wilk test. The raw swim times and percentage indices of classes were compared for each sex and event using a 1-way analysis of variance with an alpha value of 0.05. Bonferroni post hoc analysis was used to determine the source of statistical significance when required. A paired sample t test was used to compare each mean percentage index to a predicted fixed percentage variable.

Based on an analysis of the percentage indices, this arbitrary fixed variable was set at 85% for class S10 and decreased by 5% for each class down to 45% for class S2. For the classes of visually impaired athletes (S11, S12 and S13), the arbitrary fixed variable was set at 90% for class 13 and decreased by 5% for each class down to 80% for class 11. The assignment of this fixed variable was subjective, with the goal of creating equal differences between the classes.

RESULTS

Of a total of 128 mean raw times across the classes and events, 58 (45%) were found to have no significant difference to their adjacent higher class (**Table 1**). Of the classes

Table 1
Competitive swimming times (s) for medalists for each event and class

									Class				
	S2	S3	S4	S5	S6	S7	S8	S9	S10	S11	S12	S13	Olympic
50 Free													
Male	69.9 (68.4–71.3)	52.1 (50.5–53.8)	41.6 (40.1–43.0)	35.9 (34.4–37.4)	31.4[a] (29.9–32.9) S6 = S7	29.5[a] (28.1–31.0) S7 = S8	28.1[a] (26.7–29.6) S8 = S9	26.8[a] (25.3–28.2) S9 = S10	25.4[a] (23.9–Olym) S10 = Olym	26.9[a] (25.4–28.4) S11 = S12	25.5[a] (24.1–27.0) S12 = S13	25.3[a] (23.9–26.8) S13 = Olym	21.9 (20.4–23.3)
Female	85.8 (83.9–87.8)	60.2 (58.5–62.0)	51.5 (49.7–53.2)	39.1[a] (37.5–40.7) S5 = S6	37.6[a] (36.0–39.2) S6 = S7	35.4[a] (33.8–37.0) S7 = S8	33.1[a] (31.5–34.7) S8 = S9	30.8[a] (29.2–32.4) S9 = S10	29.4 (27.8–31.0)	33.2 (31.6–34.8)	29.1[a] (27.5–30.7) S12 = S13	28.6 (27.0–30.2)	24.6 (23.0–26.2)
100 Free													
Male	149.0 (147.2–150.7)	115.4 (113.5–117.3)	92.8 (91.0–94.5)	79.0 (77.3–80.8)	70.1 (68.3–71.8)	64.8[a] (63.0–66.5) S7 = S8	62.0[a] (60.2–63.8) S8 = S9	59.0[a] (57.2–60.7) S9 = S10	55.6 (53.8–57.3)	60.4[a] (58.6–62.2) S11 = S12	56.4[a] (54.7–58.2) S12 = S13	56.1 (54.3–57.8)	48.3 (46.6–50.1)
Female	183.7 (179.8–187.6)	128.0 (124.1–131.9)	109.5 (106.0–113.0)	85.0[a] (81.8–88.2) S5 = S6	81.8[a] (78.7–85.0) S6 = S7	76.5[a] (73.3–79.7) S7 = S8	72.2[a] (69.0–75.4) S8 = S9	66.2[a] (63.1–69.4) S9 = S10	63.6 (60.5–66.8)	72.9 (69.8–76.1)	64.0[a] (60.8–67.2) S12 = S13	62.3 (59.1–65.4)	54.1 (50.9–57.2)
400 Free													
Male	n/a	n/a	n/a	n/a	311.9[a] (308.1–315.8) S6 = S7	299.5 (296.4–302.6)	284.6 (281.5–287.8)	268.7[a] (265.5–271.8) S9 = S10	258.9 (255.8–262.0)	286.3 (282.4–290.1)	266.6[a] (263.5–269.8) S12 = S13	264.8 (261.7–268.0)	224.4 (221.2–227.5)
Female	n/a	n/a	n/a	n/a	352.9[a] (342.7–363.0) S6 = S7	338.4[a] (330.1–346.7) S7 = S8	319.8 (311.5–328.2)	292.4[a] (284.1–300.7) S9 = S10	286.9 (278.6–295.2)	345.0 (333.2–356.8)	296.9[a] (286.7–307.1) S12 = S13	286.1 (274.3–297.9)	245.8 (237.5–254.1)

	S4	S5	S6	S7	S8	S9	S10	S11	S12	S13	S14
100 Back											
Male	n/a	n/a	79.9[a] (78.0–81.8) S6 = S7	76.4 (74.6–78.3)	70.9[a] (69.0–72.8) S8 = S9	66.6[a] (64.7–68.5) S9 = S10	64.2 (62.3–66.1)	70.7 (68.8–72.6)	66.0[a] (64.1–67.9) S12 = S13	66.0 (64.2–67.9)	53.8 (52.0–55.7)
Female	n/a	n/a	94.3 (92.3–96.4)	89.1 (87.1–91.1)	83.2 (81.2–85.2)	74.9[a] (72.9–76.9) S9 = S10	73.8 (71.7–75.8)	84.6 (82.4–86.8)	74.7[a] (72.5–76.9) S12 = S13	73.3 (70.9–75.8)	60.2 (58.1–62.3)
100 Breast											
Male	103.7 (101.8–105.5)	95.6[a] (93.7–97.4) S5 = S6	92.8 (91.0–94.7)	86.9 (85.0–88.7)	78.6[a] (76.7–80.4) S8 = S9	74.9 (73.0–76.7)	n/a	77.2[a] (75.4–79.1) S11 = S12	73.1[a] (71.2–74.9) S12 = S13	71.3 (69.5–73.2)	60.6 (58.7–62.4)
Female	120.0[a] (116.7–123.4) S4 = S5	112.6[a] (109.5–115.6) S5 = S6	108.3[a] (105.0–111.7) S6 = S7	102.3 (99.2–105.4)	89.8[a] (86.8–92.9) S8 = S9	85.7 (82.6–88.8)	n/a	92.1[a] (86.8–97.4) S11 = S12	84.8[a] (81.7–87.8) S12 = S13	83.2 (79.9–86.6)	67.2 (64.2–70.3)
100 Fly											
Male	n/a	n/a	n/a	n/a	67.9 (66.3–69.5)	63.6[a] (62.0–65.3) S9 = S10	61.0 (59.3–62.6)	65.3[a] (63.0–67.6) S11 = S12	62.2[a] (60.5–63.8) S12 = S13	61.1 (59.5–62.7)	52.0 (50.4–53.6)
Female	n/a	n/a	n/a	n/a	82.2 (80.3–84.2)	73.7[a] (71.7–75.6) S9 = S10	71.2 (69.1–73.4)	90.3 (86.9–93.7)	68.5[a] (66.3–70.6) S12 = S13	68.4 (65.6–71.2)	57.7 (55.9–59.8)

(continued on next page)

Table 1
(continued)

								Class					
	S2	S3	S4	S5	S6	S7	S8	S9	S10	S11	S12	S13	Olympic
200 IM													
Male													
	n/a	n/a	n/a	192.6 (188.7–196.4)	175.2 (171.7–178.7)	166.8 (163.3–170.3)	156.0 (152.5–159.4)	145.0[a] (141.5–148.5) S9 = S10	139.5 (136.0–143.0)	152.4 (148.5–156.2)	141.1[a] (137.6–144.6) S12 = S13	139.1 (135.3–143.0)	118.4 (114.9–121.9)
Female													
	n/a	n/a	n/a	226.9 (219.5–234.2)	201.2[a] (195.5–206.9) S6 = S7	194.0 (188.8–199.2)	180.8 (175.6–186.0)	163.3[a] (158.2–168.5) S9 = S10	158.8 (153.6–163.9)	187.4 (181.7–193.1)	160.6[a] (155.4–165.8) S12 = S13	155.6 (150.4–160.7)	131.4 (126.2–136.6)

Data are mean (95% confidence interval).

Abbreviation: n/a, not applicable.

[a] Indicates no significant difference to the adjacent class (eg, *S2 indicates S2 = S3).

with a physical impairment (S2–S10), a total of 38 of 86 mean values (44%) across classes and events were found to have no significant difference in mean performance time compared with their adjacent higher class. Classes S5 (50%), S6 (67%), S8 (50%), and S9 (86%) were the most similar to their adjacent higher classes, whereas classes S2 (0%), S3 (0%), S4 (17%), and S10 (8%) had the least number of mean values similar to their adjacent higher classes. For the visual impairment classes (S11–S13), the S12 class showed the most similar mean values compared with the adjacent higher class, with 100% of the mean values having no significant difference from the S13 class.

There were less similar results between adjacent classes when performance times were expressed as a percentage index relative to the corresponding Olympic time (**Table 2**). When comparing the percentage indices between classes, a total of 33 of the 128 mean values (26%) were similar to their adjacent higher class. The S9 (57%) and S12 (100%) classes showed the highest number of similar mean values to their adjacent higher classes for the physical and visual impairments, respectively. Classes S2, S3, S4, S7, and S11 showed no similar mean values to their adjacent higher class when comparing the percentage indexes.

When comparing each classes' performance index with the fixed arbitrary value a total of 77 of the 128 values (60%) showed significant differences. Typically, the percentage indexes for classes S2, S3, and S13 were significantly lower than the fixed arbitrary values set for physical and visual impairments, whereas classes S6 and S7 were significantly higher than the fixed arbitrary value (see **Table 2**). All physical and visual impairment classes showed increases in the performance index (mean for events and genders) from the 1992 to 2012 Paralympic games (**Fig. 1**).

DISCUSSION

The purpose of this study was to investigate whether the functional classification system creates an equitable delineation between its classes based solely on performance outcome. The functional classification system was found to delineate performances between some classes, but failed to do so for others. This finding is in agreement with research that has found inconsistent differences in determinants of swimming performance between adjacent classes, indicating that the current functional classification system does not always differentiate clearly between swimming groups.[7] In particular, physical impairment classes S9 and S10 and visual impairment classes S12 and S13 showed the most similar swimming performances for events and genders based on both raw times and performance indices expressed relative to Olympic performances. These results highlight the shortcomings of the current functional classification system to promote fair and equitable competition, and the need for a revised, evidence-based classification system. Sports medicine can play a lead role in this process, because Paralympic swimming relies on the effectiveness of sports-specific activity limitation tests.

When examining the raw performance times for the physical impairment classes (S2-S10) the higher classes with less severe impairments (>S5) reported more similar performances to one another compared with classes S2 to S4 (see **Table 1**). This may partly be attributed to the lower number of events competed in by the more severely impaired classes. However, another contributing factor that may cause this disparity between the higher and lower classes is the impact that impairment severity has on sporting participation and training progression.

Swimmers competing in classes S2 to S5 have lower physical function than those in higher classes, and are predominately confined to a wheelchair, have little or no use of

Table 2

Competitive swimming performances for medalists expressed as a percentage index of the related Olympic performance for each event and class

	S2 (45%)	S3 (50%)	S4 (55%)	S5 (60%)	S6 (65%)	S7 (70%)	S8 (75%)	S9 (80%)	S10 (85%)	S11 (80%)	S12 (85%)	S13 (90%)
50 Free												
Male	31.6[a] (30.9–32.2)	42.6[a] (41.8–43.4)	53.2 (52.5–53.9)	61.2 (60.5–61.9)	69.7[a] (69.0–70.4)	74.1[a] (73.4–74.8)	77.9[a] (77.2–78.6)	81.6[a] (80.9–82.3)	86.3 (85.6–87.0)	81.3[a] (80.6–82.0)	85.8[b] (85.1–86.4) S12 = S13	86.5[a] (85.7–87.1)
Female	29.1[a] (27.1–31.0)	41.1[a] (39.4–42.9)	48.9[a] (47.2–50.6)	63.3[a,b] (61.7–64.9) S5 = S6	65.6 (64.0–67.2)	69.6 (68.0–71.2)	74.4 (72.8–76.0)	80.1[b] (78.5–81.7) S9 = S10	83.8[a] (82.2–85.3)	74.2[a] (72.6–75.8)	84.6[b] (83.0–86.2) S12 = S13	86.1[a] (84.5–87.7)
100 Free												
Male	32.7[a] (32.0–33.5)	42.4[a] (41.6–43.3)	52.7 (52.0–53.5)	61.5 (60.7–62.2)	69.2 (68.4–69.9)	74.7[a] (74.0–75.5)	78.1[a] (77.4–78.9)	82.0[a] (81.3–82.8)	87.2[a] (86.4–87.9)	80.1 (79.3–80.8)	85.9[b] (85.1–86.6) S12 = S13	86.3[a] (85.6–87.1)
Female	29.8[a] (27.7–31.9)	42.6[a] (40.5–44.7)	50.3[a] (48.4–52.2)	64.0[a,b] (62.2–65.7) S5 = S6	66.3 (64.6–68.0)	70.9 (69.1–72.6)	75.1 (73.4–76.9)	81.7[a,b] (80.0–83.5) S9 = S10	85.0 (83.3–86.7)	74.3[a] (72.6–76.0)	84.7[b] (83.0–86.7) S12 = S13	86.9[a] (85.2–88.6)
400 Free												
Male	n/a	n/a	n/a	n/a	71.6[a,b] (69.9–73.3) S6 = S7	75.0[a] (73.6–76.3)	78.9[a] (77.6–80.3)	83.6[a] (82.2–85.0)	86.8[a] (85.4–88.1)	78.2 (76.5–79.9)	84.3[b] (82.9–85.7) S12 = S13	84.9[a] (83.5–86.3)
Female	n/a	n/a	n/a	n/a	69.5[a,b] (67.3–71.7) S6 = S7	72.9[a] (71.1–74.7)	77.2 (75.4–79.0)	84.3[a,b] (82.5–86.1) S9 = S10	85.7 (83.9–87.5)	71.6[a] (69.1–74.1)	82.9[a,b] (80.7–85.1) S12 = S13	86.1[a] (83.5–88.6)

100 Back												
Male	n/a	n/a	n/a	n/a	67.6[a,b] (65.9–69.3) S6 = S7	70.5 (68.8–72.2)	76.1 (74.4–77.8)	80.9[b] (79.2–82.6) S9 = S10	84.0 (82.3–85.7)	76.2[a] (74.5–77.9)	82.0[a,b] (80.3–83.7) S12 = S13	82.1[a] (80.4–83.8)
Female	n/a	n/a	n/a	n/a	64.0 (62.5–65.5)	67.7[a] (66.3–69.2)	72.6[a] (71.1–74.1)	80.6[b] (79.1–82.1) S9 = S10	81.8[a] (80.3–83.3)	71.5[a] (69.9–73.1)	81.2[a,b] (79.6–82.8) S12 = S13	82.7[a] (80.9–84.5)
100 Breast												
Male	n/a	n/a	58.5[a] (57.0–60.0)	63.4[a,b] (61.9–64.9) S5 = S6	65.3 (63.9–66.8)	69.8 (68.3–71.3)	77.4 (75.9–78.8)	81.1 (79.6–82.5)	n/a	78.6 (77.1–80.0)	83.0[a,b] (81.5–84.4) S12 = S13	85.0[a] (83.6–86.5)
Female	n/a	n/a	56.2[b] (54.2–58.2)	59.9[b] (58.1–61.8) S5 = S6	62.1[a,b] (60.1–64.1) S6 = S7	66.1[a] (64.2–67.9)	75.3[b] (73.4–77.1) S8 = S9	78.7 (76.8–80.5)	n/a	72.2[a] (69.0–75.4)	79.6[a,b] (77.8–81.4) S12 = S13	81.1[a] (79.1–83.2)
100 Fly												
Male	n/a	n/a	n/a	n/a	n/a	n/a	77.0 (75.3–78.7)	81.8[a,b] (80.2–83.5) S9 = S10	85.4 (83.8–87.1)	78.5 (76.1–80.8)	83.8[b] (82.1–85.5) S12 = S13	85.2[a] (83.5–86.9)
Female	n/a	n/a	n/a	n/a	n/a	n/a	70.9[a] (69.1–72.6)	78.7[b] (76.9–80.5) S9 = S10	81.3[a] (79.4–83.3)	65.4[a] (62.3–68.5)	84.3[b] (82.3–86.3) S12 = S13	84.7[a] (82.2–87.3)

(continued on next page)

Table 2
(continued)

								Class					
	S2 (45%)	S3 (50%)	S4 (55%)	S5 (60%)	S6 (65%)	S7 (70%)	S8 (75%)	S9 (80%)	S10 (85%)	S11 (80%)	S12 (85%)	S13 (90%)	
200 IM													
Male													
	n/a	n/a	n/a	61.9[a] (60.7–63.2)	67.7[a] (66.5–68.9)	71.0[a] (69.9–72.2)	76.0 (74.9–77.2)	81.7[a] (80.5–82.9)	84.9 (83.8–86.1)	78.1[a] (76.8–79.4)	84.0[b] (82.8–85.2) S12 = S13	84.9[a] (83.6–86.2)	
Female													
	n/a	n/a	n/a	58.6 (56.3–61.0)	65.3[b] (63.5–67.1) S6 = S7	68.0[a] (66.3–69.6)	73.0 (71.3–75.6)	80.6[b] (78.9–82.2) S9 = S10	82.8[a] (81.1–84.5)	70.5[a] (68.7–72.3)	82.1[a,b] (80.4–83.7) S12 = S13	84.6[a] (82.9–86.3)	

Data are mean (95% confidence interval).
Abbreviation: n/a, not available.
[a] Indicates significant difference from fixed arbitrary value.
[b] Indicates no significant difference to the adjacent class (eg, *S2 indicates S2 = S3).

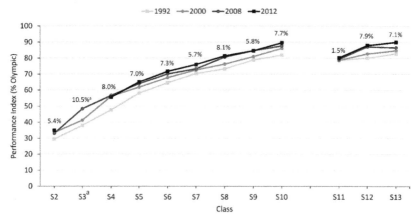

Fig. 1. Mean performance index (gender and event) for each class for the 1992 and 2012 Paralympic games. Percentages represent changes in performance index from 1992 to 2012. [a] Difference in percentage index from 1992 to 2008.

their upper and lower extremities and their trunk, have moderate to severe coordination difficulties, and/or a degree of limb loss in up to 4 limbs. These swimmers need more assistance for transportation, accessing facilities, starting races, and have considerably less training time, all of which might negatively impact their training progression compared with swimmers with higher physical function. These factors may also explain why swimmers in lower classes (S2–S4) have less consistency in their race-to-race performances; oscillations in movement and function make consistent performances more difficult to produce, thus, causing greater variances in performances within and between the lower classes.[8] Comparatively, increased participation rates and trainability of less impaired swimmers likely promotes more consistent swimming performances and greater competitiveness within these classes, causing greater progressions in performance.

Despite these barriers to participation and training for the more severely impaired classes, it is interesting to note that all of the physical impairment classes showed similar progressions in performances over competition cycles (see **Fig. 1**). From 1992 to 2012, the classes had a mean increase of $7.3 \pm 1.6\%$ of Olympic performance with no clear differences between the lower (S2 to S4 = 5.4% to 8.0%) and higher classes (S5 to S10 = 5.7% to 8.1%). These results are complimentary to the advancements of the Paralympic movement; they demonstrate that Paralympic swimming performance has progressed more so than Olympic swimming performance over the past 2 decades. However, the similarity in progression between lower and higher classes suggests that the shortcomings of the functional classification system to delineate performances between higher classes is more likely due to limitations in the classification methods, rather than greater training progression or competitiveness within the higher classes.

A key finding from this study is the lack of strong connection between impairment and swimming performance. This outcome is evidenced by the similarities in both raw times and performance indices between physical impairment classes S9 and S10, and visual impairment classes S12 and S13 (see **Tables 1** and **2**). Although swimmers in these classes have been found to have increasing "sport-specific" impairment severity (eg, from S13 to S11), the lack of difference between swimming performances between these classes suggests that the current classification methods are not effective in grouping athletes. The integration of an appropriate sports medicine test would be beneficial in addressing this issue. This finding is reinforced from earlier studies on the effectiveness of the medical bench tests against swimming kinematics.[9] In this previous study, data were collected via 3 different procedures: (i) the musculoskeletal range of motion, as per the swimming classification protocol, (ii) the 3-dimensional kinematic range of movement when simulating swimming, and (iii) the bilateral hand force the swimmer generated on a swimming ergometer. The study found that there were inconsistent and generally weak correlations (approximately three-quarters of all measures) between the musculoskeletal range of motion, the 3-dimensional kinematic range of motion, and the force output measures.

The IPC Athlete Classification Code stipulates that athletes should be grouped based on the impact of their impairment on their given sport, not simply by their impairment severity.[1] The ineffectiveness of the current functional classification system to delineate between certain classes may have resulted from issues with measurement weighting (ie, relative contribution of different impairment measures to classification outcome) and measurement aggregation (ie, aggregation of different types of impairment measures to classification outcome). It is also possible that impairment tests included in the functional classification system do not account for the greatest variance in Paralympic swimming performance. For example, research has found inconsistent and weak correlations between the current functional classification system range of motion scores, and actual 3-dimensional kinematics, and hand force production measures during simulated swimming on a swim bench ergometer.[9] Collectively, these findings demonstrate the requirement for research to define more accurately the relationship between existing impairment measures and the determinants of swimming performance,[10] as well as exploring other impairment measures that may have a greater impact on swimming performance.

The development of evidence-based classification systems in Paralympic swimming requires validated measures of impairment that are impairment specific, account for the greatest variance in swimming performance, and are as resistant to training as possible. Several of the current impairment measures used as part of the current functional classification system may be problematic because they are subjective and have high dependency on user judgment, including methods of manual muscle testing and motor coordination assessment.[9]

Instrumented tests that provide objective measures of impairment will likely provide more valid and reliable measures that allow for clearer definitions between impairment and swimming performance. Research in Paralympic track and field has defined the impact of instrumented measures of strength and motor coordination impairment on sporting performance to guide the development of evidence-based classification.[11] Similar research examining the relationship between instrumented tests of impairment and their relative impact on swimming performances is warranted in Paralympic swimming to guide the development of a new evidence-based classification system.

Another important consideration of the revised classification system is the impact that impairment has on swimming performance in different events (swimming strokes) and distances. Currently, the functional classification system does aim to account for swimming stroke (ie, S, SB, and SM) although the impact of impairment on swimming performances in each swimming stroke has not been addressed fully. The current functional classification system does not account for how different impairments may interact with swimming performances for a given swimming stroke over different distances. This study found the current functional classification system to be particularly ineffective in differentiating raw performance times between the higher classes (>S6) in the shorter distance events in comparison with the longer distance events. For example, for the higher classes (>S6) there were a greater number of similar raw mean values between adjacent classes for the 50-m freestyle (90%) compared with the 100-m freestyle (70%) and 400-m freestyle (50%; see **Table 1**).

These findings are supportive of Daly's and Vanlandewijck's[3] criticism of the functional classification system for not accounting for short and long distance events, because the physical abilities that contribute to swimming performance are likely to change for different event distances. They suggest that the contribution of the arms and legs to net propulsion changes over increased distance, and that impairment tests of the upper and lower limbs should be weighted accordingly for short and long distance events. Future research should define the impact of impairments on swimming performance for different swimming strokes and distances.

A limitation of the current study is the arbitrary fixed variable comparison of the Paralympic swimming performance with the respective Olympic swimming performance. As stated in the Methods section, this nominal ratio was set at 85% of the Olympic swimmers for Paralympic class S10 athletes. A second limitation was the nominal 5% variation in swimming performance time for the different Paralympic swimming classes. There were no relevant previous studies to establish these guidelines, so the assumption was made there should be a consistent 'difference' between each Paralympic swimming class.

SUMMARY

This study found that the current classification system delineates performances between some classes, but fails to do so for others. This inconsistency can largely be attributed to a lack of understanding of the impact that different impairment types and severities have on swimming performance. The subjective measurement of impairment is also a key concern that likely limits the validity of impairment measures as they relate to swimming performance, as well as causing inconsistencies in athletes' classification owing to a high dependency on user judgment. Impairment tests should be instrumented allowing for objective measurement, impairment specific, account for the greatest variance in sporting performance, and be as resistant to training as possible. Future research that identifies valid and reliable impairment measures as well as defining their impact on swimming performance will have significant implications for the development of a new evidence-based classification system that allows for fairer and more equitable competition than the current classification system. This information forms the blueprint for the new IPC swimming classification system.

REFERENCES

1. Tweedy SM, Vanlandewijck Y. International Paralympic Committee position stand - background and scientific rationale for classification in paralympic sport. Br J Sports Med 2009. https://doi.org/10.1136/bjsm.2009.065060.
2. Wu S, Williams T. Paralympic swimming performance, impairment, and the functional classification system. Adapted Physical Activity 1999;16(3):251–70.
3. Daly DJ, Vanlandewijck Y. Some criteria for evaluating the "fairness" of swimming classification. Adapt Phys Activ Q 1999;16(3):271–89.
4. Edmonds R, Leicht A, McKean M, et al. Daily heart rate variability of paralympic gold medallist swimmers: a 17-week investigation. J Sport Health Sci 2015;4(4): 371–6.
5. Burkett B. Contribution of sports science to performance: swimming. In: Vanlandewijck Y, Thompson W, editors. Handbook of Sports Medicine and

Science: Training and Coaching the Paralympic Athlete. International Olympic Committee Medical Commission Publication. Chapter 10. United Kingdom: Wiley-Blackwell Publication; 2016.

6. Burkett B, Malone L, Daly D. 100m race strategy comparison between Olympic and visually impaired paralympic swimmers. J Sci Med Sport 2003;(Suppl 6,4): 80.

7. Oh YT, Burkett B, Osborough C, et al. London 2012 paralympic swimming: passive drag and the classification system. Br J Sports Med 2013;47(13):838–43.

8. Fulton SK, Pyne D, Hopkins W, et al. Variability and progression in competitive performance of paralympic swimmers. J Sports Sci 2009;27(5):535–9.

9. Evershed JA, Mellifont R, Burkett B. Sports technology provides an objective assessment of the paralympic swimming classification system. Sports Tech 2012;5(1–2):49–55.

10. Lee CJ, Sanders RH, Payton CJ. Changes in force production and stroke parameters of trained able-bodied and unilateral arm-amputee female swimmers during a 30 s tethered front-crawl swim. J Sports Sci 2014;32(18):1704–11.

11. Beckman EM, Connick MJ, Tweedy SM. How much does lower body strength impact paralympic running performance? Eur J Sport Sci 2016;16(6):669–76.

Engineering and Technology in Wheelchair Sport

Rory A. Cooper, PhD[a],*, Yetsa A. Tuakli-Wosornu, MD, MPH[b],
Geoffrey V. Henderson, MD[c], Eleanor Quinby, BS[c], Brad E. Dicianno, MD[a],
Kalai Tsang, MS[a], Dan Ding, PhD[a], Rosemarie Cooper, MPT[a],
Theresa M. Crytzer, DPT, ATP[a], Alicia M. Koontz, PhD, RET[a], Ian Rice, PhD[d],
Adam W. Bleakney, BS[e]

KEYWORDS

- Wheelchair sport • Upper limb health • Technology and engineering

KEY POINTS

- As technology and engineering continue to evolve, athletes and their coaches will be confronted with selecting sports equipment that maximizes performance and safety.
- Wheelchair athletes must be cognizant of their upper limb health because injury can profoundly affect daily function and, ultimately, quality of life.
- Ideally, wheelchair systems designed to promote efficient transfer of energy to the handrims should be evaluated for their simultaneous effects on the upper limbs.
- There is enormous opportunity for the development of technologies capable of projecting injury and performance metrics to athletes and coaches.

INTRODUCTION

Goals of the Paralympics include social equality and promoting inclusion and the attainment of full potential using sport as a vehicle.[1] Wheelchair racing has been a component of Paralympic sport since the original idea was conceived. Furthermore, wheelchair racing has changed the face of adaptive sport. From the early days of racing on cinder tracks or in parking lots, to Bobby Hall completing the first Marathon, to

The authors have nothing to disclose.
[a] Human Engineering Research Laboratories, VA Pittsburgh Healthcare System, 6425 Penn Avenue, Suite 400, Pittsburgh, PA 15206, USA; [b] Yale University Orthopaedics & Rehabilitation, Yale Physicians Building, 800 Howard Avenue, New Haven, CT 06510, USA; [c] Department of Physical Medicine & Rehabilitation, University of Pittsburgh, Kaufmann Medical Building, Suite 201, 3471 Fifth Avenue, Pittsburgh, PA 15213, USA; [d] Department of Kinesiology & Community Health, University of Illinois at Urbana-Champaign, Urbana-Champaign, Illinois, Louise Freer Hall, 906 S. Goodwin Avenue, Urbana, IL 61801, USA; [e] Disability Resources & Educational Services, University of Illinois at Urbana-Champaign, Urbana-Champaign, Illinois, 1207 S. Oak Street, Champaign, IL 61820, USA
* Corresponding author.
E-mail address: rcooper@pitt.edu

wheelchair racers competing on the world stage, wheelchair racers have been demonstrating the abilities of people with disabilities in a very clear and public manner.[2,3]

As the United Nations' 2006 Convention on the Rights of Persons with Disabilities described, social and community inclusion for persons with disabilities in well-resourced and resource-scarce settings depends on access to mobility aids and assistive technologies.[4] Moreover, the rights to which all persons are entitled include full participation in economic, educational, and social dimensions of society. However, to fully exercise those rights, one needs to be mobile.[5,6] Compared with their able-bodied counterparts, those with moderate to severe disabilities in low-resource settings experience lower rates of educational attainment, higher rates of poverty, and higher rates of noncommunicable diseases, which is due, in part, to immobility.[6–8] More than 29 million people in low-income and middle-income countries need prosthetic and orthotic equipment and services, and between 20 and 100 million require wheelchairs.[7]

Wheelchair users face unique barriers to increasing and maintaining their fitness.[8,9] However, video games, Web sites, and smartphone applications (apps) can make fitness more accessible and motivating. This article provides a brief review of resources that can help a wheelchair user increase physiologic response to exercise, develop ideas for adaptive workout routines, locate facilities and outdoor areas that are physically accessible for exercise, and develop wheelchair sports-specific skills.

FUNDAMENTAL PRINCIPLES OF SPORTS WHEELCHAIR DESIGN

Current ultralight manual wheelchairs have their origin in the design of sports wheelchairs.[10] There are some basic principles that hold true for most sports wheelchair design.[11,12]

Weight

In most wheelchairs sports, especially those in which speed or agility are required, the lowest possible weight is often a design goal. Lower weight tends to reduce the force required to propel and maneuver the wheelchair, making it faster and more agile.

Stiffness and Strength

Ideally, sports wheelchairs would be very light, extremely strong, and highly stiff. This allows the energy transferred from the user to the chair to be applied to the desired motion without dissipation. However, design trade-offs need to be made to optimize stiffness, strength, and weight.

Resistance

In wheelchair sports in which mobility is critical, the goal of designing the wheelchair is to minimize resistance. The most common type of resistance that designers of sports wheelchairs attempt to control are: rolling resistance, wind resistance, and internal resistance. Rolling resistance is commonly minimized by choice of wheels, tires, and bearings, and by careful alignment of the wheels. Internal resistance is commonly referred to as flex or movement resulting from the person moving within the seat, the seat moving with respect to the frame, and bending and warping of the frame that causes wheel misalignment or user energy to be dissipated by the frame.

Ergonomics

The biomechanical and ergonomic goal of sports wheelchair design is for the device to become one with the user at a subconscious level. Simultaneously, the fitting and positioning of the user should maximize the control and motion of the wheelchair in response to volitional movement of the user, with minimal physiologic effort. The user interface and interaction is often the most complex design challenge.

These 4 factors must be weighed against the abilities (physical, physiologic, skill) of the users, the safety of the user and other participants, and the goals of the sport. The materials, manufacturing, and fitting techniques are determined by these factors, as well as the sport-specific needs, and the abilities of the user or users. Typically, manufacturers and builders tend to use a standardized set of features to manage costs, and then have some customizable aspects to fit individual users. A key to sports wheelchair design is to have the seat fit as carefully as a shoe or prosthetic socket, and to fit the geometry of the chair as carefully as a professional cyclist.

ADVANCED DESIGN AND FABRICATION TOOLS

Engineering tools have had an important impact on sports wheelchairs. Materials, manufacturing techniques, measurement tools, and design software have all been used to improve performance of sports wheelchairs. Computer-aided design (CAD) software permits engineers to create virtual models of sports wheelchairs that are accurate simulations of various designs.[13,14] CAD permits testing of various design concepts without the time and cost associated with building prototypes. Software tools can be used to test the strength, stiffness, weight, and resistance of the designs. The ergonomics, such as body position, are difficult to accurately simulate, especially propulsion. CAD software can interface with computer-aided manufacturing (CAM) software to help fabricate designs chosen for prototyping or actual production. CAM software includes tolerances, materials, and parameters to program the specific machines used to manufacture components. Sports wheelchairs are typically made in small numbers, and hence use a combination of computer numerically controlled (CNC) machines and hand fabrication. Typically, complex and precision parts are made with CNC machines, whereas components that need a high degree of personalization are hand-crafted.

Additive manufacturing (AM), also known as 3-dimensional (3D) printing, is making its way in to wheelchair sports.[15] Typically, 3D printers use plastics to make complex shapes drawn with CAD and CAM software. AM is a term to describe a set of technologies that create 3D objects by adding layer on layer of material. Materials can vary but there are some common features for AM, such as use of computers together with special 3D modeling software. AM devices read data from a CAD file and build a structure layer by layer from printing material, which can be plastic, liquid, powder filaments, or even sheets of paper. The term AM includes such technologies as rapid prototyping, direct digital manufacturing, layered manufacturing, and 3D printing. There are several AM technologies to build 3D structures and objects.

A stereolithography apparatus (SLA) converts liquid plastic into solid 3D objects. Typically, this is done by using a laser or focused light to cure a photosensitive liquid plastic. Digital light processing (DLP) is like stereolithography. DLP technology uses digital micromirrors laid out on a semiconductor chip. Both DLP and SLA work with photopolymers. SLA and DLP differ in the source of the light used in the curing processes. Fused deposition modeling (FDM) technology and fused filament fabrication functional prototypes can be printed, as well as final end-use products. FDM can use high-performance engineering-grade thermoplastic materials, allowing flexibility and utility in design. FDM technology build objects layer by layer from the bottom up by heating and extruding a thermoplastic filament. Selective laser sintering (SLS) is a technique that uses laser as power source to form solid 3D objects. The main difference between SLS and SLA is that it uses powdered material in the vat instead of liquid resin as stereolithography does. The SLS laser is powerful enough to fuse the powder; to reduce laser power the powder is often heated in an oxygen-free furnace. SLS does not use support structures because the object being printed is constantly surrounded by unsintered powder. Selective laser melting (SLM) is a technique that forms 3D objects by means of a high-power laser beam that fuses and melts metallic powders together. SLM process fully melts the metal material into solid 3D parts, unlike SLS metal parts. SLM uses a high-power laser beam as its power source, whereas Electron Beam Melting uses an electron beam, which is the main difference between these 2 methods. Laminated object manufacturing uses layers of adhesive-coated paper, plastic, or metal laminates, which are fused together using heat and pressure and then cut to shape with a computer-controlled laser or knife.

Plastic parts such as rigid gloves for wheelchair racing and mounting brackets are more commonly being 3D printed.[16] Currently, FDM and SLS are the most common AM approaches used in sports wheelchairs.

BREAKTHROUGH SPORT WHEELCHAIRS

Success in wheelchair sports is said to depend on 3 factors: the athlete, the wheelchair, and the interaction between the athlete and the wheelchair.[8] Proper use of engineering and technology has the potential to affect all 3 factors significantly. Coupled with scientifically based training systems, athletes with disabilities use technology to maximize performance and competitive success the same as any professional athlete. The following section provides examples of recent breakthrough technologies that have been adopted by athletes participating in the sport of wheelchair racing.

Successful wheelchair racing depends on an athletes' ability to generate and sustain speed through highly developed propulsion technique. Consequently, material properties and user interface characteristics dramatically influence an athlete's ability to propel effectively and maintain speed. For example, racers seek to optimize the fit, weight, stability, aerodynamics, rigidity, and rolling resistance of their equipment, in addition to maintaining superior physical conditioning. A racer's sensitivity to the fit and feel of a racing wheelchair cannot be overstated because extraneous grams or even millimeters can affect numerous performance and injury-related factors.

Consequently, manufactures continually adopt the latest technologies and engineering techniques to maximize each athlete's potential. Companies such as BMW, Honda, Nissin, and OX Engineering use exotic materials for frame construction and sophisticated techniques to ensure an optimized fit between athlete and racing wheelchair. Construction procedures involve 3D scanning of athletes' bodies, CAD, and other advanced simulation processes. For example, Honda-Yachiyo is developing a fully carbon fiber racing frame (cage) using a process that incorporates an athletes' anthropometrics and current wheelchair racing body positioning into its construction (**Fig. 1**). The athlete's previous racing chair can be superimposed over the new carbon fiber frame to ensure an equivalent fit or to help inform modifications.[17] The process can be observed here: https://www.youtube.com/watch?v=gq9JnkKWTfE&feature=youtu.be.

Nissin Medical Industries, Honda-Yachiyo, and OX Engineering (Carbon GPX)[18] build hybrid racing wheelchairs that use combinations of carbon fiber and aluminum components to achieve many of the goals. Athletes have the option of selecting a fork made of either carbon fiber or aluminum (**Fig. 2**).

Similarly, BMW of North America has designed customized racing wheelchairs for Team USA wheelchair racers competing at the 2016 Paralympic Games in Rio de Janeiro, Brazil.[19] The chairs were built by the same group that made carbon fiber bobsleds for the 2014 Winter Olympics in Sochi, Russia. The engineers have taken advantage of numerous modern technologies to optimize the fit and design of their racing

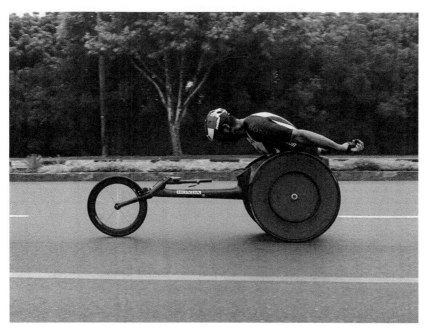

Fig. 1. Honda full carbon fiber racing wheelchair. (*Courtesy of* Ernst van Dyk, Enabled Sport, Cape Town, South Africa.)

chair, including 3D scanning of athletes' bodies. The BMW racer features modernized aerodynamic efficiencies, carbon fiber material, a complete chassis redesign, and a personalized approach for customized athlete fit (**Fig. 3**). The chair also uses a modular design with expanding foam to customize the seating interface (a process similar what is

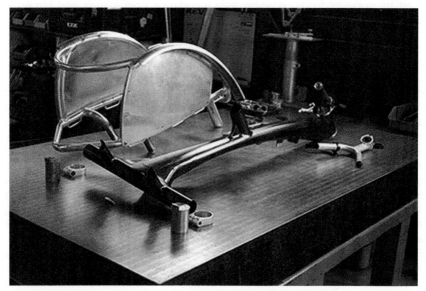

Fig. 2. OX HYBRID. (*Courtesy of* OX Engineering Group, Chiba, Japan.)

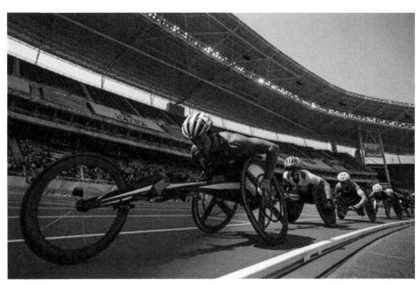

Fig. 3. BMW racing wheelchair, full carbon fiber frame. (*Courtesy of* Olympic Information Services, International Olympic Committee, Lausanne, Switzerland.)

used to interface race car drivers in their seat). Another unique element is evident in the redesigned fork and steering system that creates a seamless marriage to the main frame, increasing lateral stability and stiffness.

TECHNOLOGICAL INEQUITIES

There are substantial disparities in access to sports wheelchairs. Inequities exist in all countries but for different reasons. Cost is in many regards a common barrier in obtaining sports wheelchairs. In most countries, sports wheelchairs need to be purchased by personal funds, possibly with assistance from friends and family, and through charitable organizations. There are a few exceptions, such as the US Department of Veterans Affairs, that recognize the importance of sports and exercise in health promotion and maintenance. Hence, individuals with greater means have access to more expensive and often higher quality sports wheelchairs. This results in people training and competing with widely different wheelchairs, especially at the local and regional levels. Some people may participate in the same chair that they use for daily mobility, whereas others may have a custom-fitted sports wheelchair specifically designed for rugby, basketball, racing, or a host of other sports. Technological inequities exist in low-income countries where adaptive sports programs are limited and where manufacturers, even small manufacturers, tend not to market their products. This results in potentially talented athletes being unaware of the opportunities that may exist to help them reach their full potential. This is a missed opportunity because many people with disabilities who use wheelchairs do not attain the full health benefits of sports and exercise. Moreover, some individuals and even national sporting organizations may choose to forego participation in wheelchair sports that necessitate the use of highly customized or high-cost sports wheelchairs.

Even at the highest levels of competition, inequities exist. There are 2 primary causes: (1) athletes from some countries are not aware of or do not have access to the latest technologies and (2) corporations sponsor athletes and provide technology to a few select athletes that are unavailable to other athletes. For example, in the 2016

Paralympic Games, there were athletes competing in wheelchair racing with off-the-shelf models of racing wheelchairs that were purchased from another athlete or from a manufacturer supplier, others had custom-fitted racing wheelchairs made from readily available materials (eg, aluminum, titanium, and nylon), and a small number had highly engineered and optimized wheelchairs created by well-resourced large companies (eg, the BMW carbon racing wheelchair). This can be considered technology-doping (or techno-doping). Of course, technological progress need to be encouraged to advance sport and community integration of people with disabilities. This needs to be done within the rules of the sport and the spirit of competition.

Inequities in wheelchair sports are not new, nor are challenges to technology-based rules. Up until the 1980s, athletes competed in wheelchairs that are much like the heavy steel depot wheelchairs used for transport in hospitals.[20] Early pioneers made changes such as cutting the backrest tubes to lower their height to allow more freedom of movement for the arms, lowering the seat height and creating a higher seat angle by altering the seat upholstery, and by using smaller pushrims. In the 1980s, basketball wheelchairs began to be custom made to have rigid frames, be lighter, and have adjustable axles to be more maneuverable. Racing wheelchairs went through rapid transformations. Some of the most significant were compensators (for turning on the track and allowing the chair to track straight on cross-slopes), high-pressure tubular tires (especially for the front wheels), fenders and side guards, and wheel-mounted pushrims. The 1990s introduced even further differentiation and innovation occurred. This yielded specialized chairs for tennis and rugby, as well as further advances in basketball and racing chairs. Interestingly, there was a convergence in the ergonomics of wheelchair design in many of the sports that moved the propulsion wheel axles as close as possible to the center of gravity of the user. This tends to have multiple advantages. It generally increases propulsion efficiency by increasing access to the pushrims, improving turning, and balancing mass over the largest wheels to minimize rolling resistance. This resulted in the kneeling position in wheelchair racing, and the introduction of 6-wheel chairs for tennis, basketball, and rugby.

The inequities created by differences in wealth, access to knowledge, availability of facilities, and the influence of sponsorship tilt the playing field in wheelchair sport.[21] This creates an opportunity for investigation into whether the differences are great enough to warrant attention and, if they are, what are possible means to mitigate factors that create an imbalance. Some potential approaches include implementing stricter standards for sports wheelchairs to minimize differences, designing high-performance sports wheelchairs at low cost, creating financing models that make sports wheelchairs more accessible, and restricting competitions to sports wheelchairs that are commercially available and that have achieved a specific number of sales (eg, restricting use of high-cost 1-off devices). These and other questions need to be explored to increase participation in wheelchair sports, and to increase the equity of competition at international events.

APPROPRIATE WHEELCHAIR DESIGN AND USE IN RESOURCE-SCARCE ENVIRONMENTS

As outlined by the International Society for Prosthetics and Orthotics, wheelchairs are deemed appropriate for their user when they are "safe, durable and maintainable," meet the functional and health needs of their users under local environmental conditions, provide "proper fit and postural support based on sound biomechanical principles and can be accessed and sustained in the country at the most economical and affordable price."[22–25] Unfortunately, appropriate wheelchairs and personal mobility equipment can be difficult for daily wheelchair users in developing countries to obtain.

Although standard handrim propelled manual wheelchairs are often donated through governmental or nongovernmental organizations,[26–29] rough natural terrain (especially in rural areas); inconsistently available or prohibitively expensive maintenance materials and processes; hot, humid and rainy climates; and poorly maintained roads can make commercial chairs impractical, inefficient, and inoperable in low-resource countries.[26,30–33] Standard chairs may often go unused or are sold.[32] On the other hand, wheelchairs can also be used in unexpected ways in developing settings, such as shower chairs or to transport people and/or goods, necessitating culturally sensitive, context-appropriate design.[34]

Social Enterprise and Policy

Key governmental and nongovernmental stakeholder organizations, including Motivation, Whirlwind Wheelchair International, Center for International Rehabilitation, Handicap International, Artificial Limbs Manufacturing Corporation of India, and the Tanzania Training Center for Orthopedic Technologists, are dedicated to ensuring the provision of appropriate wheelchairs suitable for resource-limited environments. In addition, the International Society for Prosthetics and Orthotics, World Health Organization, and Landmine Survivors Network have disseminated consensus statements outlining conclusions and recommendations for the design, manufacture, and use of appropriate wheelchairs in developing countries. National health care structure, education and training, project monitoring, cost calculations, and user group domains are included in service provision recommendations. Appropriateness, quality assurance, and sustainability domains are included in technology recommendations.[22]

Design Features of Wheelchairs in Resource-Scarce Environments

In the 1960s in Uganda, Professor (Dr) Ronald Lawrie Huckstep[35] designed the first purpose-built wheelchair for a developing setting. Since then, the cardinal features of his 3-wheel design: simplicity, cost-efficiency, durability, and the potential for sustainable local manufacture and repair through basic training, have remained requisite features of a successful chair for use in low-income settings.[23,27–29,31,36–38] From rural Southeast Asia to urban sub-Saharan Africa, effective designs use sturdy but lightweight and locally available material such as wood or thin-wall steel tubing. The incorporation of prefabricated and multipurpose equipment such as universal welding equipment and bicycle wheels is common.[36–39] Bicycle inner tubes and plastic balls have been used to create pressure-relieving seat cushions functionally comparable to standard foam cushions.[40] A rapid and simple fabrication protocol is important because it creates the opportunity to train local laborers as part of a sustainability strategy.[36–41] A study in Tanzania found that a 3-wheel design with a detachable rear wheel increased maneuverability on local terrain and folding features increased portability.[26] A prototype evaluation study in Indonesia found that a longer wheelbase and alternating seat functionality worked well for ascending inclines, sitting more ergonomically at a table, and transferring.[42] In rural India, a near floor-level chair has been trialed to facilitate domestic activities traditionally performed on the floor.[43]

A qualitative assessment in Tanzania identified 5 themes that resonate throughout many resource-limited countries: tricycles and 3-wheel models tend to be more popular than 4-wheel models; most citizens with impairment rely on charitable donations to purchase and, at times, operate a mobility aid; repurposing prefabricated components and outsourcing tasks can reduce production costs; bicycle components are available in rural areas; and donated, depot-style wheelchairs are often irresponsibly distributed and poorly designed for their operating environment.[39] In diverse urban and rural low-income setting, wheelchair users of both genders consistently report improved quality of life and satisfaction with environmentally appropriate and locally manufactured wheelchairs.[44–47] However, improved quality of life, physical and psychological health, and function have also been demonstrated among 519 adults in India, Chile, and Viet Nam who used a standard, low-cost, semirigid depot style wheelchair.[44]

Sports wheelchairs have been designed for use in low-income countries as well.[21,48] Design requirements have included low-cost but high-quality prefabricated components in addition to removable anti-tippers, adjustable tension backrest, 24″ wheels, adjustable seat dump, variable camber, 4″ casters, fore-aft axle position, removable bumpers, height adjustable footrest, four wheels, single anti-tipper (pivot), cost less than $125 without wheels, 16″ seat width and backrest height, and nylon upholstery.[21]

ELECTRONIC TOOLS AND TECHNOLOGIES FOR SPORT AND PHYSICAL ACTIVITY
Wearable Technologies

Wheelchair sport performance depends on the interaction between the athlete and the wheelchair.[8] To understand the many factors involved in wheelchair sport performance, coaches and trainers have been trying to gain insights into athlete's skills and the wheelchair configuration that influence the athlete–wheelchair interaction and the overall sport performance.[9] With the advancement in microsensors, the use of wearable technology to objectively assess athlete's energy cost, skills, and performance in real-time in different wheelchair sports has become popular. Three types of wearable monitors are designed and/or validated for assessing physical activity and sports performance in wheelchair athletes: commercial monitors, commercial monitors with custom algorithms, and custom monitors.

Data from commercial monitors, such as spatial and physiologic changes of an athlete during sport, are typically processed by the manufacturer's algorithms to provide athletes and coaches meaningful information such as energy expended, number of propulsions, and distance traveled. Currently, there is 1 commercial wearable monitor in the market designed for wheelchair users: the Apple Watch (Apple, Inc, Cupertino, CA, USA); however, its accuracy has not been validated since its release in autumn 2016. Other commercial wearable devices are not designed but are validated for wheelchair athletes. The activPAL trio (PAL Technologies Ltd, Glasgow, Scotland, UK), for example, was evaluated for tracking wheel revolutions and angle of rotations, and the results showed that the absolute error for the number of wheel revolutions was 0.59% with an ICC (Inter-Class Correlation) of 1.00, and the Bland-Altman 95% limits of agreement ranged from −0.029 to 0.032 revolution when compared with the actual measurements.[49] Although some commercial monitors show good validity when compared with the criterion measures, they lack the ability to accurately estimate energy cost during sports.

The energy cost is a crucial indicator of an athlete's muscular strength and physical fitness.[50,51] Because there is a lack of commercial wearable monitors for estimating energy cost in wheelchair users, some researchers have adapted the commercial monitors designed for the ambulatory population, such as Sensewear (Bodymedia, Pittsburgh, PA, USA) and ActiGraph GT3X+ devices (ActiGraph, LLC, Pensacola, Florida, USA), for wheelchair athletes. Various algorithms have been developed to substitute the manufacturers' algorithms of the commercial monitors to better assess energy expenditure (EE). A systematic review showed that commercial monitors with custom algorithms have relative and absolute errors of EE estimation ranging from −41.0% to 50.2% and from 1.65% to 81.6%, respectively, when compared with the portable metabolic cart or the doubly labeled water.[52] Although commercial monitors with custom algorithms can estimate EE in wheelchair athletes, they do not assess the propulsion efficiency or the number of pushes that are vital for skills training and injury prevention.

Pushing economy or efficiency is essential in wheelchair sports. The ability of athletes to accelerate quickly from standstill, maintain sprinting speed, and prevent injury is critical to success.[8] Thus, researchers have designed and validated custom wearable monitors for wheelchair athletes to track speed, propulsion frequency, and number of propulsions. For speed, the custom wearable device made by Hiremath and colleagues[53] (2013) and Moss and colleagues[54] (2003) showed that the relative and absolute estimation errors ranged from −2.2% to 0.8% and from 0.03% to 2.2%,[53] respectively. For propulsion frequency, the monitor created by Washburn and Copay[55] (1999) showed that the Pearson correlation ranged from 0.26 to 0.35 between the estimated and the measured propulsion frequency, and the monitor developed by Ojeda and Ding[56] (2014) showed the absolute error ranged from 12.9% to 24.2%, with ICC ranged from 0.690 to 0.916. For the number of propulsions, the monitor made by Ojeda and Ding[56] (2014) showed the absolute errors ranged from 8.0% to 13.4% and the ICC ranged from 0.984 to 0.994. This information helps to optimize push strategies while maneuvering the wheelchair during game play and prevents shoulder-related injury.[8]

In addition to wheelchair athletes' skills, wheelchair configuration affects athletes' posture, stability, pressure distribution, and propulsion, which in turn affects the overall performance.[54] Wearable technology can be used to customize the wheelchair configuration based on individual athlete's performance in different wheelchair setups. Although wearable technology has been used in quantifying wheelchair athletes' skills and performance, its use in tracking the physical forms and the quality of movements in wheelchair athletes are still under investigation. Further research in movement quality is desired to facilitate future research and development in wheelchair design and configuration, exercise training protocols, and injury prevention.

Computer-Assisted Rehabilitation Environment

The Computer-Assisted Rehabilitation Environment (**Fig. 4**) is a virtual reality system made up of a motion platform with 6° of freedom, a dual belt force instrumented treadmill, a motion capture system, a 180° projection screen, and 5-speaker surround system, all of which are integrated through D-Flow software (Motekforce Link, Amsterdam, The Netherlands). The system at the Human Engineering Research Laboratories is specifically adapted to accommodate the needs of wheelchair users, with a wide belt treadmill (2 m long, 1.2 m wide, with 2 0.5 m wide belts) and 8 tie-down points for attaching wheelchairs with different configurations. The motion platform can be programmed to reproduce slopes (up to 20°), cross-slopes, and roughness to recreate real-world environments.

The system can accommodate both manual and electric power wheelchairs. Wheelchairs are mounted the platform using a 4-point tie down system. The ropes are given enough play so that a wheelchair user has enough room to move in the platform in the forward and backward direction. In addition, the subject is also attached to the fall safety harness, which is then attached to the safety harness attachment post on the motion platform. There are 2 different safety harnesses that have been tested for 2 differing weight capacities that can accommodate subjects weighing up to 300 lb.

The instrumented treadmill can be set up to run in a preselected speed by the operator or can be set to operate at the user's self-selected speed, using the self-paced algorithm available with the system. The self-paced functionality of the treadmill automatically adjusts the speed of the treadmill to match the movement of reflective markers placed on the wheelchair. The treadmill speeds up or slows down as needed to keep the position of the markers close to the zero position. This ability of the software to adjust based on user's propulsion allows for realistic propulsion pattern in a safe environment. The software platform (D-Flow) allows for the person to be an integral part of a real-time

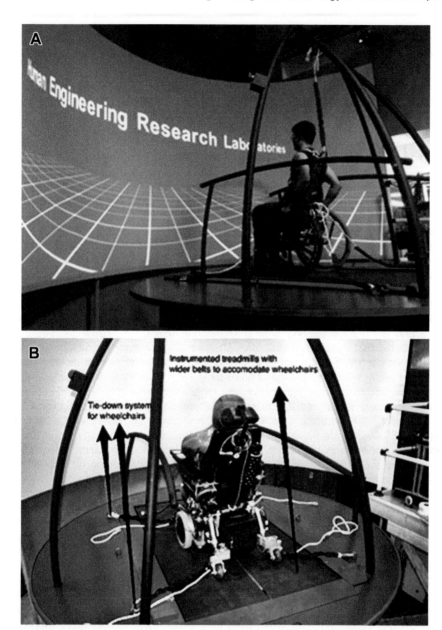

Fig. 4. The specific adaptations of the system at Human Engineering Research Laboratories. (*A*) Wheelchair user on CAREN System. (*B*) Placement of wheelchair on CAREN System. (*Courtesy of* Human Engineering Research Laboratories, Pittsburgh, PA.)

feedback loop in which multisensory input devices measure the behavior of the subject (eg, their motions, forces) and output devices (eg, virtual reality environment, platform motions, speakers), and return motorsensory, visual, and auditory feedback to the user. Performance measurements include upper body ranges of motions, joint forces and moments, muscle activity, and metabolic demands. As such, the system is being used to evaluate new wheelchair designs and concepts, to characterize differences in propulsion abilities between user populations (paraplegia and tetraplegia), and to assess the impact of wheelchair setup on slopes and cross-slopes.

Resistance Training and Vibration Exercise

Strong upper limb musculature is essential to achieving independence in activities of daily living such as wheelchair propulsion, wheelchair transfer activities, and weight-relieving maneuvers.[57] These activities place high demands on the upper extremities[58–60] and practicing them over time negatively affects upper extremity health.[61] The shoulders, elbows, and wrists are all highly susceptible to degeneration, overuse injuries, and pain.[62] The shoulder is the most common site of upper extremity pain in manual wheelchair users, with reported pain ranging from 32% to 78%.[58] A range of pathologic conditions at the shoulder have also been documented, including impingement syndrome, adhesive capsulitis, recurrent dislocations, rotator cuff tears, and tendinitis.[63] Shoulder pain has been most closely associated with transfers, weight-relieving activities, and ramp propulsion,[64] indicating that these activities may be the most demanding ones performed. Increasing the strength-generating capacity of the upper extremity muscles can improve one's ability to meet the demands of high-intensity propulsion and transfer tasks, and potentially reduce the propensity to develop shoulder pain.

Numerous studies have examined the effects of varying forms of structured resistance and endurance training among wheelchair users.[65–67] These studies have demonstrated that engaging in structured fitness training, including resistance training 2 to 3 times per week of the upper limbs leads to improvements in muscle strength, increased performance during activities of daily living, and improved quality of life.[67] Although a combination of endurance and resistance training is recommended for overall increased fitness, resistance training targets and leads to greater gains in upper extremity work capacity, muscle strength, and power compared with endurance training.[68,69] Resistance training is also recommended for combating muscle imbalances associated with overuse[57,70] and for treating shoulder pain.[71–73] A study showed that wheelchair users who concentrated on strengthening the muscles of the posterior shoulder and upper back while stretching the muscles of the anterior shoulder and chest reported greater pain relief and an easier time performing propulsion and weight-relief activities when compared with an attention control group who received video instruction on pain relief.[72] The amount of strength gain achieved through resistance training reportedly varies from study to study (10%–60%) with larger gains found in studies that involve weight lifting universal systems or equipment and frequent, progressive increases in training loads.[74]

Vibration exercise has gained recent popularity and adoption among recreational to elite athletes. This is because vibration training has been shown in numerous studies to increase muscle strength, power, and performance when integrated into a resistance training program[75,76] or when used as a supplement to alternative modes of training.[77] Vibration exercise is mostly practiced in the form of whole body vibration (WBV), in which one stands or sits on an oscillating platform.[75] Vibrating dumbbells have also been developed more recently for upper-body exercise (**Fig. 5**). Despite the controversy surrounding possible training effects with vibration, multiple studies have shown that both WBV and vibrating dumbbell use elicits greater muscle activation not only in the muscles targeted but also in the surrounding and supporting muscle groups (eg, antagonists).[78,79] Using vibration above a certain threshold frequency (12 Hz for plates, and 16 Hz for dumbbells) elicits a stretch reflex (contraction) in the muscle.[75] The number of contractions is equivalent to the vibration frequency (eg, 20 Hz = 20 contractions per second). When frequencies exceed 20 Hz for plates

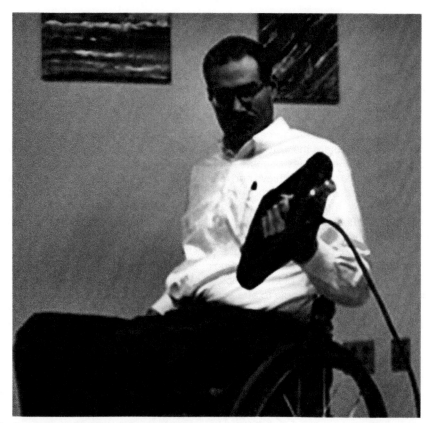

Fig. 5. Vibrating dumbbell for exercise.

(28 Hz for dumbbells), the muscle fibers activated do not have enough time to complete a full contraction and relaxation cycle[77] and are, therefore, in constant cocontraction, which results in increased muscle force and power postvibration.[79,80] Moreover, muscle electromyographic patterns observed with upper limb vibration at high frequencies (44 Hz) have indicated a more efficient and effective recruitment of high threshold motor units during fatiguing contractions.[81] The effects of vibration on the body have been extensively studied and guidelines have been developed to regulate exposure to such stimuli.[82] The frequency, amplitudes, and exposures used in previous vibration studies and the proposed study are considered acceptable and safe.[75,83] Combined results from all of these studies suggest that vibration may be an effective and safe tool for enhancing resistance training among wheelchair users.

The SmartWheel

Wheelchair racing propulsion involves highly specialized techniques that can take years for an athlete to develop. Because racers must contact the pushrim precisely at high speeds, it is easy for stroke timing and coordination errors to occur. For example, the total force a racer produces is the vector sum of the 3D component forces. These component forces can be either productive (accelerating the wheel forward) or wasteful (braking or slowing the wheel). The Racing SmartWheel (Human Engineering Research Laboratories, Pittsburgh, PA, USA) measures these forces directly and lets the athlete know where energy is being wasted during contact with the handrim. The use of repetitive wasteful forces can limit speed and performance, and may contribute to the development of upper limb repetitive strain injuries (eg, rotator cuff strain). To reduce the risk of injury, the pressure through the muscles and joints of the upper limb and the number of times the arm propels the wheelchair forward (cadence) must be kept to a minimum, which can be done by optimizing the balance of forces applied to the handrim. Racers can optimize their stroke by learning to use a higher proportion of productive forces relative to total force (cutting out wasteful forces). Decreasing wasteful forces can be accomplished by maximizing torque (the power it takes to rotate the wheel), which should be a large proportion of the total force. Additionally, if athletes become more productive on the handrim they may be able to use fewer strokes to achieve and maintain a desired speed. The Racing Smart-Wheel can help racers measure the influence of different glove styles or sitting postures. Ultimately, the information gathered from a Racing SmartWheel will help racers and their coaches devise training strategies to optimize the racing stroke, while tracking the user's progress over time.

The SmartWheel is a force and torque sensing wheel that was developed by Dr Rory Cooper, and others at the Human Engineering Research Laboratories[84] to allow for quantifying propulsion biomechanics in real-time. The unique qualities of the SmartWheel include being able to attach it to any quick-release hub without altering any aspect of the user's wheelchair or setup, such as the camber or seat angles (**Fig. 6**). Earlier studies with the SmartWheel enabled discovery of associations

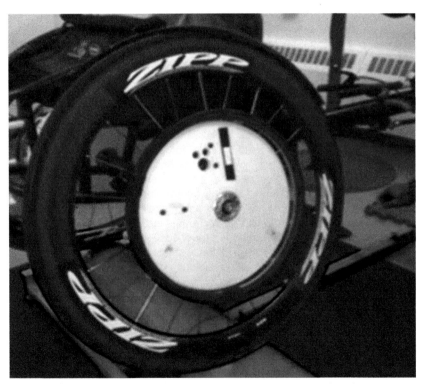

Fig. 6. The SmartWheel. (*Courtesy of* Human Engineering Research Laboratories, Pittsburgh, PA.)

between propulsion technique and the development of repetitive strain injuries at the wrist and shoulder, and understanding of how wheelchair type and setup influences technique.[57] The SmartWheel provides output similar to force plates or platforms, such as the component forces and moments measured around the hub, in addition to velocity (number of meters traveled per second) and cadence (number of strokes per unit time). The SmartWheel was originally developed for researchers and morphed into clinical application as the evidence surfaced about best propulsion techniques. The ability to measure technique with the SmartWheel in a clinic gave therapists a tool that they could use to assess their patients' technique and retrain or measure the impact of using different types of wheelchairs, seating systems, or configurations. With a company to support its development into a practical clinical tool, the SmartWheel has found wide-spread use in more than 100 clinics world-wide.

The Racing SmartWheel (**Fig. 7**) is like the SmartWheel except is built from a 28-inch diameter racing wheel that can detect and withstand the large forces that racing athletes apply to the handrim. Both wheels have sensors on the beams that measure the forces exerted on the handrim and sensors that measure the angle of the wheel. The SmartWheel and Racing SmartWheel wirelessly send the data to a computer that converts these files to Microsoft Excel, creating a report useful to rehabilitation professionals, athletes, and coaches. All athletes want to move faster, expend the least amount of energy, and avoid pain and injury. The Racing SmartWheel is a device that can help wheelchair athletes to improve their stroke mechanics to improve performance and prevent injury.

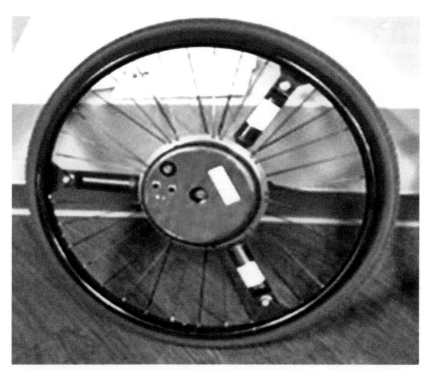

Fig. 7. The Racing SmartWheel, attached to a racing wheelchair, on a dynamometer. (*Courtesy of* Human Engineering Research Laboratories, Pittsburgh, PA.)

Video Game Motivation for Exercise

One of the key barriers people with disabilities face in maintaining and increasing their fitness is the lack of accessible exercise equipment.[85] GameWheels and GameCycle (Human Engineering Research Laboratories, Pittsburgh, PA, USA), 2 exercise systems that combine accessible equipment with video-gaming, were created to promote physical activity and enhance cardiorespiratory fitness.[86–90] GameWheels uses a portable roller system that allows users to control video-game graphics by propelling their wheelchairs.[89] GameCycle is an interface with a similar video-game design, though it is controlled using a cranking arm ergometer.[87,88] Both systems have been found to produce a physiologic response comparable to exercise, to successfully stimulate participants to workout at a high intensity, and provide a more enjoyable and motivating experience than standard exercise equipment.[86,89–91]

APPLICATIONS AND WEB SITES THAT PROVIDE WORKOUT IDEAS AND INSTRUCTION

A few smartphone apps and Web sites offer inclusive, easy-to-use exercise instructions and workout planning ideas. The National Center on Health, Physical Activity, and Disability Web site[92] offers a wealth of information on many health and exercise topics, including links to material on equipment, programs, organizations, and parks that are accessible to wheelchair users. One particularly helpful resource is their guide, *Discover Accessible Fitness: A Wheelchair User's Guide for Using Fitness Equipment*.[93] This manual provides exercise descriptions and instructions on how wheelchair users can maintain proper form by shifting their weight or using gym equipment in creative ways. This allows users to easily adapt equipment that would otherwise be difficult to use. Another Web site with beneficial information, *Physio-Therapy eXercises*,[94] allows individuals to select from more than 1000 exercises, and use these to create their own workout program. Each exercise provides the user with a visual example of how to perform it, precautions to consider, and information on the purpose of the exercise. It is also available as an app. Similarly, other apps that present accessible exercise options are *Wheelchair Exercises*,[95] *Rx for Exercise: A Physician's Toolkit*,[96] *CPF Challenge*,[97] and *SCI-Ex*.[98] SCI-Ex is particularly notable because it offers information on adapting typical fitness-center equipment for someone using a wheelchair. It also provides sample videos that demonstrate proper form and execution of the exercises.

Applications and Web Sites for Accessible Fitness Information and Resources

Several apps and Web sites can help wheelchair users locate accessible gyms, trails, and parks. For example, the National Parks system is working to make their parks more accessible, and the Web page for each park offers information on the accessible facilities, trails, and activities available.[99,100] However, users must navigate to each individual park's Web site to find this information. *All Trails*[101,102] and *TrailLink*[103,104] are Web sites that have related apps and that allow users to search for accessible trails using broader geographic filters. This enables users to see all accessible trails in a selected area. For users looking for fitness center accessibility information, the Web sites *AXS Map*,[105] *Access Earth*,[106] and *AbleRoad*[107] provide accessibility ratings for businesses in selected locations. Both *AXS Map* and *AbleRoad* also have apps that provide the same functionality.[108,109] Although these Web sites and apps provide honest, user-generated ratings, only a few businesses are rated in each city, meaning that they do not provide all-inclusive information.

Applications and Web Sites for Developing Sport-Specific Skills

Some Web sites and apps are dedicated to helping individuals learn or excel in specific sports. *Let's Roll: Learning Wheelchair Tennis with the Pros*[110] is a Web site that provides instructional videos for individuals looking to become proficient in wheelchair tennis. For users looking to discover accessible sport options, the British Paralympic Association Web site[111] offers a search-by-impairment option that displays available sports based on the user's selected disability. The site also offers information about clubs and organizations for each sport. *Gateway to Gold*[112] is an app intended to encourage Paralympic hopefuls that was launched by the US Paralympic Team in 2016.[113] It allows users to register as a possible competitor, upload videos of themselves performing qualifier skill tests, and submit these videos for review by Team USA. The app works in conjunction with their Gateway to Gold qualifying events, and is an attempt to make it easier for athletes to pursue Paralympic sports at the highest level.

SUMMARY

Mobility mitigates the health risks associated with disability-related immobility, and can transform the lives of individuals and families facing physical disability.[114] Although international mobility technology research can be challenging, continued efforts in this field are encouraged. Providing readily available information about accessible fitness options may help a population at greater risk of a sedentary lifestyle to increase and maintain their fitness goals. This information can enable wheelchair users to remain motivated, develop innovative exercise routines, find accessible facilities, and refine specific skills to compete at a professional level.

As technology and engineering continue to evolve, athletes and their coaches will be confronted with selecting sports equipment that maximizes performance and safety. Wheelchair athletes must be cognizant of their upper limb health because injury can profoundly affect daily function and, ultimately, quality of life. Ideally, wheelchair systems designed to promote efficient transfer of energy to the handrims should be evaluated for their simultaneous effects on the upper limbs. Therefore, there is enormous opportunity for the development of technologies capable of projecting injury and performance metrics to athletes and coaches. Although technology for performance improvement has evolved considerably in the past 10 years for general population athletes, handrim athletes still have little opportunity to view real-time measures beyond distance, speed, and time spent in propulsion. Like bicyclists, wheelchair racers and other handrim athletes could benefit profoundly from the inclusion of instrumentation that measures variables like power output (watts), cadence (strokes used per quantity of time), and EE. As in cycling, real-time knowledge of a cadence has many useful applications to wheelchair racers in the contexts of both training and competition. For example, athletes may vary cadence depending on training goals, form, body position, and other factors. Similarly, knowledge of the forces applied to the handrim could provide useful information related to upper limb injury, stroke technique, and fitness. Combined implementation of wearable body sensors, miniaturized data loggers, and motion-recognition technologies have great potential in the context of handrim propulsion, and may offer athletes practical solutions for monitoring performance and injury-related metrics in real-world environments.

REFERENCES

1. International Paralympic Committee. Paralympics–history of the movement. Paralympic.org. Available at: https://www.paralympic.org/the-ipc/history-of-the-movement. Accessed August 9, 2017.

2. Anderson D. The athlete in the wheelchair. The New York Times 1977;72(col. 1–2).

3. Lewis AN, Cooper RA, Seelman KD, et al. Assistive technology in rehabilitation: improving impact through policy. Rehabilitation Research, Policy, and Education 2012;26(1):19–32.

4. United Nations. Convention on the rights of persons with disabilities. New York: United Nations; 2006.

5. World Health Organization. World report on disability. Geneva (Switzerland): World Health Organization; 2011.

6. Tuakli-Wosornu YA, Haig AJ. Implementing the world report on disability in West Africa: challenges and opportunities for Ghana. Am J Phys Med Rehabil 2014; 93(1 Suppl 1):S50–7.

7. Zipfel E, Cooper RA, Pearlman J, et al. New design and development of a manual wheelchair for India. Disabil Rehabil 2007;29(11–12):949–62.

8. Goosey-Tolfrey V. Supporting the paralympic athlete: focus on wheeled sports. Disabil Rehabil 2010;32(26):2237–43.

9. Sindall P, Lenton J, Whytock K, et al. Criterion validity and accuracy of global positioning satellite and data logging devices for wheelchair tennis court movement. J Spinal Cord Med 2013;36(4):383–93.

10. Cooper RA. A perspective on the ultralight wheelchair revolution. Tech Disabil 1996;5:383–92.

11. Cooper RA, De Luigi AJ. Adaptive sports technology and biomechanics: wheelchairs. PM R 2014;6:S31–9.

12. Laferrier JZ, Rice I, Pearlman J, et al. Technology to improve sports performance in wheelchair sports. Sports Tech 2012;5(1–2):4–19.

13. Zipfel E, Olson J, Puhlman JE, et al. Design of a custom racing hand-cycle: review and analysis. Disabil Rehabil Assist Technol 2009;4(2):119–28.

14. Grindle GG, Deluigi AJ, Leferrier JZ, et al. Evaluation of highly adjustable throwing chairs for people with disabilities. Assist Technol 2012;24(4):240–5.

15. Lunsford C, Grindle G, Salatin B, et al. Innovations with 3D printing in physical medicine and rehabilitation: a review of the literature. PM R 2016;8(12):1201–12.

16. Rice I, Dysterheft J, Bleakney AW, et al. The influence of glove type on simulated wheelchair propulsion: a pilot study. Int J Sports Med 2016;37(1):30–5.

17. Yachiyo Industry Co. L. Honda yachiyo racing wheelchair. 2017. Available at: http://www.yachiyo-ind.co.jp/products/wcr/. Accessed May 11, 2017.

18. Engineering OX. 2017. Available at: http://www.oxgroup.co.jp/wc/products/gpx_cfrp/info-gpxcfrp.htm. Accessed August 9, 2017.

19. BMW Group. BMW unveils Team USA racing wheelchair for Rio 2016 paralympic games. Woodcliff Lake (NJ): BMW Group; 2016. Available at: https://www.press.bmwgroup.com/usa/article/detail/T0259516EN_US/bmw-unveils-team-usa-racing-wheelchair-for-rio-2016-paralympic-games. Accessed August 9, 2017.

20. Cooper RA. Wheelchair racing sports science: a review. J Rehabil Res Dev 1990;27(3):295–312.

21. Authier EL, Pearlman J, Allegretti A, et al. A sports wheelchair for low income counties. Disabil Rehabil Assist Technol 2007;29(11/12):963–7.

22. International Society for Prosthetics and Orthotics. ISPO consensus conference on appropriate orthopaedic technology for low-income countries: conclusions and recommendations. Prosthet Orthot Int 2001;25(3):168–70.

23. Sheldon S, Jacobs NA. ISPO consensus conference on wheelchairs for developing countries: conclusions and recommendations. Prosthet Orthot Int 2007; 31(2):217–23.

24. Eggers SL, Myaskovsky L, Burkitt KH, et al. A preliminary model of wheelchair service delivery. Arch Phys Med Rehabil 2009;90(6):1030–8.
25. Moody L, Woodcock A, Heelis M, et al. Improving wheelchair prescription: an analysis of user needs and existing tools. Work 2012;41(Suppl 1):1980–4.
26. Amosun S, Ndosi A, Buchanan H. Locally manufactured wheelchairs in Tanzania - are users satisfied? Afr Health Sci 2016;16(4):1174–81.
27. Eide AH, Øderud T. Assistive technology in low-income countries. In: Maclachlan M, Swartz L, editors. Disability & international development. New York: Springer; 2009. p. 149–60.
28. World Health Organzation, United States Agency for International Development. Joint position paper on the provision of mobility devices in less resourced settings. Geneva (Switzerland): World Health Organization; 2011.
29. World Health Organzation. Guidelines on the provision of manual wheelchairs in less resourced settings. Geneva (Switzerland): World Health Organization; 2008.
30. Rhoda A, Cunningham N, Azaria S, et al. Provision of inpatient rehabilitation and challenges experienced with participation post discharge: quantitative and qualitative inquiry of African stroke patients. BMC Health Serv Res 2015;15:423.
31. Majinge RM, Stilwell C. Library services provision for people with visual impairments and in wheelchairs in academic libraries in Tanzania. South African Journal of Libraries and Information Science 2013;79(2):39–50.
32. Mukherjee G, Samanta A. Wheelchair charity: a useless benevolence in community-based rehabilitation. Disabil Rehabil 2005;27(10):591–6.
33. Pearlman J, Cooper RA, Zipfel E, et al. Towards the development of an effective technology transfer model of wheelchairs to developing countries. Disabil Rehabil Assist Technol 2006;1(1–2):103–10.
34. Pearlman J, Cooper RA, Krizack M, et al. Lower-limb prostheses and wheelchairs in low-income countries. IEEE Eng Med Biol Mag 2008;27(2):12–22.
35. Huckstep RL. Poliomyelitis: a guide for developing countries including appliances and rehabilitation for the disabled. London: Churchill Livingstone; 1975.
36. Hotchkiss R. Independence through mobility: guide to the manufacture of the ATI-Hotchkiss wheelchair. Washington, DC: Appropriate Technology International; 1985.
37. World Health Organzation. Guidelines for training personnel in developing countries for prosthetics and orthotics services. Geneva (Switzerland): World Health Organzation; 2005.
38. Golding JS, Nathan RH. A third world wheelchair. Int Disabil Stud 1987;9(1):38–40.
39. Winter A. Assessment of wheelchair technology in Tanzania. Int J Serv Learn Eng 2006;2(1):60–77.
40. Guimaraes E, Mann WC. Evaluation of pressure and durability of a low-cost wheelchair cushion designed for developing countries. Int J Rehabil Res 2003;26(2):141–3.
41. Ozturk A, Ucsular FD. Effectiveness of a wheelchair skills training programme for community-living users of manual wheelchairs in Turkey: a randomized controlled trial. Clin Rehabil 2011;25(5):416–24.
42. Ohlson E. Increased personal mobility for wheelchair users in developing countries: a wheelchair prototype evaluation study in Indonesia. In: Lindgaard G, Moore D, editors. Proceedings of the 19th Triennial Congress of the IEA. Melbourne (Australia): IEA; 2015. p. 976.

43. Lysack JT, Wyss UP, Packer TL, et al. Designing appropriate rehabilitation technology: a mobility device for women with ambulatory disabilities in India. Int J Rehabil Res 1999;22(1):1–9.

44. Shore S, Juillerat S. The impact of a low cost wheelchair on the quality of life of the disabled in the developing world. Med Sci Monit 2012;18(9):Cr533–42.

45. Visagie S, Eide AH, Mannan H, et al. A description of assistive technology sources, services and outcomes of use in a number of African settings. Disabil Rehabil Assist Technol 2017;12(7):705–12.

46. Visagie S, Scheffler E, Schneider M. Policy implementation in wheelchair service delivery in a rural South African setting. Afr J Disabil 2013;2(1):63.

47. Jefferds AN, Beyene NM, Upadhyay N, et al. Current state of mobility technology provision in less-resourced countries. Phys Med Rehabil Clin N Am 2010; 21(1):221–42.

48. Motivation Brockley Academy. Sports wheelchairs. 2017. Available at: https://www.motivation.org.uk/Pages/Category/sports-wheelchairs. Accessed August 10, 2017.

49. Coulter E, Dall P, Rochester L, et al. Development and validation of a physical activity monitor for use on a wheelchair. Spinal Cord 2011;49(3):445–50.

50. Burnley M, Jones A. Oxygen uptake kinetics as a determinant of sports performance. Eur J Sport Sci 2007;7(2):63–79.

51. Caspersen C, Powell K, Christenson G. Physical activity, exercise, and physical fitness: definitions and distinctions for health-related research. Public Health Rep 1985;100(2):126–31.

52. Tsang K, Hiremath S, Crytzer T, et al. Validity of activity monitors in wheelchair users: a systematic review. J Rehabil Res Dev 2016;53(6):641–58.

53. Hiremath SV, Ding D, Cooper RA. Development and evaluation of a gyroscope-based wheel rotation monitor for manual wheelchair users. J Spinal Cord Med 2013;36(4):347–56.

54. Moss A, Fowler N, Goosey-Tolfrey V. A telemetry-based velocometer to measure wheelchair velocity. J Biomech 2003;36(2):253–7.

55. Washburn R, Copay A. Assessing physical activity during wheelchair pushing: validity of a portable accelerometer. Adapt Phys Activ Q 1999;16(3):290–9.

56. Ojeda M, Ding D. Temporal parameters estimation for wheelchair propulsion using wearable sensors. Biomed Res Int 2014;2014:645284.

57. Consortium for Spinal Cord Medicine. Preservation of upper limb function following spinal cord injury: a clinical practice guideline for healthcare professionals. Washington, DC: Paralyzed Veterans of America; 2005.

58. Morrow MM, Hurd WJ, Kaufman KR, et al. Shoulder demands in manual wheelchair users across a spectrum of activities. J Electromyogr Kinesiol 2010;20: 61–7.

59. Sabick MB, Kotajarvi BR, An KN. A new method to quantify demand on the upper extremity during manual wheelchair propulsion. Arch Phys Med Rehabil 2004;85:1151–9.

60. Gagnon D, Koontz AM, Mulroy SJ, et al. Biomechanics of sitting pivot transfers among individuals with spinal cord injury: a review of the current knowledge. Top Spinal Cord Inj Rehabil 2009;15:33–58.

61. Brose SW, Boninger ML, Fullerton B, et al. Shoulder ultrasound abnormalities, physical examination findings, and pain in manual wheelchair users with spinal cord injury. Arch Phys Med Rehabil 2008;89:2086–93.

62. Sie IH, Waters RL, Adkins RH, et al. Upper extremity pain in the postrehabilitation spinal cord injured patient. Arch Phys Med Rehabil 1992;73:44–8.

63. Boninger ML, Towers JD, Cooper RA, et al. Shoulder imaging abnormalities in individuals with paraplegia. J Rehabil Res Dev 2001;38:401–8.
64. Curtis KA, Roach KE, Applegate EB, et al. Reliability and validity of the wheelchair user's shoulder pain index (WUSPI). Paraplegia 1995;33:595–601.
65. Jacobs PL, Nash MS. Exercise recommendations for individuals with spinal cord injury. Sports Med 2004;34:727–51.
66. Fisher JA, McNelis MA, Gorgey AS, et al. Does upper extremity training influence body composition after spinal cord injury? Aging Dis 2015;6:271–81.
67. Valent L, Dallmeijer A, Houdijk H, et al. The effects of upper body exercise on the physical capacity of people with a spinal cord injury: a systematic review. Clin Rehabil 2007;21:315–30.
68. Dost G, Dulgeroglu D, Yildirim A, et al. The effects of upper extremity progressive resistance and endurance exercises in patients with spinal cord injury. J Back Musculoskelet Rehabil 2014;27:419–26.
69. Jacobs PL. Effects of resistance and endurance training in persons with paraplegia. Med Sci Sports Exerc 2009;41:992–7.
70. Burnham RS, May L, Nelson E, et al. Shoulder pain in wheelchair athletes. The role of muscle imbalance. Am J Sports Med 1993;21:238–42.
71. Curtis KA, Tyner TM, Zachary L, et al. Effect of a standard exercise protocol on shoulder pain in long-term wheelchair users. Spinal Cord 1999;37:421–9.
72. Mulroy SJ, Thompson L, Kemp B, et al. Strengthening and optimal movements for painful shoulders (STOMPS) in chronic spinal cord injury: a randomized controlled trial. Phys Ther 2011;91:305–24.
73. Van Straaten MG, Cloud BA, Morrow MM, et al. Effectiveness of home exercise on pain, function, and strength of manual wheelchair users with spinal cord injury: a high-dose shoulder program with telerehabilitation. Arch Phys Med Rehabil 2014;95:1810–7.
74. Nash MS, van de Ven I, van Elk N, et al. Effects of circuit resistance training on fitness attributes and upper-extremity pain in middle-aged men with paraplegia. Arch Phys Med Rehabil 2007;88:70–5.
75. Rittweger J. Vibration as an exercise modality: how it may work, and what its potential might be. Eur J Appl Physiol 2010;108:877–904.
76. Osawa Y, Oguma Y, Ishii N. The effects of whole-body vibration on muscle strength and power: a meta-analysis. J Musculoskelet Neuronal Interact 2013; 13:380–90.
77. Mueller SM, Aguayo D, Zuercher M, et al. High-intensity interval training with vibration as rest intervals attenuates fiber atrophy and prevents decreases in anaerobic performance. PLoS One 2015;10:e0116764.
78. Mischi M, Cardinale M. The effects of a 28-Hz vibration on arm muscle activity during isometric exercise. Med Sci Sports Exerc 2009;41:645–53.
79. Bosco C, Cardinale M, Tsarpela O. Influence of vibration on mechanical power and electromyogram activity in human arm flexor muscles. Eur J Appl Physiol Occup Physiol 1999;79:306–11.
80. Cochrane DJ, Stannard SR, Walmsley A, et al. The acute effect of vibration exercise on concentric muscular characteristics. J Sci Med Sport 2008;11:527–34.
81. McBride JM, Porcari JP, Scheunke MD. Effect of vibration during fatiguing resistance exercise on subsequent muscle activity during maximal voluntary isometric contractions. J Strength Cond Res 2004;18:777–81.
82. Griffin MJ. Minimum health and safety requirements for workers exposed to hand-transmitted vibration and whole-body vibration in the European Union; a review. Occup Environ Med 2004;61:387–97.

83. Rubin C, Pope M, Fritton JC, et al. Transmissibility of 15-hertz to 35-hertz vibrations to the human hip and lumbar spine: determining the physiologic feasibility of delivering low-level anabolic mechanical stimuli to skeletal regions at greatest risk of fracture because of osteoporosis. Spine 2003;28:2621–7.

84. Asato KT, Cooper RA, Robertson RN, et al. SmartWheels: development and testing of a system for measuring manual wheelchair propulsion dynamics. IEEE Trans Biomed Eng 1993;40:1320–4.

85. Cooper R, Vosse A, Robertson R, et al. An interactive computer system for training wheelchair users. Journal of Biomedical Engineering - Applications, Basis and Communications 1995;7(1):52–60.

86. Crytzer TM, Dicianno BE, Fairman AD. Effectiveness of an upper extremity exercise device and text message reminders to exercise in adults with spina bifida: a pilot study. Assist Technol 2013;25(4):181–93.

87. Fitzgerald SG, Cooper RA, Thorman T, et al. The GAME(Cycle) exercise system: comparison with standard ergometry. J Spinal Cord Med 2004;27(5):453–9.

88. Guo S, Grindle GG, Authier EL, et al. Development and qualitative assessment of the GAME(Cycle) exercise system. IEEE Trans Neural Syst Rehabil Eng 2006; 14(1):83–90.

89. O'Connor TJ, Cooper RA, Fitzgerald SG, et al. Evaluation of a manual wheelchair interface to computer games. Neurorehabil Neural Repair 2000;14(1): 21–31.

90. O'Connor TJ, Fitzgerald SG, Cooper RA, et al. Kinetic and physiological analysis of the GAME(Wheels) system. J Rehabil Res Dev 2002;39(6):627–34.

91. O'Connor TJ, Fitzgerald SG, Cooper RA, et al. Does computer game play aid in motivation of exercise and increase metabolic activity during wheelchair ergometry? Med Eng Phys 2001;23(4):267–73.

92. The Board of Trustees of the University of Alabama. Building Inclusive Communities. National Center on Health, Physical Activity and Disability (NCHPAD). Available at: http://www.nchpad.org/. Accessed May 12, 2017.

93. The Board of Trustees of the University of Alabama. Discover accessible fitness. National Center on Health, Physical Activity and Disability (NCHPAD). Available at: http://www.nchpad.org/1247/5933/Discover ~ Accessible ~ Fitness. Accessed May 12, 2017.

94. NSW Department of Health. PhysioTherapy eXercises. PhysioTherapy eXercises for people with injuries & disabilities. Available at: https://www.physiotherapyexercises. com/. Accessed May 15, 2017.

95. *Wheelchair Exercises* [computer program]. Version 2.0. Euless, TX: Preferred Mobile Applications, LLC; 2015.

96. *Rx for Exercise* [computer program]. Version 1.0.2. Chicago, IL: Connections Marketing; 2017.

97. *CPF Challenge* [computer program]. Version 1.02. New York, NY: The Cerebral Palsy Foundation; 2017.

98. *SCI-Ex* [computer program]. Version 1.0029.b0029. Atlanta, GA: Shepherd Center; 2017.

99. U.S. National Park Service. U.S. National Park Service homepage. U.S. National Park Service. Available at: https://www.nps.gov/index.htm. Accessed May 12, 2017.

100. U.S. National Park Service. Accessibility for Visitors. U.S. National Park Service. Available at: https://www.nps.gov/aboutus/accessibilityforvisitors.htm. Accessed May 12, 2017.

101. AllTrails, Inc. AllTrails homepage. Alltrails. Available at: https://www.alltrails. com/. Accessed May 12, 2017.

102. *AllTrails-Hiking, Running and Biking Trails* [computer program]. Version 7.5.0. San Francisco, CA: AllTrails, Inc; 2017.

103. Rails-to-trails conservancy. Bike trails, walking trails & trail maps. TrailLink. Available at: https://www.traillink.com/. Accessed May 12, 2017.

104. *TrailLink-Trails & Maps* [computer program]. Version 1.4.1. Washington, DC: Rails-to-Trails Conservancy; 2016.

105. AXS Map. AXS map homepage. AXS map. Available at: https://www.axsmap. com/. Accessed May 12, 2017.

106. Access Earth. Access Earth homepage. Access Earth. Available at: http:// access.earth/. Accessed May 12, 2017.

107. AbleRoad™ Associates Inc. AbleRoad™ - disability access. AbleRoad™. Available at: http://ableroad.com. Accessed May 12, 2017.

108. *AbleRoad* [computer program] Version 3.04. Waltham (MA): AbleRoad Associates Inc; 2014.

109. *AXS Map* [computer program] Version 2.9.2. Austin (TX): Alice Cook; 2015.

110. Hall D, Berman R. Let's roll: learning wheelchair tennis with the pros. Let's roll wheelchair tennis. Available at: http://letsrollwheelchairtennis.com/. Accessed May 12, 2017.

111. British Paralympic Association. Find a sport. Parasport. Available at: http:// parasport.org.uk/find-a-sport/. Accessed May 18, 2017.

112. *Gateway to Gold* [computer program]. Version 1.1.6. Colorado Springs, CO: United States Olympic Committee Coaching Education; 2017.

113. US Paralympics. U.S. Paralympics launches gateway to gold app. Colorado Springs (CO): US Paralympics; 2016. Available at: http://www.teamusa.org/US-Paralympics/Features/2016/July/15/US-Paralympics-Launches-Gateway-To-Gold-App. Accessed August 10, 2017.

114. Ommaya AK, Adams KM, Allman RM, et al. Research Opportunities in Rehabilitation Research. J Rehabil Res Dev 2013;50(6):vii–xxxii.

Sport-Specific Limb Prostheses in Para Sport

Lara Grobler, PhD[a,b,*], Wayne Derman, MBChB, MSc (Med) (Hons), PhD, FFIMS[a]

KEYWORDS

• Para sport • Prostheses • Amputation • Performance • Sport-Specific prostheses

KEY POINTS

- Prostheses are an integral part of life for most individuals with amputation.
- Modern technology has made the participation in sport significantly easier for individuals with amputation and has reduced some of the risks that may occur with the use of non sport-specific prostheses for sport.
- Sport-specific prostheses facilitate peak performance by aiming to satisfy the requirements of the sport.
- The influence of these technological advances are still not always understood.

INTRODUCTION

Prostheses have been used to facilitate participation in sport for individuals with amputation since 1976, when athletes with amputation took part in sprint events at the Paralympic Games for the first time.[1] In that edition of the Paralympic Games, athletes made use of nonsport-specific prostheses, which consisted of rigid keel prostheses with no flexion ability in the ankle joint. Since then, the prostheses used in sporting activities have changed significantly, to sport-specific prostheses designed and manufactured according to the specific requirements of the sport. To design the optimal prosthesis for an athlete, multiple factors must be considered. These factors include the anatomic limb amputated; the site of amputation; the requirements and regulations of the sport; medical factors relating to the cause of the amputation; and, most importantly, the comfort of the prosthesis during use. With regard to the characteristics of the prostheses, factors such as prosthesis length, stiffness, and attachment site should also be considered because these may have an impact not only on comfort but also on performance.

The authors have nothing to disclose.
[a] Institute of Sport and Exercise Medicine, Faculty of Health and Medical Sciences, Stellenbosch University, Francie van Zijl Drive, Tygerberg, Cape Town 7505, South Africa; [b] Department of Sport Science, Faculty of Education, Stellenbosch University, Suidwal Street, Coetzenburg, Stellenbosch 7600, South Africa
* Corresponding author.
E-mail address: Lgrobler@sun.ac.za

Physical activity is an important factor in maintaining health and preventing non-communicable disease for all individuals but especially those with impairment or disability.[2] However, lifestyle and behavioral factors often change with amputation, which lead to decreased participation in physical activity[3] despite that physical fitness is an integral part of the rehabilitation process. Thus, a better understanding of the factors associated with amputation, the prostheses used, and barriers and facilitators to sport and physical activity may be crucial in the endeavor to improve physical fitness and performance of individuals following amputation.

AMPUTATION

The International Paralympic Committee (IPC) defines an amputation as the partial or total absence of bones or joints as the result of congenital or acquired (traumatic or due to illness) medical conditions. A review of the literature relating to the incidence of lower limb amputation on a global scale found greater incidence of lower limb amputation in individuals with diabetes (46.1–9600 per 10^5 in the population) in comparison with individuals without diabetes (5.6–600 per 10^5 in the population).[4] This indicates a significantly greater occurrence of amputation due to vascular dysfunction and similar diseases related to inactivity.

Upper Limb Amputation

Upper limb amputations can take place at any of the following anatomic positions: transphalangeal, transmetacarpal, transcarpal, wrist, transradial, elbow, transhumeral, shoulder, or forequarter.[5] For participation in Para sport, there are minimum eligibility criteria with which the athlete needs to comply. For example, a minimum eligibility criterion is usually an amputation at least through the wrist (www.paralympic.org/classification).

Lower Limb Amputation

As with upper limb amputations, there is an array of amputation levels for individuals with lower limb amputation. These include partial toe, toe disarticulation, partial foot resection, transmetatarsal, Lisfranc, Chopart, Syme, transtibial (long and short), through-knee disarticulation, transfemoral (long and short), hip disarticulation, hemipelvectomy, and hemicorporectomy.[5] Similar to upper limb amputations, there is a minimum eligibility criterion for participation in classified Para sport, which, in the case of lower limb amputees, is specified as an ankle disarticulation (www.paralympic.org/classification).

CLASSIFICATION

In competitive sport for individuals with impairment, athletes are classified into smaller, more homogenous groups. This system has been adopted by the IPC to maintain fairness in the sport.[6] Each sport has its own classification system determined by medical and/or functional criteria. In the medical classification system, the athlete is classified according to the medical diagnosis, whereas a functional classification system is based on the impact that a specific impairment may have on performance of a sport.[6] In sports for athletes with amputations, the athletes are often classified according to medical classification; therefore, the level of amputation. In track and field (T/F), for example, athletes with unilateral or bilateral transfemoral (above-knee) amputations are classified into class T/F42, whereas bilateral (T/F43) and unilateral (T/F44) transtibial amputees are classed separately although they compete in a combined T/F44 class. Individuals with upper limb amputations will be classified as T/F45 to T/F47, depending on the extent of the impairment. Athletes with a T/F45 classification have impairments of both arms similar to a transhumeral amputation, whereas athletes with a T/F46 classification include those with unilateral transhumeral amputations or bilateral transradial amputations. Finally, athletes in the T/F47 classification include unilateral transradial amputations. In other sports, such as swimming, a functional classification system is used throughout and athletes with amputations are classified alongside athletes with other impairments and similar abilities. In these cases, athletes with amputations may compete against other impairment types in a combined class.

PROSTHETIC COMPONENTS

There are 2 main types of prostheses. The first is nonsport-specific prostheses that function as every-day prostheses. This prosthesis allows the wearer to complete functions of daily living with greater ease, such as nonsport-specific walking prostheses that allows the individual to walk. In the case of an upper limb amputee, a nonsport-specific upper limb prosthesis allows the individual to hold or grasp objects. The second type of prostheses are sport-specific prostheses. These are prostheses designed specifically for the requirements of the sport. A very well-known example of sport-specific prostheses is the running specific prostheses or blades that sprinters use in the Paralympic Games. Sport-specific prostheses often do not mimic the shape of a biological limb; however, they aim to return the required function that was lost due to the amputation and optimize the performance of the athlete.

Upper Limb Prostheses

Scant literature is available regarding upper limb prostheses in sport. A systematic review found only 4 studies relating to athletes with upper limb amputation,[7] of which 2 studies were focused on the biomechanical characteristics of swimmers,[8,9] 1 on the cardiopulmonary function of alpine skiers,[10] and another on sports injuries in soccer players.[11] However, prostheses are not used in Para swimming or Para soccer and, therefore, this research is not reviewed here.

Most sports in which individuals with upper limb amputations participate do not require the use of prostheses. In Para cycling, individuals with upper limb amputations make use of prostheses purely for steering and gear changes.[12] These prostheses must be designed specifically for an athlete's anatomy and functional requirements. One aspect to consider when designing an upper limb prosthesis for Para cyclists, is that different Para cycling disciplines may require different handlebars. Therefore, different attachments between the socket and the handlebars may be required.[13] For Para athletics (track), upper limb prostheses are used mainly to assist the athlete in the sprint starts, as well as to create better symmetry in the athletes' running gait.

Lower Limb Prostheses

Typically, lower limb amputation results in the use of prostheses for locomotion. Individuals with lower limb amputation may also choose to use such prostheses for land-based sport or physical activity. A nonsport-specific lower limb prosthesis for individuals with transtibial or comparable amputation may be made up of a foot, pylon, and socket; whereas the lower limb prostheses for individuals with transfemoral or comparable amputation may include a prosthetic knee (**Figs. 1** and **2**). The specific components used in the complete prostheses may vary in terms of technological advancement and depend on the requirements and comfort of the athlete.

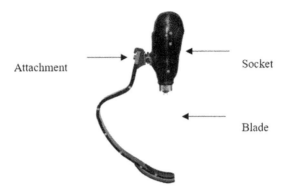

Attachment   Socket

Blade

Fig. 1. Components of a running-specific prosthesis.

Sport-specific prostheses, on the other hand, are prostheses specifically designed to facilitate the participation in specific sporting codes and to adhere to the requirements that the sport may place on both the athlete and the prostheses. The 3 Para sports codes for which the most literature relating to the prostheses used are cycling, long jump, and sprinting.

Cycling prostheses
The use of a prosthesis in Para cycling is to facilitate the connection between the residual limb and the bicycle crank; therefore, it is an important part of the bicycle's

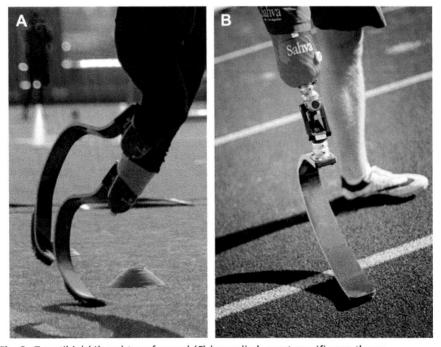

Fig. 2. Transtibial (*A*) and transfemoral (*B*) lower limb sport-specific prostheses.

propulsion system. Para cyclists with unilateral lower limb amputations have a choice of whether they want to use a prosthesis for propulsion or whether they want to compete with propulsion purely from the sound limb, whereas Para cyclists with bilateral lower limb amputations have a choice of whether they want to use lower limb prostheses or revert to hand cycling. It is common for cyclists with transtibial amputations to use a prosthesis; however, transfemoral amputees often do not use a prosthesis due to discomfort, as well as inefficient power production with the prosthesis.[14] Instead, they often propel themselves purely with the sound limb or revert to hand cycling. With regard to prostheses selection, recreational cyclists usually make use of nonsport-specific prostheses for cycling, whereas elite Para cyclists make use of specifically-designed, aerodynamic carbon fiber prostheses. These cycling-specific prostheses pose significant aerodynamic benefits to the cyclist in comparison with nonsport-specific prostheses.[15] This aerodynamic benefit is due to the aerodynamic design of the prosthesis in comparison with nonsport-specific prostheses. This benefit, however, does not outweigh the power production deficit associated with amputation, which is a result of the loss of muscle mass and effective mechanical contribution by the residual limb to total power production.[16] Consequently, the power output and overall performance of Para cyclists is lower than that of their able-bodied counterparts.

Although recreational Para cyclists may use nonsport-specific prostheses, these prostheses are inadequate to meet the performance requirements of elite Para cyclists. This is mostly due to the importance of prosthesis stiffness in power transfer for Para cyclists. Nonsport-specific prostheses are mostly designed to achieve some degree of ankle flexion to achieve a gait pattern that better resembles able-bodied walking.[16] Therefore, during the down stroke (power phase) of the cycle rotation, a nonsport-specific prosthesis will compress, thereby wasting muscular power in the compression of the prosthesis rather than applying it to the propulsion of the bicycle. On the other hand, the recoil of a nonsport-specific prosthesis during the recovery phase of the cycle rotation will produce torque that does not contribute to the propulsion of the bicycle.[17] Further evidence of the importance of the stiffness of the prosthesis can be found in the improvement of pedaling symmetry in unilateral transtibial amputees with increased prosthesis stiffness.[16]

Bicycle setup considerations Bicycle setup refers to the anatomic position of the athlete on the bicycle, and plays an important role in both performance and susceptibility to injury. There seems to be a significant correlation between incorrect bicycle setup and overuse injury. One study found that a deviation from the optimal anatomic distance between the saddle and the pedals put cyclists at a higher risk of knee pain.[18] Furthermore, if the distance between the saddle and the handlebar is too short, kyphotic posture can result. If this distance is too great, chronic lumbar pain may occur.[18] Athletes with lower limb amputation have additional bicycle setup considerations to take into account.

First, athletes with unilateral amputation have a leg-length discrepancy, which, in addition to decreased musculature in the affected limb, can lead to asymmetry in the power production of the 2 lower limbs.[17] Some literature has indicated that the reduced power production observed in the affected limb is compensated for by the sound limb[19]; however, the overall power output is significantly lower in comparison with able-bodied cyclists.[16] With regard to bicycle setup, leg-length discrepancy in unilateral amputees poses a significant challenge. Para cyclists often attach a prosthesis to the residuum of the affected limb to create symmetric hip height while standing. However, if prosthesis length is selected according to the standing leg length of the sound limb, the pedal stroke of the affected limb is negatively affected. This is due to the prosthesis not being able to flex and extend to the same degree as a biological ankle would. Therefore, if the prosthesis is set up to mirror the sound limb, the limb might be too long at the top of the pedal stroke and too short at the bottom of the pedal stroke. It has been suggested that this can be addressed by shortening the pedal crank arm on the affected limb side.[17] However, although this technique improves kinematic (joint angle and range of motion) symmetry, it does not improve kinetic (work and force production) symmetry.[20] On the contrary, it exaggerates the force production and subsequent joint moments in the sound hip and knee joints,[20] which could potentially lead to injury or chronic degeneration of the joints.

Second, the leg length of bilateral amputees can be adapted according to the preference of the athlete. However, by lengthening the prosthesis, the resultant center of mass of the athlete may be raised further from the ground, which could cause instability. Shortening the prosthesis length, on the other hand, increases knee range of motion[17] and may cause pain. Communication between the coach, athlete, and prosthetist is very important because this allows for the correct prosthetic setup to prevent injury and improve performance.

Regulations regarding prostheses Although very few regulations regarding cycling prostheses are set by the world cycling governing body, *Union Cycliste Internationale* (UCI), these regulations must be kept in mind when designing prostheses for Para cyclists. Current UCI guidelines require athletes to submit a document for approval regarding their competition prostheses, including information regarding any alterations. Prostheses are not allowed to include any energy storage or assistance systems that allow for greater propulsion energy (microprocessor or bionic-assisted prostheses). Furthermore, for cyclists with transfemoral amputation, the position of the knee is required to be in the position that a sound knee would have been in. Thus, for unilateral amputees the prosthesis knee height should be at the height of the sound knee, whereas for bilateral amputees the expected knee height needs to be determined via other anatomic measurements.

Long jump prostheses

Both transtibial and transfemoral amputees participate in long jump. The aim of long jump is to jump as far as possible by accelerating along the approach run before planting the foot on the take-off board. The athlete then propels himself or herself forward to achieve maximal horizontal projection by the combination of optimal speed, take-off angle, and height.[21] During the approach run, near maximal horizontal velocity is achieved. Horizontal velocity is used for the development of horizontal distance during flight, with some horizontal velocity being transferred to vertical velocity. This enables flight, commencing during the contact time with the foot or prosthesis striking the take-off board.[22] The ability to transfer horizontal velocity to vertical velocity stems from the athlete's ability to pivot her or his center of gravity around the planted foot in the sagittal plane. In the case of lower limb amputation, limb dominance usually shifts to the sound, biological limb (unilateral amputees); therefore, the takeoff has historically been taken from the sound limb. Recently, there has been a change toward taking off from the affected limb. This trend may be related to performance-related technological developments in sport-specific prostheses.[23]

Athletes with lower limb amputation participating in the long jump participate with the same sport-specific prosthesis as sprinters; namely, a running-specific prosthesis (RSP). The RSP is an energy storage and return prosthesis that functions mechanically as a spring. Due to the spring property of RSPs, the force on the stump during ground contact has decreased, allowing athletes to take off from the affected limb with greater ease. As technology has improved, and athletes have become more inclined to take off from the affected limb, long jump performances have improved significantly. **Fig. 3** shows the long jump results at the Olympic and Paralympic Games for the past 20 years. A recent study on the differences between taking off from the affected and unaffected limb has shown that taking off from the prosthesis may provide performance benefit to the athlete.[24]

Recently, there has been debate about whether individuals with amputation should be allowed to participate in able-bodied competitions, such as the Olympic Games. More specifically, there is debate about whether the use of a prosthesis on the take-off leg would lead to an unfair performance advantage. The debate originated with a similar situation in which the use of prostheses during sprinting events was questioned as potentially unfair. In that case, there was no scientific basis for prohibiting the athlete from taking part in the Olympic Games. When, in 2016, the case was made for an athlete with a unilateral transtibial amputation to take part in the long jump event at the Olympic Games, the athlete was prohibited from competing. This was because the athlete could not produce any evidence to suggest that the prosthesis did not give him an advantage over his competitors. It was later suggested that it will always be difficult to assess the validity of allowing prosthesis users to participate in able-bodied sport. There is an inherent difference between able-bodied athletes and athletes with lower limb amputation. This between-group difference makes it challenging to determine whether the prosthesis has an ergogenic effect on performance in athletes with lower limb amputation.[25]

Differences in jump techniques between amputees and able-bodied athletes To date, biomechanical research has focused on the technical differences between athletes with lower limb amputation and able-bodied athletes. Among the key performance indicators in the long jump technique of able-bodied athletes is the degree to which the center of mass is lowered on the second-to-last step before takeoff. Able-bodied athletes can achieve this by effectively widening the step; this lowering ensures that the vertical impulse is maximised.[21] The literature indicates that athletes with both transtibial (17.0%) and transfemoral (12.6%) amputations lower their center of mass to a lesser extent than able-bodied athletes (17.9%)[26] but that there may not be a statistically significant difference between the center of mass displacement of transtibial and transfemoral amputees during the approach to takeoff.[22]

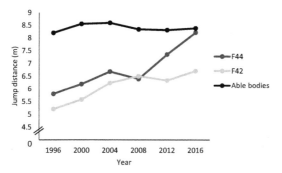

Fig. 3. First place results for the long jump event at the Olympic and Paralympic Games ranging from 1996 to 2016. F42, above-knee amputees; F44, below-knee amputees.

The inability of athletes with amputation to significantly decrease their center of mass on the second-to-last step may be due to the constraints imposed by the prosthesis.[26] For transfemoral amputees, for example, the knee needs to be in the locked position to support the weight of the athlete during takeoff.[27] Therefore, lowering the center of mass requires some adjustment from the techniques used by able-bodied athletes, such as the strategy of widening the step (see previous discussion). Another technique applied is to lower the center of mass on the last step rather than the second-to-last step[27]; however this technique creates more negative vertical velocity during the take-off phase, which is a less efficient movement pattern for the long jump. Furthermore, unilateral amputees may need to maintain their center of mass at a greater height in comparison with able-bodied athletes to ensure ground clearance by the prosthesis during the swing phase.[27]

It is postulated that by taking off from the prosthesis, the athlete could lower the center of mass to a greater extent than athletes taking off on the sound limb. However, it has been found that, in the event of the athlete taking off on the affected limb, the center of mass at touchdown of the take-off step is higher than takeoff from a biological limb. This enables the prosthesis to be loaded sufficiently for maximal propulsion.[28] This is because the prosthesis has the properties of a spring. For the spring to unload maximally, the prosthesis needs to be loaded maximally. Therefore, by touching down with a high center of mass, the athlete can compress the prosthesis (spring) to a greater extent.

With regard to the velocity achieved during the approach, athletes with lower limb amputations are not able to achieve the same speed at the take-off board as able-bodied athletes.[22] This is similar to what has been reported in the literature relating to sprinting with a prosthesis.[22]

Running-specific prostheses

The modern-day RSP was introduced in 1988 as the first flexible keel prosthesis specifically designed for running.[23] It aimed to rectify the discrepancies between running with a prosthesis and running with a biological limb. These discrepancies included (1) compensation by the sound limb in unilateral amputees, (2) force and impulse asymmetries between the affected and sound limbs of unilateral amputees, and (3) hip extensors becoming the major source of energy generation instead of ankle plantarflexors in both unilateral and bilateral amputees.[29–31] These discrepancies were attributed to the inability of the running prosthesis to flex and mimic natural plantarflexion and dorsiflexion of a biological ankle. They were also attributed to the inability of the prosthesis to absorb and generate energy to the same extent that a biological limb would. A marked improvement in the performances of athletes with lower limb amputation competing in the 100 m sprint has been found since the introduction of the modern RSP. This improvement is significantly greater than that of both able-bodied athletes and athletes with other types of impairment (cerebral palsy or visually impaired).[1,23] It is clear that there is a marked difference between the biomechanics of athletes with lower limb amputation and able-bodied athletes. However, the performances of athletes with amputation are improving at a rapid rate. There is currently only a 1.03 second difference in the 100 m performance between athletes with transtibial amputation and able-bodied athletes.

The RSP is a carbon fiber spring that stores and releases energy during the compression and release experienced during running. This more closely mimics the natural motion of the biological ankle[32] because energy absorption and return is an important part of the biomechanics of running propulsion. The biological ankle has been found to return 241% of energy that it absorbs during running.[29] To date, no literature exists to indicate that an RSP is able to produce similar levels of energy return as a biological ankle. Various investigators have also mentioned that the stiffness of an RSP is not variable during a single race as is the case with biological lower limbs.[33] During the course of running over any distance, leg stiffness will vary according to the demands on the body at a given time, such as running speed[33] and running surface.[34] This then begs the question: which prostheses would be most suitable for the different events in which an athlete may be competing?

Prosthesis selection is a complex problem, especially because very little research has focused on characterizing the differences between prostheses models and categories. The literature that has focused on the stiffness of prostheses and has indicated that the stiffness varies during the course of the contact phase due to changes in the ground contact deflection.[35] Because there are different phases of a sprint (acceleration, speed maintenance, and deceleration), it has been suggested that the average stiffness of the prosthesis is the variable that can be prescribed to guide selection of the RSP.[36] Although the stiffness is usually recommended according to the body mass of the athlete, it is common for athletes to use a category other than the category recommended by the manufacturer. Distinctions between RSP models are made for the various sprint race differences. These differences were found to relate to the contact time and ground reaction forces during athlete independent testing.[37]

Unilateral versus bilateral prostheses In unilateral amputees, symmetry has been hypothesized to be the most important factor for both performance and injury prevention. Unilateral amputees experience significant gait asymmetries. These asymmetries are present during regular walking and are exacerbated in running when lower extremity joint forces and moments are significantly higher. This places strain not only on the affected limb of the body but also on the sound limb owing to compensatory strategies. One study investigating the occurrence of step asymmetries during competition indicated that prosthesis technology might be responsible for the occurrence of step asymmetries; however, poor starts, fatigue, falls, or torso lunging were also implicated as factors that cause step asymmetries.[38] Similarly, significant differences have been found in the ground reaction forces of the affected and sound limbs in unilateral transtibial amputees running with RSPs, with the sound limb side experiencing significantly greater ground reaction forces.[39,40] The significantly lower ground reaction force with an RSP has been speculated to be among the biggest detriments to performance in athletes with amputation.[41] This is primarily related to the stiffness and deformation of the RSP during running. Technological advances in creating RSPs that can modulate stiffness according to the requirements of a specific phase of running may improve on these problems; however, strict regulation of such technology is necessary to maintain fairness among participants.

The problems relating to asymmetry are largely circumvented in athletes with bilateral amputations. However, as is evident in sprint running, these athletes are at a disadvantage in the initial stages of racing when inertia has to be overcome. Due to the lack of the propulsive musculature of the lower limb, specifically the calf muscles, these athletes are slow at the start. Some research has indicated that the simple harmonic motion of an RSP can be used to improve performance in the latter stages of a race, specifically in athletes with bilateral amputations.[42] The efficacy of this is determined by the ability of the athlete to mimic the natural resonant frequency of the prostheses. By doing this, the athlete can then improve the energy output of the prostheses with minimal energy put into it, therefore conserving energy and running more efficiently.[43] Owing to the difficulty of distributing energy to the RSP in the early stages of the race, this phenomenon is more pronounced in the latter stages when the athlete is in the maximal speed phase rather than acceleration phase. The synchronization required for this may also prove to be difficult for a unilateral amputee due to the asymmetries they experience during running. Although bilateral amputees may benefit from the use of 2 RSPs, stability is a significantly greater problem in bilateral amputees compared with unilateral amputees. A study investigating medial-lateral foot placement during running found that bilateral amputees had on average 89% greater variability in foot placement compared with unilateral amputees.[44] This indicates greater instability in athletes with bilateral amputations, for which compensation is required by placing both feet in a wider placement while running to increase the base of support.

Comparing athletes with bilateral transtibial amputation with able-bodied sprinters, investigators found a separation between biomechanical and physiological performance. Surprisingly, the amputee athlete was able to maintain similar Physiological performances to that of able-bodied athletes by significantly different biomechanical means.[41,45] This may indicate that there is a similar physiological profile between athletes with amputation and able-bodied athletes. However, some literature has indicated that there are differences in metabolic energy required when using different prostheses, specifically in the difference between rigid keel prostheses and energy storage and return prostheses.[46] That amputee athletes are physiologically similar to able-bodied athletes enables coaches to adopt similar training strategies and principles to those they would use with an able-bodied sprinter.

Transtibial versus transfemoral amputees Although the literature relating to transtibial amputee athletes has been growing, little academic literature can be found regarding transfemoral amputees. Traditionally the T/F42 class (transfemoral amputees) has been smaller than the T/F44 class (transtibial amputees). This could be the reason for the paucity of literature focused on this class. Technological changes have had a significant influence on the running gait patterns of athletes with transfemoral amputation. Before the invention of sport-specific prostheses, transfemoral amputees would run with rigid keel prostheses that had little to no flexion and shock-absorption properties. The use of these prostheses led to unilateral transfemoral amputees adopting a hop-skip movement pattern to decrease the impact on the residual limb.[47] Prostheses are now able to absorb more shock during running; therefore, athletes no longer make use of this movement pattern. However, unilateral transfemoral amputees still exhibit asymmetrical hip movement, specifically during the swing phase of running.[48] Although transtibial amputees cannot modulate the stiffness of their affected leg with increased speed, transfemoral amputees do increase leg stiffness, due to the hydraulic action of the prosthetic knee.[49]

The current trend in competitive sprinting with transfemoral amputation is for bilateral amputees to compete without a knee joint, whereas unilateral amputees compete with a knee joint. This leads to very different running gait patterns and biomechanical differences in comparison with both able-bodied and transtibial amputee sprinters. There are some concerns regarding susceptibility to injury, specifically degenerative changes in the hip joint, in these athletes. However, no literature to date has addressed this issue. More empirical research is required to define this problem, and to prevent injury and pain in later life.

FACTORS INFLUENCING PARTICIPATION SPORT AND PHYSICAL ACTIVITY

There are various factors that influence participation in sport for individuals with lower limb amputation. Participation in sports before amputation is a predictor of participation in sport after amputation.[50] In contrast, however, age, level of amputation, and cause of injury do not seem to predict sport participation.[50] Furthermore, the perception of mastery of tasks and the rehabilitation environment (rehabilitation facilities), as well as environmental barriers (physical environment), influence amputees' participation in sport and physical activity.[50,51]

Incompatibility of the prosthesis used for the desired sport may be a barrier to participation. Scientists have found that the ability to perform an activity was greater with the use of a prosthesis than without, therefore making participation easier.[52] However, the ease of participation can be improved by decreasing the energy spent to complete the task at hand. Studies have investigated the influence of residual limb length in lower limb amputees in relation to the metabolic cost of movement. For individuals with transtibial amputations, the residual limb length did not have a significant influence on the energy cost of walking.[53] This result, however, is not true in the case of individuals with transfemoral amputations because there is a moderate but positive relationship between residual limb length and energy cost of walking[54] Also, the properties of the prosthesis have been shown to influence the metabolic cost of movement.[46]

MEDICAL FACTORS RELATED TO AMPUTEES

As many as 50% to 80% of all amputees may experience chronic pain. The chronic pain most often experienced in amputees is characterized by either phantom limb pain or stump pain. Phantom limb pain is defined as neuropathic pain experienced in the missing limb,[55] whereas stump pain is mostly nociceptive pain in the residual limb brought about by increased inflammation.[55] The management of these chronic pain conditions is important because of the influence that pain may have on participation in physical activity, as well as on quality of life. Pharmacologic treatment of phantom limb pain and stump pain may include but is not limited to botulinum toxin, opioids, N-methyl-D-aspartate (NMDA) receptor antagonists, anticonvulsants, antidepressants, anti-inflammatories, calcitonin, paracetamol, and local anesthetics.[56]

The use of pharmacologic treatment in competitive Para athletes needs to be managed carefully to prevent the use of banned substances. If the need for regulated medication is significant, the athlete may be able to use the substance by applying for a Therapeutic Use Exemption from the IPC. A more conservative approach is found in non-pharmacological treatments such as Farabloc,[57] mirror therapy,[58] visuotactile illusions,[59] virtual reality treatment,[60] and hypnotic therapy.[61] These treatments, specifically mirror therapy, have been found to be very effective in the treatment of chronic phantom limb pain.[62] As stipulated in the recent International Olympic Committee consensus document on pain management, pain is influenced by biological, psychological, and contextual domains; therefore, all these domains must be addressed.[63] This makes non-pharmacological therapies specifically effective in the treatment of athletic pain.

Stump ulcers often hinder amputee athletes' prosthesis use and participation in physical activity and sport.[64] Skin problems on the stump are related to the skin and soft tissue not being adapted for loadbearing like the palms and soles of the hands and feet. The compressive and shear forces derived from ambulation and/or running on a prosthesis regularly leads to tissue damage. Furthermore, environmental conditions could lead to excessive sweating in the socket of the prosthesis, causing skin irritation.[65] It is important that the athlete dries off and cleans the stump often, especially during sport, to prevent skin irritation. Furthermore, it is essential that the socket be optimized to reduce shear and compressive forces on susceptible areas of the stump. It is widely understood that the most important factor in the comfort of prosthesis use is the fit of the socket.[66] To achieve better stump-socket comfort and reduce problems related to socket fit, the pressure profile between the stump socket and the residual limb should be such that the loadbearing areas are areas of thick tissue, whereas the more sensitive areas or areas where the bone is very superficial are non load-bearing.[66]

Another factor that may have a negative impact on the health and well-being of an athlete with amputation is the ability to thermoregulate. Insufficient thermoregulation might occur due to the decreased surface area, through which thermoregulation can take place. Furthermore, in vascular-related amputation in individuals with type 2 diabetes mellitus, there may be associated thermoregulatory problems due to metabolic, cardiovascular, and neurologic dysfunction.[67–69] Athletes, coaches, and the team medical staff should keep this in mind, particularly when participating in hot and humid conditions. Extra precautions should be taken, such as increased access to water and cold fluids, as well as monitoring of the athlete to prevent the onset of heat-related illness.

SUMMARY

Prostheses form an integral part of life for most individuals with amputation. Modern technology has made the participation in sport significantly easier for individuals with amputation and has reduced some of the risks that may occur with the use of non sport-specific prostheses for sport. Furthermore, sport-specific prostheses facilitate peak performance by aiming to satisfy the requirements of the sport. However, the influence of these technological advances is still not always understood. To encourage participation in sport and physical activity, it is essential that the prostheses and the impact that they may have on the athlete be further investigated. Although technological advances may assist the individual by allowing for easier participation in sport, there are medical challenges that accompany participation, such as phantom limb pain, stump ulcers, and inadequate thermoregulation. These factors should be monitored to promote the health, safety, and performance of amputee athletes.

REFERENCES

1. Dyer B. The progression of male 100 m sprinting with a lower-limb amputation 1976-2012. Sports 2015;3(1):30–9.
2. Lee I-M, Shiroma EJ, Lobelo F, et al. Effect of physical inactivity on major non-communicable diseases worldwide: an analysis of burden of disease and life expectancy. Lancet 2012;380(9838):219–29.
3. Burger H, Marincek C. The life style of young persons after lower limb amputation caused by injury. Prosthet Orthot Int 1997;21(1):35–9.
4. Moxey PW, Gogalniceanu P, Hinchliffe RJ, et al. Lower extremity amputations-a review of global variability in incidence. Diabet Med 2011;28(10):1144–53.
5. Cuccurullo SJ. Physical medicine and rehabilitation board review. New York: Demos Medical Publishing; 2014.
6. Tweedy SM, Vanlandewijck YC. International Paralympic Committee position stand—background and scientific principles of classification in Paralympic sport. Br J Sports Med 2011;45(4):259–69.
7. Bragaru M, Dekker R, Geertzen JH, et al. Amputees and sports. Sports Med 2011;41(9):721–40.
8. Osborough CD, Payton CJ, Daly DJ. Relationships between the front crawl stroke parameters of competitive unilateral arm amputee swimmers, with selected anthropometric characteristics. J Appl Biomech 2009;25(4):304–12.
9. Osborough CD, Payton CJ, Daly DJ. Influence of swimming speed on inter-arm coordination in competitive unilateral arm amputee front crawl swimmers. Hum Mov Sci 2010;29(6):921–31.

10. Alaranta H, Niittymaki S, Karhumaki L. Physische belastungstest bei amputierten skilaufern. Med Sport 1988;28:112–6.

11. Kegel BMD. Incidence of injury in amputees playing soccer. Palaestra 1994; 10(2):50–4.

12. Bragaru M, Dekker R, Geertzen JH. Sport prostheses and prosthetic adaptations for the upper and lower limb amputees: an overview of peer reviewed literature. Prosthet Orthot Int 2012;36(3):290–6.

13. Riel L-P, Adam-Côté J, Daviault S, et al. Design and development of a new right arm prosthetic kit for a racing cyclist. Prosthet Orthot Int 2009;33(3):284–91.

14. Gailey R, Harsch P. Introduction to triathlon for the lower limb amputee triathlete. Prosthet Orthot Int 2009;33(3):242–55.

15. Dyer B. The importance of aerodynamics for prosthetic limb design used by competitive cyclists with an amputation: an introduction. Prosthet Orthot Int 2015;39(3):232–7.

16. Childers WL, Gallagher TP, Duncan JC, et al. Modeling the effect of a prosthetic limb on 4-km pursuit performance. Int J Sports Physiol Perform 2015;10(1):3–10.

17. Childers WL, Kistenberg RS, Gregor RJ. The biomechanics of cycling with a transtibial amputation: recommendations for prosthetic design and direction for future research. Prosthet Orthot Int 2009;33(3):256–71.

18. Sabeti-Aschraf M, Serek M, Geisler M, et al. Overuse injuries correlated to the mountain bike's adjustment: a prospective field study. Open Sports Sci J 2010; 3:1–6.

19. Childers WL, Gregor RJ. Effectiveness of force production in persons with unilateral transtibial amputation during cycling. Prosthet Orthot Int 2011;35(4):373–8.

20. Childers WL, Kogler GF. Symmetrical kinematics does not imply symmetrical kinetics in people with transtibial amputation using cycling model. J Rehabil Res Dev 2014;51(8):1243.

21. Lees A, Graham-Smith P, Fowler N. A biomechanical analysis of the last stride, touchdown, and takeoff characteristics of the men's long jump. J Appl Biomech 1994;10:61–78.

22. Nolan L, Lees A. The influence of lower limb amputation level on the approach in the amputee long jump. J Sports Sci 2007;25(4):393–401.

23. Grobler L, Ferreira S, Terblanche E. Paralympic sprint performance between 1992 and 2012. Int J Sports Physiol Perform 2015;10(8):1052–4.

24. Nolan L, Lees A. Prosthetic limb versus intact limb take-off in the amputee long jump. In: ISBS-Conference Proceedings Archive. Vol. 1. 2008.

25. Beckman EM, Connick MJ, McNamee MJ, et al. Should Markus Rehm be permitted to compete in the long jump at the Olympic Games? Br J Sports Med 2017;51(14):1048–9.

26. Nolan L, Lees A. Touch-down and take-off characteristics of the long jump performance of world level above- and below-knee amputee athletes. Ergonomics 2000;43(10):1637–50.

27. Nolan L, Patritti BL, Simpson KJ. A biomechanical analysis of the long-jump technique of elite female amputee athletes. Med Sci Sports Exerc 2006;38(10): 1829–35.

28. Nolan L, Patritti BL, Simpson KJ. Effect of take-off from prosthetic versus intact limb on transtibial amputee long jump technique. Prosthet Orthot Int 2012; 36(3):297–305.

29. Czerniecki JM, Gitter A, Munro C. Joint moment and muscle power output characteristics of below knee amputees during running: the influence of energy storing prosthetic feet. J Biomech 1991;24(1):63–75.

30. Prince F, Allard P, Therrien R, et al. Running gait impulse asymmetries in below-knee amputees. Prosthet Orthot Int 1992;16(1):19–24.

31. Czerniecki JM, Gitter A. Insights into amputee running: a muscle work analysis. Am J Phys Med Rehabil 1992;71(4):209–18.

32. Buckley JG. Sprint kinematics of athletes with lower-limb amputations. Arch Phys Med Rehabil 1999;80(5):501–8.

33. McGowan CP, Grabowski AM, McDermott WJ, et al. Leg stiffness of sprinters using running-specific prostheses. J R Soc Interface 2012;9(73):1975–82.

34. Schütte KH, Aeles J, De Beéck TO, et al. Surface effects on dynamic stability and loading during outdoor running using wireless trunk accelerometry. Gait Posture 2016;48:220–5.

35. Dyer B, Sewell P, Noroozi S. How should we assess the mechanical properties of lower-limb prosthesis technology used in elite sport?—An initial investigation. J Biomed Sci Eng 2013;6(02):116.

36. Dyer BT, Sewell P, Noroozi S. An investigation into the measurement and prediction of mechanical stiffness of lower limb prostheses used for running. Assist Technol 2014;26(3):157–63.

37. Grobler L, Ferreira S, Vanwanseele B, et al. Characterisation of the responsive properties of two running-specific prosthetic models. Prosthet Orthot Int 2017; 41(2):141–8.

38. Dyer B, Noroozi S, Sewell P. Sprinting with an amputation: some race-based lower-limb step observations. Prosthet Orthot Int 2015;39(4):300–6.

39. Engsberg J, Lee A, Tedford K, et al. Normative ground reaction force data for able-bodied and trans-tibial amputee children during running. Prosthet Orthot Int 1993;17(2):83–9.

40. Grabowski AM, McGowan CP, McDermott WJ, et al. Running-specific prostheses limit ground-force during sprinting. Biol Lett 2010;6(2):201–4.

41. Weyand PG, Bundle MW, McGowan CP, et al. The fastest runner on artificial legs: different limbs, similar function? J Appl Physiol (1985) 2009;107(3):903–11.

42. Noroozi S, Sewell P, Rahman AGA, et al. Performance enhancement of bi-lateral lower-limb amputees in the latter phases of running events: an initial investigation. Proc Inst Mech Eng P J Sports Eng Tech 2012;227(2):105–15.

43. Noroozi S, Rahman AG, Khoo SY, et al. The dynamic elastic response to impulse synchronisation of composite prosthetic energy storing and returning feet. Proc Inst Mech Eng P J Sports Eng Tech 2014;228(1):24–32.

44. Arellano CJ, McDermott WJ, Kram R, et al. Effect of running speed and leg prostheses on mediolateral foot placement and its variability. PLoS One 2015;10(1): e0115637.

45. Brown MB, Millard-Stafford ML, Allison AR. Running-specific prostheses permit energy cost similar to nonamputees. Med Sci Sports Exerc 2009;41(5):1080–7.

46. Hsu M-J, Nielsen DH, Yack HJ, et al. Physiological measurements of walking and running in people with transtibial amputations with 3 different prostheses. J Orthop Sports Phys Ther 1999;29(9):526–33.

47. Mensch G, Ellis PE. Running patterns of transfemoral amputees: a clinical analysis. Prosthet Orthot Int 1986;10(3):129–34.

48. Burkett B, Smeathers J, Barker T. Walking and running inter-limb asymmetry for Paralympic trans-femoral amputees, a biomechanical analysis. Prosthet Orthot Int 2003;27(1):36–47.

49. Mauroy G, De Jaeger D, Vanmarsenille J, et al. The bouncing mechanism of running in a transfemoral amputee wearing a blade prosthesis. Comput Methods Biomech Biomed Engin 2012;15(supp1):357–9.

50. Kars C, Hofman M, Geertzen JH, et al. Participation in sports by lower limb amputees in the Province of Drenthe, The Netherlands. Prosthet Orthot Int 2009; 33(4):356–67.

51. Deans S, Burns D, McGarry A, et al. Motivations and barriers to prosthesis users participation in physical activity, exercise and sport: a review of the literature. Prosthet Orthot Int 2012;36(3):260–9.

52. Legro MW, Reiber GE, Czerniecki JM, et al. Recreational activities of lower-limb amputees with prostheses. J Rehabil Res Dev 2001;38(3):319.

53. Gailey RS, Wenger MA, Raya M, et al. Energy expenditure of trans-tibial amputees during ambulation at self-selected pace. Prosthet Orthot Int 1994;18(2): 84–91.

54. Boonstra A, Schrama J, Fidler V, et al. The gait of unilateral transfemoral amputees. Scand J Rehabil Med 1994;26(4):217.

55. Siddiqui S, Sifonios AN, Le V, et al. Development of phantom limb pain after femoral nerve block. Case Rep Med 2014;2014:238453.

56. Alviar MJM, Hale T, Dungca M. Pharmacologic interventions for treating phantom limb pain. Cochrane Database Syst Rev 2011;(12):CD006380.

57. Conine TA, Hershler C, Alexander SA, et al. The efficacy of Farabloc in the treatment of phantom limb pain. Canadian Journal of Rehabilitation 1993;6:155.

58. Foell J, Bekrater-Bodmann R, Diers M, et al. Mirror therapy for phantom limb pain: brain changes and the role of body representation. Eur J Pain 2014;18(5):729–39.

59. Schmalzl L, Ragnö C, Ehrsson HH. An alternative to traditional mirror therapy: illusory touch can reduce phantom pain when illusory movement does not. Clin J Pain 2013;29(10):e10–8.

60. Cole J, Crowle S, Austwick G, et al. Exploratory findings with virtual reality for phantom limb pain; from stump motion to agency and analgesia. Disabil Rehabil 2009;31(10):846–54.

61. Oakley DA, Whitman LG, Halligan PW. Hypnotic imagery as a treatment for phantom limb pain: two case reports and a review. Clin Rehabil 2002;16(4):368–77.

62. Foell J, Bekrater-Bodmann R, Flor H, et al. Phantom limb pain after lower limb trauma origins and treatments. Int J Low Extrem Wounds 2011;10(4):224–35.

63. Hainline B, Derman W, Vernec A, et al. International Olympic Committee consensus statement on pain management in elite athletes. Br J Sports Med 2017;51:1245–58.

64. Salawu A, Middleton C, Gilbertson A, et al. Stump ulcers and continued prosthetic limb use. Prosthet Orthot Int 2006;30(3):279–85.

65. Hagberg K, Brånemark R. Consequences of non-vascular trans-femoral amputation: a survey of quality of life, prosthetic use and problems. Prosthet Orthot Int 2001;25(3):186–94.

66. Sewell P, Noroozi S, Vinney J, et al. Static and dynamic pressure prediction for prosthetic socket fitting assessment utilising an inverse problem approach. Artif Intell Med 2012;54(1):29–41.

67. Johnstone MT, Creager SJ, Scales KM, et al. Impaired endothelium-dependent vasodilation in patients with insulin-dependent diabetes mellitus. Circulation 1993;88(6):2510–6.

68. Veves A, Akbari CM, Primavera J, et al. Endothelial dysfunction and the expression of endothelial nitric oxide synthetase in diabetic neuropathy, vascular disease, and foot ulceration. Diabetes 1998;47(3):457–63.

69. Caballero AE, Arora S, Saouaf R, et al. Microvascular and macrovascular reactivity is reduced in subjects at risk for type 2 diabetes. Diabetes 1999;48(9): 1856–62.

Para Sport Athletic Identity from Competition to Retirement

A Brief Review and Future Research Directions

Michelle Guerrero, PhD[a], Jeffrey Martin, PhD[b],*

KEYWORDS

- Identity • Athlete identity • Elite athletes • Paralympics • Sport participation
- Disability identity

KEY POINTS

- Athletes with disabilities describe their disability and sport participation in diverse ways, and different factors contribute to one's athletic identity development.
- Quantitative research on Para sport athletic identity suggests that possessing a strong athletic identity can have both positive and negative effects, whereas qualitative research on Para sport athletic identity reveals that sport participation serves as a catalyst for athletes with disabilities to develop positive identities and to challenge disablist attitudes.
- Although individuals with congenital and acquired disabilities both experience identity-related challenges, those with acquired permanent disabilities face an additional challenge of acknowledging a forever lost past self (or selves).
- Future researchers might consider examining athletes with acquired disabilities' perceptions of their past, present, and future selves through the lens of narrative identity and identifying the capabilities (eg, compassion, courage) of those who acknowledge loss but embrace current and future selves.

My identity is not disability sport. How do you practice disability sport? Do you injure yourself a bit more or what? (…) I can play basketball, swim, play table tennis – but how do you practice disability sport? It doesn't exist.[1(p157)]

—Lennart

INTRODUCTION

Self-concept is a multidimensional structure that comprises individuals' thoughts and feelings about the self across various aspects of life.[2] These varying dimensions of

---

Disclosure Statement: The authors have nothing to disclose.

[a] Department of Kinesiology, University of Windsor, 401 Sunset Avenue, Windsor, Ontario N9B 3P4, Canada; [b] Division of Kinesiology, Health and Sport Studies, Wayne State University, FAB Building, Detroit, MI 48202, USA
* Corresponding author.
E-mail address: aa3975@wayne.edu

Phys Med Rehabil Clin N Am 29 (2018) 387–396
https://doi.org/10.1016/j.pmr.2018.01.007
1047-9651/18/© 2018 Elsevier Inc. All rights reserved.

self-concept allow people to present themselves differently depending on the situation. Athletic identity is one dimension of self-concept and refers to the degree to which an individual identifies with the athletic role.[3] It is considered to serve a cognitive structure (schema) and a social role. From the cognitive structure perspective, athletic identity offers a framework for processing information, coping in various situations, and influencing behavior. From a social role perspective, athletic identity may be influenced by the degree to which significant others emphasize the athletic dimensions of the individual. Athletic identity has received ample attention by sport psychology researchers[4–8] and has shown to be important for health and fitness outcomes, global self-esteem, social relationships, and commitment to sport and physical activity.[9] Similarly, a Para sport athletic identity is the degree to which an athlete with a disability (either congenital or acquired) identifies as an athlete.

The purpose of this article is to review what is currently known about Para sport athletic identity and to offer avenues for future research directions by drawing from underused theoretic orientations about identity. The current body of literature, with some exceptions, tends to divide itself into 2 categories: quantitative research examining potential antecedents, correlates, and outcomes of an athletic identity[6] and qualitative research using interviews to learn how athletes feel about being an athlete and having a disability. Although both lines of research have broadened our understanding of Para sport athletic identity, a gap in the qualitative research pertains to how participating in sport and developing a Para sport athletic identity can help athletes with acquired disabilities adapt to a lost past self and embrace current and future selves. For instance, a lost past self, after acquiring a disability, would be an identity as an able-bodied person. A future self might be a vision and anticipatory thoughts (eg, satisfaction) and feelings (eg, pride) of being a Paralympian in 2 years.

Quantitative Research

Athletic Identity Measurement Scale

Traditionally, athletic identity among athletes with disabilities has been explored using the Athletic Identity Measurement Scale (AIMS[3]), which was developed to assess the athletic portion of a multidimensional self-concept. After examining athletic identity with a sample of nonathletic male and female college students, Brewer and colleagues[10] initially thought the AIMS was unidimensional. However, later research with intercollegiate male soccer players led Brewer and colleagues[3] to conclude that the construct of athletic identity is multidimensional, comprising 3 factors: social identity (the extent to which the athletes identify with their athletic role), exclusivity (the extent to which athletes solely identify as an athlete while minimizing other life roles), and negative affectivity (the extent to which athletes experience negative emotional responses due to injury, retirement, not being able to make a team, and so forth **Fig. 1**). Among able-bodied athletes, this 3-factor structure has generally found support.[3,11] In contrast, there is conflicting evidence that the 3-factor structure is maintained when the AIMS is used among athletes with disabilities.[6,7,12] Martin and colleagues[7] tested the multidimensionality of the AIMS in a sample of adolescent swimmers with

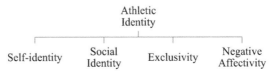

Fig. 1. Four-factor structure of the AIMS.

disabilities and found support for a 4-factor structure. Three of these factors paralleled those found in Brewer colleagues's[10] study (ie, social identity, exclusivity, and negative affectivity); but a fourth factor, labeled self-identity, also emerged. This finding suggests that although athletes with disabilities perceive themselves as legitimate, serious athletes (ie, self-identity), others (ie, social identity) do not. Other researchers using the AIMS among athletes with disabilities report support for a 3-factor structure[12] and even a single-factor structure in a sample of athletes and nonathletes with disabilities.[13] Despite ongoing controversy regarding the appropriate factor structure of the AIMS when used among athletes with disabilities, our knowledge of Para sport athletic identity has advanced.

Correlates of athletic identity

Para sport athletic identity tends to be stronger among men (vs women[14]), older athletes (vs younger athletes[3]), and more elite athletes (vs less elite athletes[15]). A strong athletic identity is also related to various psychological factors. For instance, athletic identity was positively associated with perceived competence in a sample of children with visual impairment,[16] quality of life in a sample of athletes with cerebral palsy,[17] and physical self-confidence in elite Flemish Paralympic athletes.[18] Martin and colleagues[8] examined athletic identity in a sample of adolescent swimmers and found positive correlations between: (1) self-identity and competitiveness, win orientation, and goal orientation; (2) social identity and competitiveness and win orientation; and (3) exclusivity and competitiveness. In general, these findings suggest that athletes with strong athletic identities not only reported achievement-related goals but also the motivation to attain those goals. Of interest, although there are many benefits to identifying with the athlete role, data also suggest that having a strong, exclusive athletic identity can lead to negative physical and psychological outcomes, such as post-injury depression[19] and difficulties transitioning from Para sport to retirement.[20]

Athletic identity and Para sport participation

Athletic identity both predicts and results in Para sport participation. Perrier and colleagues[13] used the Health Action Process Approach (HAPA[21]) model to predict sport participation and found that athletic identity explained additional variance in both intentions to engage in Para sport (3%) and sport participation (3%), beyond the variance accounted for by HAPA constructs (eg, instrumental expectancies, affective expectancies, maintenance self-efficacy). Tasiemski and Brewer,[22] however, found that the current amount of Para sport participation positively predicted athletic identity in addition to other variables (eg, amount of sport participation before spinal cord injury). Findings from both of these studies suggest the relationship between Para sport participation and athletic identity is likely bidirectional in nature and substantiates the value of an athletic identity for people with disabilities.

Qualitative Research

Athletic identity among persons with acquired disability

When researchers ask former able-bodied individuals with acquired permanent disabilities what it means to be an athlete or to have a disability, responses typically fall into 1 of 3 categories: those who identify as an athlete and reject the term *disability*, those who embrace a Para sport athletic identity, and those who do not attempt to develop an athletic identity and likely never will. The following 3 quotes illustrate each of these categories, respectively:

> *I am 100% an athlete, that's who I am, totally. I train hard, I lift weights, I cover hundreds of miles, go out in all weathers...I am an athlete, and want to be seen as one,*

not disabled, but an athlete outright, a winner. I don't even think of myself as disabled. I'm a Paralympian and for me that is all about being an athlete, not disability.[23(p142)]

—Emma

I'm disabled, and that defines me. I'd describe myself as a disabled athlete, in that order. I'm an athlete, for sure. But I'm more than an athlete. I'm first and foremost a disabled person ... Disability isn't just about me, my body, or Paralympic sport, or winning a medal. It's political because when your disabled society often treats you like a second-class citizen, as if being disabled is a horrible, abnormal thing, and we should be grateful for help or pity. That's wrong. It needs challenging, and if I can use my status as an athlete to do this, to bring disability rights to people's attention, then that's as good as any gold medal ... I'm proud to be disabled. I'm disabled and then an athlete, a disabled athlete. Unfortunately I don't see too many of us about in sport like this.[23(p142)]

—Mark

I definitely miss having that kind of body [pause], strength, that comes from being athletic and getting a lot of exercise...I just miss feeling that strength, that athleticism of my body and I'll never, I'll never feel that way again...[24(p112)]

—Alexandra

Various models and theories have been used to explain Para athletes' beliefs about their disability. Some investigators argue that athletes who reject a disability identity do so because they want to avoid being seen as incompetent (a characteristic that is antithetical to being an athlete and having a strong athletic identity) and resist multiple stereotypical and discriminatory labels, such as different, not normal, and less-than relative to able-bodied athletes. Furthermore, the rationale for why some athletes might embrace, rather than refute, a disability identity lies within the affirmative model.[25]

Affirmative model challenges disablist attitudes
The affirmative model is a nontragic view of disability. Instead, it focuses on positive experiences and social identities for people with disabilities. An athlete who possesses an affirmative identity is proud to be disabled and experiences benefits of living with a disability. Embracing an affirmative identity, male and female athletes with congenital and acquired disabilities from Smith and colleagues's[23] study described themselves as a *disabled athlete* as a way to express their pride in being disabled and to challenge negative discourses of disability. This point is illustrated in the aforementioned quote by Mark. Finally, adhering to a narrow definition of what it means to be an athlete and constantly comparing one's past able-bodied self with one's current self with a disability may be responsible for why some persons with acquired permanent disabilities do not identify as athletes.[24]

Athletic identity is correlated with personal and social identities
Persons with congenital disabilities who develop a weak athletic identity, or who do not develop an athletic identity at all, are less likely to adopt active, healthy lifestyles.[5] Paradoxically, one way to develop a strong athletic identity is through sport participation. Pack and colleagues[26] interviewed Paralympic swimmers on their swimming careers, perceptions of self, and impairment and found swimming experiences facilitated athletes' positive personal and social identities and, thus, supported the affirmative model.

A cohort of elite Para athletes reported that being part of a select subculture (Para-lympian) increased their sense of pride, helped normalize their physical appearances to the greater society, and catalyzed personal empowerment in nonsport contexts. These findings are similar to those noted in Swartz and colleagues'[27] study, wherein national and international South African Para athletes with both congenital and ac-quired disabilities described sport participation as a means to repair and redefine the self. These athletes also noted that participating in national and international com-petitions provided them with the opportunity to see themselves differently (abled and physically competent rather than less than and inadequate), to resist disablist atti-tudes (ie, negative views toward people with disabilities), and to feel like they belonged. Tellingly, when comparing themselves with other people with disabilities, athletes at times displayed unhelpful disablist attitudes, describing nonathletes with a disability as "lazy scroungers who are not willing to apply themselves."[23(p5)] From the foregoing, it is clear that athletes with disabilities have complex contradictions regarding the way they describe their participation in competitive sport. More research is needed to explore how athletes with disabilities may be refuting dominant stereo-types about disability.

Para Sport Athletic Identity: Future Research Directions

Identity development in Para athletes with congenital and acquired disabilities

All people, including athletes, face developmental challenges related to identity over the course of a lifetime. Significant life events, such as leaving sport, getting married, becoming a parent, or retiring from a cherished career, are often catalysts for identity changes and challenges. More than 30 years ago, Markus and Nurius[28] remarked that self-concept researchers had neglected to examine possible selves. Ten years ago, King and Hicks[29] reiterated the value of examining how individuals respond to lost selves and potential possible selves. People with disabilities face unique identity chal-lenges related to the lost, current, and possible self, as illustrated next.

A child with a congenital disability (ie, born with a disability such as cerebral palsy) is often viewed, relative to someone acquiring a disability, as having minimal identity adjustment issues. The rationale is that they have always lived with disability, have not known a life without disability, and have not faced sudden and unexpected trauma leading to acquired disability. This reasoning ignores a host of developmental tasks and associated challenges. Cognitive development during adolescence plays a signif-icant role in self-representations and identity development. Contradictions, para-doxes, anomalies, and life surprises are particularly challenging for the developing cognitive abilities of adolescents.[30] For instance, as children with disabilities become more self-aware with age and their social circles widen (eg, they attend school), they become much more aware of how their disability differentiates them from nondisabled children. Via increased social comparison processes, they become increasingly cognizant of how their physical disability (eg, spasticity from cerebral palsy) may influ-ence physical capabilities and success in sport. At the same time, they may also realize how the social (eg, teasing) and built (eg, steep stairs) environments also influ-ence their quality of life. This gradually increasing awareness of how their impairment, and society's reaction to their impairment, may result in a narrowing of their vision for future possible selves. In brief, a congenital disability does not make someone immune from disability-related identity challenges.

For individuals with acquired permanent disabilities, the same set of challenges can occur overnight, rather than gradually, particularly in the case of a traumatic event (eg, car accident). There is an additional challenge children with acquired disability face: in addition to contemplating possible future selves (eg, Paralympian) and how the number of possibilities may now be narrowed, an important past self (or selves) may be seen as suddenly and irrevocably lost (eg, able-bodied runner) and mourned. The quote appearing next by Levins and colleagues,[31] although not expressed in the possible-selves jargon, expresses the identity-related challenges experienced when a disability is acquired.

Rebuilding the embodied self after such a disruption is an extremely difficult task. A person's self-image has been developed over a lifetime in relation to particular social ideas and in terms of a body with certain skills, abilities and appearances. To confront, and to gradually let go of, those aspects of self-identity that now can never be consummated is the most difficult task of rehabilitation.[31(p506)]

In one of the few studies done from the possible-selves paradigm, Perrier and colleagues[13] reported that participants with strong postinjury athletic identities were able to focus on a present and future self and did not ruminate about lost distant past selves. Coaches, fellow athletes, and sport-focused goals (eg, training goals) were important supports for developing athletic identities after injury. Other participants ruled out possible future athletic selves because they equated being an athlete with being able bodied. Perrier and colleagues[13] suggested that participants' former able-bodied functional abilities and current limitations jointly conspired to produce a mindset that being an athlete and having an athletic identity was impossible for someone with a disability.

Self- and society-imposed definitions of what it means to be an athlete can impact athletic identity and the possibility of an athletic future self after injury, sometimes negatively. For instance, a former elite athlete reentered sport but failed to recapture a past athletic identity, as expressed next.[32]

I used to be very coordinated and my body would work in poetry to do things I wanted to do... now I spend most of my time trying not to fall on my face... Playing sports is not graceful and it is not poetic and beautiful. It is ugly...[32(p12)]

Some athletes, as the preceding quote captures, have no future self that they aspire to. After injury, even the present self can be empty of meaningful content and motivation, a nonidentity, as Sparkes and Smith[33] illustrate:

Life moves on without me, but, then, I just survive. I don't have ambitions or a future. ... I don't do anything of importance. ... Nothing [five-second pause]. A void, just existing. Then, well, life has stopped. Just, I don't know. Exist in the present, no tomorrow, nothing.[33(p311)]

The prior two quotes illustrate what are likely to be unsurprising, predictable perspectives to readers, met without alarm or disbelief. Indeed, an active literature suggests that many able-bodied adults assume (incorrectly) that most people with disabilities have a poor quality of life.[34,35] The notion that individuals with disabilities can have a good to excellent quality of life is grounded in our poor emotional forecasting ability[35] and an underestimation of our ability to cope with negative events.[36] Poor emotional forecasting is the idea that people often assume that potential negative future events, such as acquiring a disability, will be more devastating than it eventually turns out to be. Similarly, people also overestimate how good they think a positive future event (eg, winning a sporting event) will make them feel. Part of the dynamic involved in poor emotional forecasting is that people underestimate their coping skills and their ability to find meaning in other areas of life. Readers might also be surprised that people experiencing ostensibly tragic events (eg, losing the ability to walk) can gain in maturity and life quality[29] as exemplified in narrative identity research, discussed next.

Narrative identity

Narrative identity is a growing and evolving story of one's life that combines the past, present, and future and helps provide coherence, meaning, and stability.[30] Germane to the current review, McAdams and McLean[30] have found that individuals who find meaning in adversity (eg, acquiring a disability) experience greater well-being compared with individuals who struggle with finding meaning in adversity. King and Hicks[29] link narrative identity to both maturity and personal growth. Maturity is reflected in 2 distinct elements: subjective well-being and ego development. They argue that people experiencing lost possible selves (eg, acquiring a disability) who can acknowledge the loss, resist being emotionally consumed by it and focus on a best future possible self can be happy. King and Hicks[29] also suggest that ego development is facilitated by acknowledging loss and the ability to richly articulate past valued lost goals. An interesting paradox is hinted at the following: maturity is facilitated by developing a detailed and complex understanding of a lost self but at the same time an absence of dwelling on that loss. Preliminary research with gay individuals and divorced women have provided support for the aforementioned premises.[37,38] Additionally, King and Hicks[29] note that a prominent coping mechanism that facilitated ego development and subjective well-being was humor. A second mechanism is a sense of compassion for others and the lost possible self. A final perspective among mature individuals able to fully know and acknowledge a lost self without dwelling on it was gratitude. Other capacities that seem to be associated with personal growth are the ability to acknowledge surprise (ie, we cannot always predict life events), a sense of humility (ie, acknowledging one's inadequacies), and courage.[29]

The role of sport and developing a Para sport athletic identity as an important current and future possible self, after acquiring a disability, has rarely been investigated. A recent review of narrative and discursive research in athletic identity indicated only 2 studies in disability sport.[39] In one study, Sparkes and Smith[40] found that 4 men who acquired a spinal cord injury playing rugby struggled to let go of a past athletic identity that was inextricably linked to a masculine identity. All 4 men focused on obtaining a restored self or their past able-bodied self as exemplified next:

> I can't do any of those things I used to really enjoy, like work, play rugby, football, pop out for a drink. That is why I want my old life back. This is not me." "I hate being quadriplegic and I am still trying for a cure. I still see myself as able bodied...[40(p271)]

Sparkes and Smith[40] examined athletes struggling to develop future possible selves. Future research might consider examining athletes with disabilities who have embraced current and future selves and if the factors elucidated by King and Hicks,[29] such as compassion, humility, and courage, helped them adapt to a lost past self and embrace current and future selves. Identity construction and the value of understanding the ramifications of a disability sport athletic identity does not end when sport ends as discussed next.

Identity implications of leaving sport

Yeah. I don't think I would have retired unless I had a job. Cause we had a baby so I wouldn't have been able to—I would have carried on doing sport until I had a job or income so that I could retire.... When I was competing I was quite well paid.... If you're in that position it is quite difficult to retire. (Retired Paralympian[41]).

The aforementioned quote is unique to disability sport; it suggests that an athlete might continue playing sport because of financial reasons (well-paying career), despite their desire to retire. The quote also reflects the professionalization of elite-level disability sport for selected elite-level Paralympians while simultaneously pointing the way to a unique research goal: what happens to athletic identity when athletes continue to play but psychologically disengage? One hint of the ramifications of disinvesting in an athletic identity while still performing can be found in the work of Martin and Ridler,[42] who examined the performance of Para World Championship swimmers stratified by retirement status (ie, retiring for sure, will retire in the future, or contemplating but unsure of retirement). A full 45% of Para swimmers who did not plan to retire finished within 1 second of their swimming time goal. Only 17% of Para swimmers considering retiring were within 1 second of their goal. Those considering retiring also had lower athletic identities compared with those who did not plan to retire. Of note, the sample was quite small ($N = 17$), so certainly caution is in order when considering results. Nonetheless, one might speculate that athletes naturally disinvested in their athletic identities in order to adjust to postsport life whereby sport plays a much smaller role. At the same, it is conceivable that disinvesting in athletic identity preceded poorer performance (eg, resulted in less effective training and preparation).[42] A focus on postsport life may also have contributed to less-than-ideal performance preparation. The aforementioned musings clearly need rigorous investigation.

SUMMARY

In summary, 3 conclusions are apparent. First, athletes with disabilities describe developing a Para sport athletic identity in 2 mutually exclusive ways. Some athletes reject a Para sport athletic identity because they view Para sport and a Para sport identity in a negative light. Other athletes embrace Para sport and see the various benefits (eg, renewed purpose in life) associated with it and with becoming an athlete and adopting a Para sport athletic identity. Second, quantitative findings on Para sport athletic identity suggest that possessing a strong athletic identity can have both positive and negative effects. One positive effect is increased self-esteem, whereas a negative effect might be depression when unable to participate in sport because of an injury. Qualitative findings reveal that sport participation serves as a catalyst for athletes with disabilities to develop positive identities and to challenge people who might marginalize them by dismissing their engagement in Para sport. Third, using narrative identity to explore athletes with acquired disabilities' perceptions of past, present, and future selves in sport holds promise as a future research line. For example, identifying capacities (eg, compassion, courage) of athletes with acquired disabilities who acknowledge a past characterized by loss, but who are also deeply engaged in their present and future selves, can help guide intervention work. Another avenue for future research is the need for researchers to better understand athletes who continue to participate in sport but are, to some extent, psychologically disengaged.

REFERENCES

1. Wickman K. "I do not compete in disability": how wheelchair athletes challenge the discourse of able-ism through action and resistance. Eur J Sport Sci 2007; 4:151–67.
2. Carver C, Reyonlds S, Scheier M. The possible selves of optimists and pessimists. J Res Pers 1994;28:131–41.
3. Brewer B, Van Raalte J, Linder D. Athletic identity: Hercules' muscles or Achilles heel? Int J Sport Psychol 1993;24:237–54.
4. Martin J. Psychological considerations for Paralympic athletes. In: Acevedo EO, editor. Oxford encyclopedia of sport, exercise, and performance psychology. New York: Oxford University Press; 2017. p. 99–114.

5. Martin J. Disability, sport, & psychological well-being. In: Horn TS, Smith AL, editors. Advances in sport and exercise psychology. 4th edition. Champaign (IL): Human Kinetics; 2017. p. 244–65.

6. Martin J, Eklund R, Adams-Mushett C. Factor structure of the athletic identity measurement scale with athletes with disabilities. Adapt Phys Activ Q 1997;14: 74–82.

7. Martin J, Mushett C, Eklund R. Factor structure of the Athletic Identity Measurement Scale with adolescent swimmers with disabilities. Brazilian Journal of Adapted Physical Education Research 1994;1:87–99.

8. Martin J, Mushett C, Smith K. Athletic identity and sport orientation of adolescent swimmers with disabilities. Adapt Phys Activ Q 1995;12:113–23.

9. Horton R, Mack D. Athletic identity in marathon runners: functional focus or dysfunctional commitment? J Sport Behav 2000;23:101–19.

10. Brewer B, Boin P, Petitpas A. Dimensions of athletic identity. Paper presented at: American Psychological Association annual conference. Toronto (Canada), August 8–13, 1993.

11. Hale B, James B, Stambulova N. Determining the dimensionality of athletic identity: a 'Herculean' cross-cultural undertaking. Int J Sport Psychol 1999;30:83–100.

12. Groff D, Zabriskie R. An exploratory study of athletic identity among elite alpine skiers with physical disabilities: issues of measurement and design. J Sport Behav 2006;29:126–41.

13. Perrier M, Sweet S, Strachan S, et al. I act, therefore I am: athletic identity and the health action process approach predict sport participation among individuals with acquired physical disabilities. Psychol Sport Exerc 2012;13:713–20.

14. Brewer B, Cornelius A. Norms and factorial invariance of the athletic identity measurement scale. Academic Athletic Journal 2001;16:103–13.

15. Tasiemski T, Kennedy P, Gardner B, et al. Athletic identity and sports participation in people with spinal cord injury. Adapt Phys Activ Q 2004;21:364–78.

16. Shapiro D. Athletic identity and perceived competence in children with visual impairments. Palaestra 2007;19:6–7.

17. Groff D, Lundberg N, Zabriskie R. Influence of adapted sport on quality of life: perceptions of athletes with cerebral palsy. Disabil Rehabil 2009;31:318–26.

18. Van de Vliet P, Van Biesen D, Vanlandewijck Y. Athletic identity and self-esteem in Flemish athletes with a disability. European Journal of Adapted Physical Activity 2008;1:9–21.

19. Brewer B. Self-identity and specific vulnerability to depressed mood. J Pers 2008; 61:343–64.

20. Grove J, Lavallee D, Gordon S. Coping with retirement from sport: the influence of athletic identity. J Appl Soc Psychol 1997;9:191–203.

21. Schwarzer R. Self-efficacy in the adoption and maintenance of health behaviors: theoretical approaches and a new model. In: Schwarzer R, editor. Self-efficacy: thought control of action. Washington, DC: Hemisphere; 1992. p. 217–42.

22. Tasiemski T, Brewer B. Athletic identity, sport participation, and psychological adjustment in people with spinal cord injury. Adapt Phys Activ Q 2011;28:233–50.

23. Smith B, Bundo A, Best M. Disability sport and activist identities: a qualitative study of narratives of activism among elite athletes with impairment. Psychol Sport Exerc 2016;26:139–48.

24. Perrier M, Smith B, Strachan S, et al. Narratives of athletic identity after acquiring a permanent physical disability. Adapt Phys Activ Q 2014;31:106–24.

25. Swain J, French S. Toward an affirmation model of disability. Disabil Soc 2000;15: 569–82.

26. Pack S, Kelly S, Arvinen-Barrow M. "I think I became a swimmer rather than just someone with a disability swimming up and down:" Paralympic athletes' perceptions of self and identity development. Disabil Rehabil 2017;39(20):2063–70.

27. Swartz L, Bantjes J, Knight B, et al. "They don't understand that we also exist:" South African participants in competitive disability sport and the politics of identity. Disabil Rehabil 2018;40(1):35–41.

28. Markus H, Nurius P. Possible selves. Am Psychol 1986;41:954–69.

29. King L, Hicks J. Whatever happened to "what might have been?": regrets, happiness, and maturity. Am Psychol 2007;62:625–36.

30. McAdams D, McLean K. Narrative identity. Curr Dir Psychol Sci 2013;22:233–8.

31. Levins S, Redenbach D, Dyck I. Individual and societal influences on participation in physical activity following spinal cord injury: a qualitative study. Phys Ther 2004;84:496–509.

32. Crawford J, Gayman A, Tracey J. An examination of post-traumatic growth in Canadian and American ParaSport athletes with acquired spinal cord injury. Psychol Sport Exerc 2014;15:399–406.

33. Sparkes A, Smith B. Men, sport, spinal cord injury and narrative time. Qual Res 2002;3:295–320.

34. Albrecht G, Devlieger P. The disability paradox: high quality of life against all odds. Soc Sci Med 1999;48:977–88.

35. Ubel P, Loewenstein G, Schwarz N, et al. Misimagining the unimaginable: the disability paradox and health care decision making. Health Psychol 2005;24: S57–62.

36. Wilson T, Gilbert D. Affective forecasting knowing what to want. Curr Dir Psychol Sci 2005;14:131–4.

37. King L, Raspin C. Lost and found possible selves, subjective well-being, and ego development in divorced women. J Pers 2004;72:603–32.

38. King L, Smith N. Gay and straight possible selves: goals, identity, subjective well-being, and personality development. J Pers 2004;72:967–94.

39. Ronkainen N, Kavoura A, Ryba T. Narrative and discursive perspectives on athletic identity: past, present, and future. Psychol Sport Exerc 2016;27:128–37.

40. Sparkes A, Smith B. Sport, spinal cord injury, embodied masculinities, and the dilemmas of narrative identity. Men Masc 2003;4:258–85.

41. Project PRISM. Para-athlete retirement: insights, support and management. Available at: http://www.lboro.ac.uk/media/wwwlboroacuk/content/peterharrisoncentre/downloads/resources/PRISM%20Summary%20(Final%20copy).pdf. Accessed June 14, 2017.

42. Martin L, Ridler G. The impact of retirement status on athletic identity and performance expectations: a study of Paralympic swimmers at a major international competition. In: Abstracts of the 28th International Congress of Applied Psychology. International Association of Applied Psychology (IAAP). Paris (France), July 8–13, 2014.

The Social Empowerment of Difference

The Potential Influence of Para sport

Carla Filomena Silva, BA, BSc, MSc, PhD[a],
P. David Howe, BSc, MA, PhD[b],*

KEYWORDS

• Ableism • Difference • Disability studies • Empowerment • Para sport

KEY POINTS

• The recognition, acceptance, and valuing of difference within Para sport cultures must naturally drive the emergence of new sports and sporting ethos that are more attuned with this attitude and understanding.

• In attempting to critically educate wider society on the value of difference and pluralism, Para sport culture needs to proactively promote the participation of all people with disabilities.

• Fostering an empowering understanding of the difference associated with disability demands increased participation of people with disabilities as the active creators of Para sport cultures, rather than as mere recipients of services for them.

• All athletes, including athletes with impairments, should be considered differently abled, rather than disabled, because neither difference nor disability are absolute categories.

INTRODUCTION

A year after the 2012 London Paralympic Games, the *Guardian* newspaper brought to public attention the failure of Paralympic Games in changing how society views so-called disabled people, "British Paralympians' success in 2012 brought celebrity status but has done little for the daily life of the disability community."[1] This assertion is hardly surprising; despite claims made by the International Paralympic Committee (IPC) regarding the empowering potential of sport, which have mostly have been unsubstantiated.[2–4] It is, of course, extremely difficult to evaluate to what extent sport events ignite social change, let alone the potential of empowerment, due to both conceptual and methodological weaknesses. Conceptually, it is difficult to clearly define

Disclosure Statement: The authors have nothing to disclose.
a Social Science of Sport, School of Science and Technology, Nottingham Trent University, Nottingham NG1 4FQ, UK; b Social Anthropology of Sport, School of Sport Exercise and Health Science, Loughborough University, Loughborough LE11 3JE, UK
* Corresponding author.
E-mail address: p.d.howe@lboro.ac.uk

Phys Med Rehabil Clin N Am 29 (2018) 397–408
https://doi.org/10.1016/j.pmr.2018.01.009
1047-9651/18/Crown Copyright © 2018 Published by Elsevier Inc. All rights reserved.

pmr.theclinics.com

the sphere of influence of mega sport events and to theoretically support the causal relationship with social change. Methodologically, the difficulty lies in defining indicators of empowerment, as well as in using reliable methods to measure the extent of those outcomes, asserting a relation of causality between them.[5,6]

The potential of sport for social good is limited because the scope of interventions and evaluations fail to consider the multidimensional nature of social exclusion, the structural cause of systemic systems of social inequality.[7] Thus, it is very rare that significant social change can be correlated with specific sport events or programs in isolation from concerted interventions in other dimensions of social life, such as welfare, employment, or education.[8] As such, to assume that the Paralympic Games should be any different is misguided. Although the authors believe in the social power of sport, the uncritical view that positive social change is intrinsic to sport detracts from realizing this potential. Believing in the magical power of sport prevents the active drive toward positive change in the form of well-designed, purposeful action that effectively reduces the social exclusion of people identified as socially marginal, such as participants in Para sports. Para sport culture refers to the practice community[9] of disability sport, from the grassroots to high-performance levels, which engages in sport as governed by the rules and regulations of the IPC.[10] We believe that to effect sustainable positive social change, it must be initiated within the grassroots of Para sport culture if the rhetoric of the IPC around empowerment is to be achievable.

This article draws on disability studies literature to identify the most significant sources of disability exclusion and discrimination, and discusses to what extent Para sport culture replicates or challenges this status quo. It examines whether Para sport culture has the potential to truly contribute to the social empowerment not only of athletes but of people with disabilities more generally. Central to this reflection, should be a recognition, acceptance, and valorization of difference. The focus on difference is critical in any effort to foster the social emancipation of groups identified as socially marginal because the source of all discrimination lies in the social cultural meanings ascribed to difference. In alignment with Iris Young[11(p163)], in our vision, a good society does not eliminate or transcend group difference. Rather, there is equality among socially and culturally differentiated groups who mutually respect each other and affirm each other in their differences.

The goal of this article is to urge actors to engage with Para sport culture critically and reflect on their own system of beliefs and associated practices, searching for signs of engrained discrimination. This difficult process demands a willingness to suspend old beliefs and be open to self-appraisal, criticism, and pluralist democratic discussion within its own boundaries. It is simply impossible for an institution, such as the IPC, to promote positive change in the lives of people with disabilities without addressing its own responsibility in the perpetuation of their social disadvantage. After recognizing the existence of cultural traits that work against the IPCs self-proclaimed goal of empowerment, it is essential to promote and enact the necessary changes in ideologies and practices so that these are more attuned to achieving this aim for all people with disabilities. We hope this work offers useful guidance to initiate this process of self-reflection and regeneration.

Ableism is the primary source of social disadvantage for people with disabilities. Because the process of dismantling ableism presupposes a reconceptualization of difference, this article draws on various authors' theorization of difference to explore some of the ways in which Para sport culture can promote this emancipatory shift.

This article concludes with recognition of the challenge that our suggestion to invest in difference as a positive and fundamental tenet of Para sport identity imposes on the IPC and the whole Para sport community. This challenge, using Minow's[12] term "dilemma of difference," can be overcome by deconstructing its dilemmatic nature. Thus, this article constitutes an explicit invitation for Para sport culture to courageously embrace a politics of difference[11] as an essential condition to enhance the lives of their constituency and positively affect society more broadly.

THE HEGEMONIC POWER OF ABLEIST NORMS

If sporting cultures are to socially emancipate athletes and people with disabilities, this influence will only be significant and long-lasting if it challenges the systemic sources of oppression causing social oppression. Disability studies illuminate ideology as the most essential and harmful source of discrimination toward people with disabilities. One of the founding fathers of disability studies, Michael Oliver[13(p44)] suggests that:

> *The hegemony that defines disability in capitalist society is constituted by the organic ideology of individualism, the arbitrary ideologies of medicalisation underpinning social intervention and personal tragedy theory underpinning much social policy.*

In reaction against the dominance of an individualistic, medicalized view of disability, disability scholars and activists started, in the last quarter of the twentieth century, to defend a social understanding of disability, diverting from understanding it as an individual problem to illuminating the multiple ways in which social structures and environments create avoidable disadvantage and exclude people who experience disability.[14] In this sense, disability is more the product of social injustice than the consequences of a biological impairment. This understanding became known as the social model of disability. Within this model, the ideology of disablism, "a set of assumptions (conscious or unconscious) and practices that promote the differential or unequal treatment of people because of actual or presumed disabilities"[15(p4)] has been instrumental in shifting the so-called disability problem from the individual impairment to the inadequate social environment. This concept has been instrumental in the politicization of disability and, concomitantly, in the creation and implementation of legislation and social policies with visible impact on the lives of people with disabilities. Notwithstanding, although disablism illuminates the social plight of people with impairments, the concept has limitations: it fails to challenge the assumption of disability experience as a problem and, crucially, it fails to identify the primary location of disability oppression in the engrained, naturalized belief in able-bodiedness as the only viable and valid way of being fully human. From that point of view, "impairment or disability (irrespective of 'type') is inherently negative and should the opportunity present itself, be ameliorated, cured or indeed, eliminated!"[15(p5)] In essence, ableism is:

> *A network of beliefs, processes and practices that produce a particular kind of self and body (the corporal standard) that is projected as the perfect, species-typical and essential and fully human. Disability then is cast as a diminished state of being human.[15(p44)]*

By focusing solely on the attenuation of the manifestation of disablism (eg, limited opportunities for participation in sport) and neglecting its structural causes (eg, ableism), disability advocates reinforce their position as marginal, undermining their proactive role as co-creators of social realities. Thus, disablist perspectives, despite being well-intentioned, continue to generate social responses to disability that attempt to determine what can be done for the disabled, the so-called Other. Within this paradigm, social responses and interventionist strategies, although important, are not sufficient to foster social emancipation because they only mask the symptoms of a harmful social malady, the ideology that being able is the only valuable way of being.

In sporting contexts, for instance, a supposedly emancipatory response to disablism is to expand access to the sporting activities that are highly regarded by the able-bodied world, including individual sports, such as athletics and swimming, and team sports, such as basketball. These are designed in the image of a normalized view of athletic bodies. The problem is, against the hegemonic power of this able-bodied ideal of athleticism, the disabled athletic body will continue to be seen as lacking elite sporting prowess, except for those individuals seen as supercrips, who are highly functioning athletes who have undergone the process of cyborgification.[16–18] The treatment of disabled athletes who cannot go through the process of cyborgification and be transformed into supercrips is not at all surprising because "The level of literacy about disability is so low as to be non-existent, and the ideology of ability is so much a part of every action, thought, judgment, and intention, that its hold on us is difficult to root out."[19(p9)] It is not surprising that the athletes whose impairments situate them farther from the able-bodied norm[20] receive less support, recognition, and media attention, and seem to be intentionally excluded from the Paralympics.[16,18] In other words, in fighting disablism, emancipation and empowerment in Para sport translates to emulation of able-bodiedness[15,21] and encourages athletes to hide their disability and pass as normal.[19,22] It equates with the ability to overcome one's impairment and display able-like qualities and to be successful per normal standards; for instance, athletes who equal or outperform Olympic athletes.[23]

In contrast to fighting ableism, empowerment in Para sport reformulates the parameters of success from the perspective that sporting performances by impaired bodies are intrinsically valid, without the need for comparative assessments with mainstream sport. Para sport culture is not a paradox and, therefore, success and respect are granted to both the athlete who runs a specific distance in a time comparable to an able-bodied athlete and the bocce player whose skills of precision, focus, and willpower transcends her or his competitors.

It is fundamental to unveil the mechanisms and expressions of this ideology of ableism and to critically examine them, acknowledging their harmful effects, before advancing to designing emancipatory strategies. It is absolutely essential for the Para sport community to introspectively examine the multiple ways in which it fails to challenge ableism or, even worse, reinforces it. By anchoring this critical reflection of its emancipatory potential in the concept of ableism, Para sport cultures can challenge oppression at its root by stimulating a new, more positive, and realistic social and cultural understanding of the lives of people with impairments.

For Para sport culture to challenge ableism, it is important to consider that this ideological perspective is maintained essentially by the working of 2 elements: first, "the notion of the normative (and normate individual) and secondly, the enforcement of a constitutional divide between perfected naturalised humanity and the aberrant, the unthinkable, quasi human hybrid and therefore non-human."[15(p6)] Both mechanisms are as powerful as they are invisible. The notion of the normative leads to an authoritative naturalized acceptance of able-bodiedness. Also, the divide between able or disabled as an ontological, material, and sentient dichotomy enforces an internalized surveillance system to which almost all respond with attempts to conform to the hegemonic norm so that they may belong to the able-bodied world in a process of "compulsory able-bodiedness."[24(p93)] As it stands, because the able-bodied norm is, for many people, unattainable, challenging this ideology will result in the liberation not only of the disabled minority but of all citizens. Alongside other authors,[11,25] we propose that the best way to challenge the hegemonic power of ableism is to recognise, accept, and value impairment and the experience of disability as valid and valuable expressions of humanness; that is, to celebrate the merit inherent in difference as an enrichment of humanness.

Thus, the core of the fight against ableism is located in the concept of difference. Difference entails a disruptive power that ought to be exploited by Para sport culture if its political influence is to be exercised. As Young[11(p167)] states, "the assertion of a positive sense of group differences provides a standpoint from which to criticize prevailing institutions and norms." Furthermore, the dissolution of the constitutional divide between the able majority (Us) and the disabled minority (Them) demands a fluid understanding of difference "not as absolute otherness"[11(p98)] but as the "relatedness of things with more or less similarity in a multiplicity of possible respects."[11(p99)] In this sense, all athletes (including athletes with impairments) may be considered "differently abled"[26(pxiii)] rather than disabled because neither difference nor disability are absolute categories. Can Para sport culture drive this cultural shift?

WHY DIFFERENCE MUST MATTER IN PARA SPORTS

It is now established that ableism is the most important cause of oppression and inequality of opportunities for people identified as disabled. It then follows that a positive account of the difference expressed in Para sport culture holds the power to destabilize the core precepts of ableism and the power of the normative, and to dilute the constitutional divide between abled and disabled. The authors assert that a reflexive and productive management of difference within and by the Para sport community is paramount to counteracting ableism. We draw on Hall,[27] Young,[11] and Minow[12] and their theories of difference.

Perspectives on difference from Hall[27] derive from linguistics and are intrinsically connected to the way cultures are structured. He states, "difference matters because it is essential to meaning; without it, meaning could not exist,"[27(p225)] and this meaning arises from the interpreted differences between oppositions (white or black; day or night; feminine or masculine). The problem is that binary oppositions of this type oversimplify and reduce the complexity of reality, often with harmful consequences. For instance, by creating the constitutional divide between Us (able) and Them (disabled), essentializes and dichotomizes difference: "Difference, as the relatedness of things with more or less similarity in a multiplicity of possible respects, here congeals as the binary opposition a/not-a."[11(p99)] An individual is either abled or disabled.

Another harmful feature of these dichotomies is that they are seldom neutral, with the first side of the binary being "elevated over the second, because it designates the unified, the self-identical, whereas the second side lies outside the unified as the chaotic, unformed, transforming, that always threatens to cross the border and break up the unity of the good."[11(p99)] These categories of meaning usually reflect existent social hierarchies. In this sense, an able-bodied dominant majority defines disability in the same way that blackness is defined by the dominant white people. The antidote for these harmful effects is to counteract the understanding of difference as essential and absolute by exposing its relational nature. In other words, "making the taken-for-granted character of normalcy visible and thus open to both exploration and change."[28(p6)] This shift implies challenging the need for binary oppositions by proposing an understanding of difference as value-neutral, fluid, nuanced, continuous, and (culturally and historically) contingent. In so doing, it is recognized that difference solely names the differently similar or similarly different, denying the possibility of absolute differences between human beings. When the difference that disability makes is understood in these terms, athletes with disabilities will be less reluctant to expose and accept their (partial) difference, and actors within sport communities (including the public) will be less quick to judge and stigmatize them. These athletes will cease to be the Other; that is, difference is always relational, a product of a purposeful comparative exercise based on the selection of selected traits rather than an essential attribute.[12] How can this shift in perspective be practiced and showcased by Para sport communities?

Hall[27] first highlights that difference is relational rather than absolute. When Para sports were being developed, it was organized by impairment-specific groups. The International Organisations of Sport for the Disabled (IOSDs) each developed their own classification systems designed specifically to create a level playing field for competition.[16,29] At this point in its development, Para sport culture was illuminating medical differences between groups of people with impairment. With the advent of the IPC in 1989, there was a push toward a functional classification system, which is still used in the sport of swimming.[30] The benefit of this system is that it takes bodies with distinctive impairments and groups them together for competition based on their degree of function in the swimming pool. Although the IOSDs classification systems used in the sport of swimming explicitly highlight difference between impairment groups as essential, the IPC functional classification systems acknowledge the similarity between impairment groups as they relate to swimming proficiency, therefore showcasing the relational character of difference. Thus, the possession of different types of impairments may not constitute a fundamental, absolute difference between athletes, in the same way it does not constitute an absolute difference between people with and without impairments.

The second linguistic theoretic perspective closely links with the previous by emphasizing the dialogical character of difference: "we need 'difference' because we can only construct meaning through a dialogue with the 'Other'"[27(p225)] and so "The 'Other', in other words, is essential to meaning."[27(p225)] Because the meaning of difference is necessarily dialogic, this opens way to its renegotiation, an opportunity to "enter a struggle over meaning."[27(p225)]

Ableism reinforces its cultural dominance through a process of widespread dissemination of the able-bodied experience and culture as a universal perspective, representative of all humanity. This is accomplished by rendering the difference of disability experiences invisible, silencing the perspective of this minority, and compromising the dialogic nature of difference. Yet, as Hall[27] defends, the meaning of difference can be challenged, negotiated, and reconstructed. Its meaning is never fully fixed nor does it belong to a specific group; thus the negotiation of what disability means is a never-ending cultural endeavor to be performed dialogically by a multiplicity of voices. From this follows that ableist views of disability as inferior and deviant do not have to be passively accepted.

Para sport culture is highly instrumental in providing an environment in which the meanings of ability and disability, and concomitantly of athleticism, can be negotiated as long as it allows for the free expression of heterogeneity of voices, within a culture of democratic pluralism. However, as Hahn[21] stresses, Para sports can serve to emulate able-bodiedness rather than to subvert it. With this caveat in mind, we prefer to emphasize the potential for Para sports to become an active agent in the dialogic process of constructing difference associated with disability. How and why can Para sport culture step up to this role?

Collectively, the Para sport community must cultivate an ethos of multicultural dialogue, open to alternative views and creativity. To do so in a socially emancipatory manner, it must embrace the heterogeneity of the public it proclaims to serve. That is, it must represent the diversity of human embodiment. Given the marginal position of athletes with high support needs and the tendency to exclude them from the Paralympic Games,[18] special attention must be granted to the expansion and promotion of opportunities for these athletes. There also must be increased awareness of the additional disadvantage faced by women, particular ethnicities, lower social economic classes, and those of marginal sexualities, and to the possible amplifying effects of the intersection of these categories. For real opportunities, the range of obstacles that particular groups within Para sports may face must be considered. To subvert the dominant and universalizing ableist discourse, Para sport culture needs to value and embrace diversity of voices. The potential to negotiate dominant views of difference depends on the opportunities granted to the oppressed minority to participate and disseminate counter-dominant views. Currently, Para sports are still governed and managed mostly by nondisabled people for the disabled, perpetuating dependency and powerlessness.[31,32] This power imbalance within Para sports needs to be urgently addressed.

Third, Hall[27] presents an anthropological account of difference as essential in the making of cultures. He suggests "[t]he argument here is that culture depends on giving things meaning by assigning them to different position within a classificatory system. The marking of 'difference' is thus the basis of that symbolic order, which we call culture."[27(p226)] All cultures are framed within symbolic boundaries that promote stability by keeping the defined categories pure. Hall[27] continues, "Stable cultures require things to stay in their appointed place."[27(p226)] Although these symbolic boundaries are responsible for stigmatizing and expelling what does not fit, "it also makes 'difference' powerful ... threatening to cultural order."[27(p226)] As such, the ideology of ableism is the symbolic boundary that defines disability as deviance.

The IPC and Para sport culture more generally celebrate difference in part because it makes the general public feel uneasy. The United Kingdom's Channel 4 campaign of Paralympics awareness entitled "Freaks of Nature," which includes the documentary "Inside Incredible Athletes," is an exemplar of this because they were designed to celebrate and exacerbate the difference associated with Para sport bodies. Media campaigns such as these are designed to draw the able public toward attending the Paralympic Games, which is the flagship event of Para sports. Jönsson[33(p230)] has suggested "that describing [the] Paralympics as a 'freak show' reinforced the Paralympic identity, an identity that in some ways can be used as a political weapon against ableist politics." Although some scholars criticized the use of this theme because of the able–disabled dichotomy it reinforces,[34,35] we concur with Bogdan[36(pxi)] that, "Freak is not a quality that belongs to the person on display. It is something we created; a perspective, a set of practices—a social construction." In this way, the celebration of Paralympians as freaks is designed to get the public to engage with the Paralympic Games and Para sport more generally and can be used to subvert the cultural premises that created those same images, enacting a form of transgressive appropriation.[19]

Finally, Hall[27(p227)] emphasizes the psychoanalytical role that difference plays in the constitution of the Self: "Our subjectivities are formed through this troubled, never-completed, unconscious dialogue with-this internalisation of - the 'Other'." At the individual level, participation in Para sports can function as a critical pedagogy. Ethnographic research[37] within a national sitting volleyball community has shown how participation in the sport was the catalyst for people with acquired and congenital impairments to progress from a state of "internalised ableism" to a state of "double consciousness," "when the oppressed subject refuses to coincide with these devalued ... visions of herself or himself."[11(p60)] An interviewee from sitting volleyball suggested, "When I meet people and I tell them what I have done, they say: 'Oh, you're such an inspiration!' Why am I an inspiration? Why? Because I have a metal leg? Why does that make me an inspiration? I am just doing something that I class as normal. I don't class myself as being disabled because I can do everything you can."

This positive subjectivity stems from the confrontation with alternative perspectives on disability. Another sitting volleyball athlete suggested, "Seeing so many people with so many disabilities, how different people moved around was a massive turning point for me … I remember sitting, watching a man, a whole match watching just one man that had a similar disability to mine. And just seeing how he moved and began to think, if he can do that, I can also do it. It was amazing!"[37(p142)]

As a nonexclusionary community, sitting volleyball also presents the opportunity for people with and without impairments to interact and collaborate in a context of performative play; that is, it provides the opportunity for both the able and the disabled to construct their selves in differentiation to an Other. The outcome of this can be a more enlightened account of the Other as differently abled rather than absolutely different. One nonimpaired player reflected, "It makes you think about your own life and how fast you can go from being able bodied to disabled. On the other hand, these people are not unhappy … If you become disabled, you can still have a good life. My initial apprehension came from not knowing. Not being confronted with that before."[37(p143)]

This psychoanalytical quality of difference can be instrumental in emphasizing the relevance of empathy in the acceptance of difference; that is, the ability to understand and feel what it is to be the Other, from their perspective, while keeping a clear sense of one's own distinctive self.[38] Para sport culture can promote this empathetic understanding if it resists the temptation to enclose itself in disability ghettos and harnesses its power toward the dissolution of the divide between the able and the disabled.

All these perspectives collude to illuminate the productive power of difference as a political mechanism through Para sports. We agree with Hall[27] that the political power of difference should welcome the participation of multiple and divergent voices; in this case, the able and the disabled. Therefore, we reject the idea that the empowerment potential of Para sports is solely predicated on the activism of athletes and people with disabilities, while interdicting the involvement of nondisabled people. Traditional identity politics is paradoxic in the sense that it incurs the same exclusionary and essentializing practices that led to marginalization. If the empowerment potential of Para sport culture is to be actualized through the acknowledgment, valuing, and acceptance of difference, the sporting community itself ought to embody this celebration of difference.

THE CHALLENGE DIFFERENCE IMPOSES ON PARA SPORTS

What we propose is, no doubt, a daring enterprise. The ideology of ableism and the practices that sustain it continuously reinforce and each other, in a continuous symbiosis that is very difficult to break. To realize its empowerment mission, Para sport culture faces a serious challenge deriving from the ambivalent character of difference in Western societies, which Minow[12(p20)] articulates as the dilemma of difference: "When does treating people differently emphasize their differences and stigmatize or hinder them on that basis? and when does treating people the same become insensitive to their differences and likely to stigmatize them or hinder them on that basis?"

The answer to this question is that sensitive attention to relevant difference can only harm when and if difference is essentialized and understood as otherness. When understood as a relational, dialogical, anthropological, and psychological concept, difference will instead support the positive affirmation and liberation of athletes and people with disabilities.

In the quest for cultural recognition as legitimate sport and for wide public acceptance, Para sport culture, and the IPC in particular, have often chosen to shy away from difference (as a fluid, relational category) to invest in the most culturally recognisable and already accepted sporting practices and values, prioritizing the panoply of dominant sports and competitive values, imposed in part by its close relation to the International Olympic Committee.[39] This IPC strategy, however, largely operates from a standpoint of able-bodiedness to earn mainstream social legitimacy; recognition; and, concomitantly, secure financial viability. Going back to ableism, not only does this strategy emulate able-bodied norms, it also reinforces the constitutional divide between the abled or the disabled.

The alternative path, we propose, is recognition, acceptance, and valuing of difference (and similarity) inherent to impaired bodies. This path would expand the cultural boundaries of athleticism and sport by exploring the active and positive potentialities of impaired moving bodies, and harness the development of more inclusive, creative, and plural sporting cultures, as DePauw[40] anticipated in 1997. The dilemma of difference[12] surfaces in the sense that investing in difference is not without risk because institutions such as the IPC are likely to face strong cultural resistance at all levels of sporting cultures, which may be the reason that this most significant institution in Para sports has celebrated difference in its public rhetoric but has failed to put it into action in practice.

SUMMARY

The assumption that the Paralympic Games can ignite positive social change in the lives of people with disabilities has been received with skepticism by disability activists[21,41] and researchers[42–45] alike. The short-term nature of the Paralympic Games and its political allure opens the door for its political manipulation by governments, with the rhetoric of empowerment not always reaching the everyday lives of people with disabilities. Para sport communities and cultures can drive change in a much more meaningful, sustainable, and long-lasting fashion by forging the emergence of stable, committed, and cohesive communities of practice in which a critical pedagogy can develop. In other words, the hegemony of ableism can be actively counteracted by an awareness of its artificiality and coerced nature, and by the cultivation of values such as empathy, openness, acceptance of difference, and political consciousness. At the root of this pedagogy is a perception and embodiment of difference as a relational (rather than absolute) quality through sporting practices within heterogeneous communities. Understood in its relativeness and contingency, difference need not be negated because to do so reinforces able-bodied sameness as the ideal to which everyone should aspire. Thus, the path toward a more empowering society for people with disabilities ought to be grounded in a cultural understanding of difference as nonabsolute (everything and everyone is at the same time, similarly different and differently similar). We propose that only by enacting a politics of difference[11]; that is, a politics grounded in sporting habitus in which difference is accepted and valued, can Para sports make a real impact on the lives of athletes and people with disabilities, more generally.

Drawing ideas on difference from Hall,[27] Young,[11] and Minow,[12] the arguments developed in this article highlight how the situation can improve in the future:

1. The recognition, acceptance, and valuing of difference within Para sport cultures must naturally drive the emergence of new sports and sporting ethos that is

more attuned with this attitude and understanding. Because mainstream sports were created to respond to an embodiment ideal defined by ableism, this transformation is very much needed. At the Paralympic level, for instance, this may result in an increased promotion of specific Para sports such as bocce, goalball, and sitting volleyball. New sporting cultures, in which movement practices and the interaction between differently embodied participants are creatively exercised, are very much needed.

2. In attempting to critically educate wider society on the value of difference and pluralism, Para sport culture needs to proactively promote the participation of all people with disabilities, paying particular attention to the exponential disadvantage inherent in the intersection of disability with other categories of difference (eg, gender, class, race, ethnicity, sexuality, religion), which hinder access to apparently accessible opportunities.

3. Fostering an empowering understanding of the difference associated with disability demands increased participation of people with disabilities as the active creators of Para sport cultures, rather than as mere recipients of services. The heterogeneity of the Para sport public needs to be replicated in the representation of people with disabilities at all levels of governance and practice (IPC, management of clubs and associations, coaching, education), with particular emphasis on decision-making processes and structures.

To close, the political potential of Para sport cultures[45] ought to be embraced by everyone involved. Politics does not necessarily involve the display of grandiose gestures of political activism but rather an attitude and aligned practice of openness toward difference, which overflows the boundaries of sporting communities to permeate all dimensions of social life. Following Gandhi's and Michael Jackson's words ("Man in the Mirror"), Para sport culture ought to be the change it wants to see in the world.

REFERENCES

1. Walker P, Topping A. Paralympics legacy fails to shift attitudes to disabled people. The Guardian 2013. Available at: https://www.theguardian.com/sport/2013/aug/29/paralympics-legacy-disabled-people. Accessed August 10, 2017.

2. Braye S, Dixon K, Gibbons T. The 2012 Paralympics and perceptions of disability in the UK. In: Dixon K, Gibbons T, editors. The impact of the 2012 Olympic and Paralympic games: diminishing contrasts, increasing varieties. Basingstoke (UK): Palgrave Macmillan; 2015. p. 15–34.

3. Hodges C, Jackson D, Scullion R, et al. Tracking changes in everyday experiences of disability and disability sport within the context of the 2012 London Paralympics. 2014. Available at: http://eprints.bournemouth.ac.uk/21596/. Accessed July 10, 2017.

4. Howe PD, Silva CF. The fiddle of using the Paralympic Games as a vehicle for expanding [dis]ability sport participation. Sport and Soc 2018;21(1):125–36.

5. Coalter F. A wider social role for sport: who's keeping the score? London: Routledge; 2007.

6. Coalter F. Sport-for-change: some thoughts from a sceptic. Social Inclusion 2015; 3(3):19–23. Available at: http://www.cogitatiopress.com/socialinclusion/article/view/222. Accessed August 13, 2017.

7. Spaaij R, Magee J, Jeanes R. Sport and social exclusion in global society. London: Routledge; 2014.

8. Collins M, Kay T. Sport and social exclusion. London: Routledge; 2014.

9. Morgan WJ. Leftist theories of sport: a critique and reconstruction. Urbana (IL): University of Illinois Press; 1994.
10. Howe PD, Jones C. Classification of disabled athletes: (Dis)empowering the Paralympic practice community. Sociol Sport J 2006;23(1):29–46.
11. Young IM. Justice and the politics of difference. Princeton (NJ): Princenton University Press; 1990.
12. Minow M. Making all the difference: inclusion, exclusion, and American law. New York: Cornell University Press; 1990.
13. Oliver M. The politics of disablement. London: Macmillan Education; 1990.
14. Shakespeare T. Disability rights and wrongs. London: Routledge; 2006.
15. Campbell FK. Contours of ableism: the production of disability and abledness. New York: Palgrave Macmillan; 2009.
16. Howe PD. The cultural politics of the Paralympic movement. London: Routledge; 2008.
17. Howe PD. Cyborg and supercrip: the Paralympics technology and the (Dis) empowerment of disabled athletes. Sociol 2011;45(5):868–82.
18. Purdue DEJ, Howe PD. Who's in and who is out? Legitimate bodies within the Paralympic games. Sociol Sport J 2013;30(1):24–40.
19. Siebers T. Disability theory. Ann Arbor (MI): University of Michigan Press; 2008.
20. Deal M. Disabled people's attitudes toward other impairment groups: a hierarchy of impairments. Disabil Soc 2003;18(7):897–910.
21. Hahn H. Sports and the political movement of disabled persons: examining nondisabled social values. Arena Rev 1984;8(1):1–15.
22. Goffman E. Stigma: notes on the management of spoiled identity. Englewood Cliffs (NJ): Prentice-Hall; 1963.
23. Wolbring G. Paralympians outperforming Olympians: an increasing challenge for Olympism and the Paralympic and Olympic movement. Sport Ethics Philos 2012; 6(2):251–66.
24. McRuer R. Crip theory: cultural signs of queerness and disability. Albany: NYU Press; 2006.
25. Michalko R, Titchkosky T. Rethinking normalcy: a disability studies reader. Toronto (Canada): Canadian Scholars' Press; 2009.
26. Davis LJ. Enforcing normalcy disability, deafness, and the body. New York: Verso; 1995.
27. Hall S. The spectacle of the "other". In: Hall S, Evans J, Nixon S, editors. Representation: cultural representation and signifying practices. 2nd edition. London: Sage; 2013. p. 215–71.
28. Michalko R, Titchkosky T. Rethinking normalcy: a disability studies reader. Toronto: Canadian Scholars' Press; 2009.
29. Sherrill C. Disability sport and classification theory: a new era. Adapt Phys Activ Q 1999;16(3):206–15.
30. Jones C, Howe PD. The conceptual boundaries of sport for the disabled: classification and athletic performance. J Philos Sport 2005;32(2):133–46.
31. Purdue D, Howe PD. Empower, inspire, achieve: (dis)empowerment and the Paralympic games. Disabil Soc 2012;27(7):1–14.
32. Howe PD, Parker A. Celebrating imperfection: sport, disability and celebrity culture. Celebr Stud 2012;3(3):270–82.
33. Jönsson K. Paralympics and the fabrication of "freak shows": on aesthetics and abjection in sport. Sport Ethics Philos 2017;11(2):224–37.
34. Peers D. Patients, athletes, freaks: paralympism and the reproduction of disability. J Sport Soc Issues 2012;36(3):295–316.

35. Silva CF, Howe PD. The (In) validity of supercrip representation of paralympian athletes. J Sport Soc Issues 2012;36(2):174–94.

36. Bogdan R. Freak show: presenting human oddities for amusement and profit. Chicago: University of Chicago Press; 1988.

37. Silva CF. Forbidden to stand: the impact of sitting volleyball participation on the lives of players with impairments [doctoral thesis]. Loughborough (United Kingdom): Loughborough University; 2014. Available at: https://dspace.lboro.ac.uk/2134/14178.

38. Howe D. Empathy: what it is and why it matters. Basingstoke (UK): Palgrave Macmillan; 2012.

39. Purdue DEJ. An (In) convenient truce? Paralympic stakeholders' reflections on the Olympic–Paralympic relationship. J Sport Soc Issues 2013;37(4):384–402.

40. DePauw KP. The (In) visibility of DisAbility: cultural contexts and sporting bodies. Quest 1997;49:416–30.

41. Braye S, Dixon K, Gibbons T. "A mockery of equality": an exploratory investigation into disabled activists' views of the Paralympic games. Disabil Soc 2013; 28(7):984–96.

42. Brittain I, Beacom A. Leveraging the London 2012 Paralympic games: what legacy for disabled people? J Sport Soc Issues 2016;40(6):499–521.

43. Darcy S. The politics of disability and access: the Sydney 2000 games experience. Disabil Soc 2003;18(6):737–57.

44. Lane P. Legacy: generating social currency through Paralympic excellence. In: Legg D, Gilbert K, editors. Paralympic legacies. Champaign (IL): Common Ground; 2011. p. 191–8.

45. Wedgwood N. Hahn versus Guttmann: revisiting "sports and the political movement of disabled persons". Disabil Soc 2014;29(1):129–42.

Social Inclusion Through Para sport

A Critical Reflection on the Current State of Play

Jason Bantjes, D Lit et Phil*, Leslie Swartz, PhD

KEYWORDS

- Social inclusion • Para sport • Paralympics • Disability
- International Paralympic Committee (IPC)

KEY POINTS

- The Paralympic movement has done much to promote social inclusion, challenge stereotypes, and change unhelpful attitudes toward disability.
- There are many challenges that the movement faces if it seeks to continue its sociopolitical agenda of promoting social inclusion.
- Sports physicians can contribute to lively debate about how to overcome these challenges, so that Para sport continues to promote the inclusion of all disabled people.

INTRODUCTION

Medicine has played an integral role in both the inception and development of Para sport, and sports physicians are well positioned to continue to influence the development of the Paralympic movement. The origins of the Paralympic Games can be traced back to the work of neurologist, Dr Ludwig Guttmann, who used sport as an integral component of the rehabilitation of paraplegic patients at Stoke Mandeville Hospital in Buckinghamshire.[1] A Para sport competition was held at Stoke Mandeville Hospital to coincide with the opening ceremony of the London Olympic Games in July 1948,[2] thus aligning the event with the Olympic movement. Initially the Para sport competition at Stoke Mandeville Hospital was little more than an event for disabled ex-servicemen and women, but it nonetheless became an annual event that attracted international participation in 1952.[2] The first Olympic-style Para sport tournament, convened in Rome in 1960, was a modest event with 400 athletes from 23 countries participating.[3] Since then, the Paralympic Games have grown in both stature and prominence; they are now firmly aligned with the Olympic Games and have expanded

Disclosure Statement: The authors have nothing to disclose.
Department of Psychology, Stellenbosch University, Private Bag X1, Matieland 7602, South Africa
* Corresponding author.
E-mail address: jbantjes@sun.ac.za

Phys Med Rehabil Clin N Am 29 (2018) 409–416
https://doi.org/10.1016/j.pmr.2018.01.006
1047-9651/18/© 2018 Elsevier Inc. All rights reserved.

to include a wide range of sports and disabilities.[4] The Rio 2016 Paralympic Games were a large and spectacular event; 2.15 million spectators witnessed the performance of 4328 athletes from 159 countries participating in 22 sports.[5] As the Paralympic Games have grown, it has been transformed from an event which embraced sport as a means of rehabilitation, to become an elite event, a public spectacle, and a socio-political movement that explicitly seeks to promote social inclusion. Please see David Legg's article, "Paralympic Games: History and Legacy of a Global Movement," in this issue, for a full history of the Paralympic Games. This article describes the importance and value of Para sport and its potential to promote social inclusion. It critically considers the claims that have been made about the role of the Paralympic Games in promoting social inclusion, and highlights the challenges that the movement might face as it continues to advance its agenda as a socio-political movement committed to promoting social inclusion. The article concludes by turning its attention to the question of what role sports medicine might play in the future of the Paralympic movement.

THE IMPORTANCE AND VALUE OF PARA SPORT

The considerable benefits of organized sport and physical activity are well documented. Sport promotes the physical and psychological health of individuals.[6,7] Participating in physical activity promotes social interaction, reduces feelings of isolation, and promotes a sense of belonging, particularly for young people.[8,9] At a societal level, sport has the potential to promote social cohesion, social development, and peace.[10] The fact that most governments consider the promotion of sport to be one of their responsibilities is evidence of the widespread belief that sport has substantial public, personal, and political benefits.

Sport has particular value for persons with disabilities; in addition to the general health benefits of physical activity, sport can serve as a means of physical rehabilitation[11] and an arena in which to promote social interaction and achieve social inclusion. Positive correlations have been demonstrated between participation in sport and quality of life among persons with disabilities.[12] The United Nations has affirmed that "Sport can integrate people with disabilities into society, providing an arena for positive social interaction, reducing isolation and breaking down prejudice. Sports programs for the disabled are also a cost-effective method of rehabilitation. They are highly therapeutic, improving motor skills and increasing mobility, self-sufficiency and self-confidence."[13(p12)]

The Paralympic Games have been heralded for their ability to promote political transformation and social inclusion by:

- Challenging unhelpful societal stereotypes about people with disabilities[14,15]
- Changing attitudes about disability by emphasizing achievement rather than impairment[4]
- Providing a stage on which athletes with disabilities can resist social oppression[16]
- Creating an arena in which athletes with disabilities can participate in the formation of their own social identities[17]

Considerable advances toward social inclusion have been achieved through the Paralympic movement. Gould and Gould have affirmed that, "Few developments have challenged existing ways of thinking about sport and disability more than the rise of the Paralympic Games."[4(p133)] Claims have been made that the Paralympic Games have been a major force in "accelerating the agenda of inclusion and by helping to promote the concept of a barrier-free environment within town planning and architectural discourse."[4(p133)] The press coverage that the Paralympic Games enjoy has helped create the impression (at least in the media) that access to sport is available to all. In spite of the considerable progress that has been made to promote social inclusion through sport, there are still a number of challenges that the Paralympic movement face as it seeks to advance its socio-political agenda. Chief among these challenges are:

- Tensions that exist in the relationship between the Paralympic Games and the Olympic Games
- Issues about fairness and inequality within the Paralympic Games
- Questions about the extent to which the Paralympic Games actually promote participation in Para sport among nonelite athletes
- Concerns about the extent to which the Paralympic Games perpetuate unhelpful stereotypes of disability that work against true inclusion
- Contradictions that exist between the medical model of disability and the social model of disability with respect to the manner in which Paralympic athletes are classified and assigned to different classes

Each of these challenges is briefly discussed.

SEPARATE AND UNEQUAL?

For the first time, at the Seoul 1988 Summer Olympics the Paralympic Games and Olympic Games were held in the same venue, although they were convened as separate events.[1] This practice continues today with the Paralympic Games and Olympic Games being run as separate, but supposedly equal, competitions. Gold and Gold have questioned whether this arrangement truly assists in the promotion of social inclusion or simply perpetuates difference, segregation, and inequality.[4] Several authors have dubbed the Paralympic Games a "sideshow" to the Olympic Games and pointed out how the status quo subordinates the Paralympic movement and Paralympic athletes.[18,19] It is hard to argue that the Paralympic Games and Olympic Games are equal when there are such stark inequalities in terms of funding for the events, financial support and sponsorship for the athletes, media coverage, and the competitors' status and prestige as elite athletes. It would certainly seem that current practices perpetuate what Goggin and Newell have described as "social apartheid,"[20] thus reinforcing social exclusion for persons with disabilities.

It is patently apparent from the organizational structures and mission statements of the International Paralympic Committee (IPC) and International Olympic Committee (IOC) that the 2 institutions are distinct and different entities; the IPC is not actually a member of the IOC and has its own vision, mission, goals and roles. The motto of the IOC is "Swifter, Higher, Stronger" which implies a focus on pushing the limits of human physical capabilities. By contrast the IPC's motto is "Spirit in Motion," which seems to imply something different from the Olympic Games' focus on celebrating physical achievement. As Blauwet[21] has noted, the Olympic movement seeks to develop elite sport, while the Paralympic movement explicitly aims to promote "the concepts of health and human rights for athletes with a disability," which is a much more inclusive political agenda.[21(p2)]

Although there are those who argue that it is time for the Paralympic Games and Olympic Games to come together in a single arena under a single organizing committee, there are others who contest that the ideals and values of the Olympic Games are problematic and at odds with a rights-based approach to disability. Scholars have argued that the Olympic Games as an institution is tied up in problematic imagery of the perfect athletic body and that Olympic mythology and culture have been under-pinned by fantasies about bodily perfection.[18] The focus in the Olympic Games on icons of bodily perfection does not sit comfortably with contemporary theories about disability, which reject hegemonic ideas about typical and atypical bodies. There are those who argue that the Paralympic Games, far from joining more closely with the Olympic Games, need to distance themselves as far as possible from the IOC. This argument emphasizes the potential role of the Paralympic Games in disrupting domi-nant ideas about the body, in a similar way that disability scholars are playing a key role in transforming museums as sites of observing bodies. These scholars are aware of the history of what has been termed the "enfreakment," the transformation of the disabled body into an image of titillation and spectacle,[22] and advocate for creating museums that allow for a respectful and engaged politics of looking at a range of bodies, including disabled bodies.[23] For similar ideas to be taken up in the Paralympic movement, there would need to be a reconceptualization of the relationship between the Paralympic Games and the Olympic Games.

Although it is unclear how to resolve the tensions that exist in terms of inequality and segregation between the Paralympic Games and Olympic Games, it is clear that more debate is needed on this issue before decisions are made about complete integration or radical separation of the 2 movements. Decisions that are made about how to resolve these tensions will have important implications for how the Paralympic Games are positioned to promote their agenda of social inclusion in the future and how they aligned with contemporary ideas about disability.

HOW FAIR AND INCLUSIVE ARE THE PARALYMPIC GAMES?

In their empirical analysis of levels of participation and achievement at The Doha 2015 Paralympic Athletic Championships, Swartz and colleagues[24] showed how both levels of participation and achievement in Paralympic competitions continue to be pro-foundly influenced by economic factors. The data suggested that The Doha Para-lympic Athletics Championships were dominated by high-income countries, while Para athletes from the majority world continue to be marginalized.[24] Similarly Buts and colleagues[25] have shown that the factors that determined a country's success at the Summer Paralympic Games of 1996, 2000, 2004, and 2008, were: gross domes-tic product (GDP) per capita, population size, having many participants per million in-habitants, being a former communist country, and having previously hosted the Paralympic Games.[25] These findings raise important questions about the politics of global fairness in Para sport and the extent to which the Paralympic movement is really inclusive.

DO THE PARALYMPIC GAMES INCREASE PARTICIPATION IN PARA SPORT?

There is some evidence to suggest that the growing prominence of the Paralympic Games has resulted in important attitudinal changes toward disability, inclusion and Para sport.[14,15,26] Nonetheless it remains to be seen whether these attitudinal changes have contributed, on any significant scale, to prompting participation in physical activ-ity among persons with disabilities. It is clear that attitudinal changes are really impor-tant to promote physical activity among persons with disabilities, but in the majority world it will certainly take more than changing attitudes to promote access to physical activity. Several studies have shown that there are a range of factors that serve as both barriers and facilitators to participation in physical activity among persons with disabil-ities.[27,28] These factors include resources, infrastructure, transport, adequate coach-ing, recognition, and opportunities to participate and exercise choice.[29] It is not clear how the Paralympic movement can, or whether indeed it should, be actively engaged in helping to overcome these barriers, particularly in resource scarce environments such as low- and middle-income countries, where most disabled people reside.

Research is needed in order to understand what changes in behavior are facilitated by the growing prominence of the Paralympic Games. But at the same time, one must be cautious not to over-reach by making exaggerated claims about the Paralympic movement's ability to transcend the concrete (nonattitudinal) barriers that impede participation in sport and physical activity for many people with disabilities.

DO THE PARALYMPIC GAMES PERPETUATE UNHELPFUL IMAGES AND STEREOTYPES?

Several critical scholars have noted that in spite of the apparent good achieved by the Paralympic Games, there is a danger that aspects of the event "reinforce outdated notions about the abilities, status and place of sports people with disabilities in society and sport."[18(p65)] There are real dangers that the position of the Paralympic Games and the portrayal of Paralympic athletes in the media, "perpetuates outdated stereotypes about ability and disability and reinforces a paternalism and devaluation of the achievements of Paralympians."[18(p65)]

The Paralympic movement is characterized by a supercrip discourse; that is the phenomenon by which people with disabilities are seen to go beyond what is human. For example, the slogan of The Doha 2015 Paralympic Athletic Championships was beyond incredible. This framing of Para athletes as superhuman is positive in 1 sense, but it also has the power to reinforce the unhelpful view that superhuman performances are a requirement from people with disabilities before they are seen positively as people.[17,30] Inspiration porn, a term popularized by the Australian disabled comedian Stella Young, refers to the ways in which the achievements of people with disabilities are used to entertain and inspire people without disabilities, as a form of display and titillation.[31] Inspiration porn has historical links with freak shows,[32] in which the public paid to see both what was presented as gruesome bodies and displays of extraordinary strength and prowess. In the current media age, many aspects of the freak show have gone digital, some operating through reality television.[33] These portrayals interact with and provide a context for how disability sport may be perceived by a global television-viewing audience and may in fact work against the attainment of social inclusion.

TENSIONS BETWEEN BIOMEDICAL AND SOCIAL MODELS OF DISABILITY

In its pursuit of fairness, the IPC employs an elaborate system of classification to assign athletes to particular categories or classes based on the nature of their physical impairments. Integral to the assignment of athletes to these different classes is a medical assessment to determine how far the athlete deviates from what is considered a normal body. This classification system is profoundly influenced by medical models of disability and is reliant on ideas about deficits and deviations from the norm in order to classify athletes.[18] This classification system is designed to make competition as fair as possible, so that people with similar bodies compete against one another.[34] Despite a considerable amount of work on classification, the particular mechanics of classification change over time, and there are commonly arguments that particular classifications at a particular time are not the best way of achieving fairness.[35] The way forward with this process is to increasingly refine and improve the classification system.[36] There is, however, another level of critique that undercuts the principles of classification (and hence of a key pillar of the Paralympic Games) in their entirety. Disability scholars argue that to promote social inclusion one needs to move away from models of disability that focus on bodily difference and impairment (so-called medical models) and instead embrace models of disability that assert that people are disabled not by their impairments in themselves but by their social contexts and environments. In these models, which have a variety of names, but link to the so-called social model, the emphasis is on social exclusion and on the rights of all people with non-normative bodies (and not just those who excel, as in the Paralympic Games) to be included in mainstream society and to participate in society equally with others.[37,38] There is no easy way to resolve the tensions between the focus on the body in current IPC classification system, on the 1 hand, and on the emphasis on social exclusion in contemporary disability politics on the other. This issue is at the heart of tensions around the role of the Paralympic Games in promoting social inclusion or, paradoxically, reinforcing stereotypes and dominant ideas about difference.

WHAT ROLE WILL SPORTS MEDICINE PLAY IN THE FUTURE OF THE PARALYMPIC GAMES?

Since its inception as an event that embraced sport as physical therapy, the Paralympic Games have become increasingly competitive and claimed their space as an elite athletic event. This raises questions about the extent to which there will be growing pressure on sports physicians and sports scientists to fall in and support the movement by providing technologies that promote peak performance. It is possible that in the future, sports medicine will position itself primarily to support Paralympic athletes in their pursuit of "swifter, higher, stronger" particularly if Paralympic athletes seek to align themselves with Olympic athletes. By actively and uncritically supporting Paralympic athletes in their pursuit of elite competition, sports medicine may position itself further and further away from the primary responsibility of physicians to promote health (not only the health of their individual patients but also public health). Disabled people are at risk for a range of lifestyle-related diseases and would benefit from participating in regular physical activity; there is thus a public health imperative to promote activities that engage and include disabled people in sport. Although sports physicians clearly have a role to play in supporting the physical achievements of Paralympic athletes, they might also have an important role to play by exercising their influence and status to keep the IPC focused on the goal of sport as therapy and the promotion of mass participation in Para sport. Sports physicians can, if they choose to, promote the Paralympic Games as a distinctly different kind of competition from the Olympic Games, an event that is oriented to the needs of the broader disabled sporting community and focuses, not on elite performances, but rather on values such as participation and inclusion.

SUMMARY

There is little doubt that the Paralympic Games can play, and have played, an important role in promoting social inclusion and in changing popular perceptions of disability. It is, however, inevitable that any social intervention or social movement, while challenging and changing aspects of the status quo, also reproduces aspects of it. This is certainly the case with the Paralympic movement. There are real dangers that the Paralympic Games may promote sport as a way of excluding and stigmatizing the vast majority of people with disabilities who are not elite athletes. The Paralympic Games have achieved a great deal; the challenge now is to increase the access of all people with disabilities to the benefits of physical activity. This is a challenge that cannot be sidestepped by sports physicians who are genuinely concerned with promoting the wellbeing of all persons with disabilities in all parts of the world.

REFERENCES

1. International Paralympic Committee. History of the paralympic movement. Official website of the Paralympic Movement. 2006. Available at: https://www.paralympic. org/sites/default/files/document/120209103536284_2012_02_History%2Bof% 2BParalympic%2BMovement.pdf. Accessed November 18, 2017.
2. DePauw KP, Gavron SJ. Disability sport. Leeds (United Kingdom): Human Kinetics; 2005.
3. International Paralympic Committee. Summer games overview. 2009. Available at: http://www.paralympic.org/release/Main_Sections_Menu/Paralympic_Games/ Past_Games/Summer_Games_Overview.html. Accessed November 20, 2017.
4. Gold JR, Gold MM. Access for all: the rise of the paralympic games. J R Soc Promot Health 2007;127(3):133–41.
5. International Paralympic Committee. Rio 2016. Official website of the Paralympic Movement. 2016. Available at: https://www.paralympic.org/rio-2016. Accessed November 21, 2017.
6. Eime RM, Young JA, Harvey JT, et al. A systematic review of the psychological and social benefits of participation in sport for children and adolescents: informing development of a conceptual model of health through sport. Int J Behav Nutr Phys Act 2013;10:98.
7. Warburton DE, Nicol CW, Bredin SS. Health benefits of physical activity: the evidence. CMAJ 2006;174(6):801–9.
8. Hansen D, Larson R, Dworkin J. What adolescents learn in organized youth activities: A survey of self-reported developmental experiences. J Res Adolesc 2005;13(1):25–56.
9. Holt NL, Neely KC. Positive youth development through sport: a review. Revista iberoamericana de psicologia del ejercicio y el deporte 2011;6(2):299–316.
10. Beutler I. Sport serving development and peace: achieving the goals of the United Nations through sport. Sport Soc 2008;11(4):359–69.
11. Klapwijk A. Persons with a disability and sports. In: Vermeer A, editor. Sports for the disabled. Haarlem (Netherland): Uitgeverij de Vrieseborch; 1986. p. 1–14.
12. Groff DG, Lundberg NR, Zabriskie RB. Influence of adapted sport on quality of life: Perceptions of athletes with cerebral palsy. Disabil Rehabil 2009;31(4): 318–26.
13. United Nations. Sport for development and peace: towards achieving the millennium development goals. Report from the United Nations Inter-agency Task Force on Sport for Development and Peace. Geneva (Switzerland): United Nations; 2005.
14. Hodges CE, Jackson D, Scullion R, et al. Tracking changes in everyday experiences of disability and disability sport within the context of the 2012 London Paralympic Games. Dorset (United Kingdom): Bournemouth University; 2014.
15. Wood C. One year on: a review of the cultural legacy of the Paralympic Games. London: Demos; 2013.
16. Smith B, Sparkes AC. Changing bodies, changing narratives and the consequences of tellability: a case study of becoming disabled through sport. Sociol Health Illn 2008;30(2):217–36.
17. Swartz L, Bantjes J, Knight B, et al. "They don't understand that we also exist": South African participants in competitive disability sport and the politics of identity. Disabil Rehabil 2016;40(1):35–41.
18. Kell P, Kell M, Price N. Two games and one movement? The Paralympic Games and the Olympic movement. In: Kell P, Vialle W, Konza D, et al, editors. Learning

and the learner: exploring learning for new times. Wollongong (Australia): University of Wollongong; 2008. p. 65–77.

19. Gilbert K, Schantz O. The Paralympic Games: empowerment or side show? Sydney (Australia): Verlag: Meyer & Meyer; 2008.

20. Goggin G, Newell C. Disability in Australia: exposing a social apartheid. Sydney (Australia): UNSW; 2005.

21. Blauwet C. Promoting the health and human rights of individuals with a disability through the paralympic movement. Bonn (Germany): International Paralympic Committee; 2005.

22. Garland-Thomson R. Freakery: cultural spectacles of the extraordinary body. New York: NYU Press;; 1996.

23. Sandell R, Dodd J, Garland-Thomson R. Representing disability: activism and agency in the museum. New York: Routledge; 2010.

24. Swartz L, Bantjes J, Divan R, et al. "A more equitable society": the politics of global fairness in paralympic sport. PLoS One 2016;11(12):e0167481.

25. Buts C, Du Bois C, Heyndels B, et al. Socioeconomic determinants of success at the summer paralympic games. J Sports Econom 2013;14(2):133–47.

26. Panagiotou AK, Evaggelinou C, Doulkeridou A, et al. Attitudes of 5th and 6th grade Greek students toward the inclusion of children with disabilities in physical education classes after a paralympic education program. European Journal of Adapted Physical Activity 2008;1(2):31–43.

27. DeFazio V, Porter HR. Barriers and facilitators to physical activity for youth with cerebral Palsy. Ther Recreation J 2016;50(4):327.

28. Rimmer JH, Riley B, Wang E, et al. Physical activity participation among persons with disabilities: barriers and facilitators. Am J Prev Med 2004;26(5):419–25.

29. Conchar L, Bantjes J, Swartz L. Barriers and facilitators to participation in physical activity: The experiences of a group of South African adolescents with cerebral palsy. J Health Psychol 2016;21(2):152–63.

30. Silva CF, Howe PD. The (in)validity of supercrip representation of Paralympian athletes. J Sport Soc Issues 2012;36(2):174–94.

31. Grue J. The problem with inspiration porn: a tentative definition and a provisional critique. Disabil Soc 2016;31(6):838–49.

32. Garland-Thomson R. Feminist disability studies. Signs (Chic) 2005;30(2):1557–87.

33. Williams JL. Media, performative identity, and the new American freak show. New York: Palgrave Macmillan; 2017.

34. Tweedy SM, Vanlandewijck YC. International Paralympic Committee position stand—background and scientific principles of classification in Paralympic sport. Br J Sports Med 2011;45(4):259–69.

35. Howe PD, Jones C. Classification of disabled athletes: (Dis) empowering the paralympic practice community. Sociol Sport J 2006;23(1):29–46.

36. Beckman EM, Tweedy SM. Towards evidence-based classification in paralympic athletics: evaluating the validity of activity limitation tests for use in classification of paralympic running events. Br J Sports Med 2009;43(13):1067–72.

37. Goodley D. Disability studies: an interdisciplinary introduction. London: Sage; 2016.

38. Shakespeare T. Critiquing the social model. In: Emens EF, Stein MA, editors. Disability and equality law. Surrey (United Kingdom): Ashgate Publishing Limited; 2013. p. 67.

Paralympic Games
History and Legacy of a Global Movement

David Legg, PhD

KEYWORDS

- Paralympic games • Legacy • Para sport • Disability sport • Paralympic history

KEY POINTS

- Para sport began with World War II when returning war veterans with spinal injuries benefitted from improved evacuation techniques and the invention of penicillin.
- As a result of the newly extended life span and a desire to assist in the return to normalcy for injured veterans, the focus on rehabilitation took on greater urgency.
- Like most minority groups, people with disabilities have historically sought ways to be more included in the broader society. For these reasons, Para sport, since its inception, has been influenced, affected, and intricately linked by a desire to be included into the larger and more dominant able-bodied sport culture and system.

The 2016 Summer Paralympic Games held in Rio de Janeiro, Brazil, were the second largest multisport event held that year, second only to the 2016 Summer Olympic Games held 2 weeks prior.[1] At the Paralympic Games, 4342 athletes representing 159 National Paralympic Committees competed in 22 sports. This was a far cry from the humble beginnings of the Games and movement that began during World War II at rehabilitation centers. It was at these Centers where returning war veterans and their medical leaders used sport as a means of rehabilitation both for the body and mind. On the hospital grounds, small competitions evolved into regional, national, and eventually international events with the result being what is now known as the Paralympic Games.

DISABILITY SPORT

Before moving forward on the Paralympic Games' history and legacy, it is worthwhile acknowledging that disability sport is different than Paralympic or Para sport. The word "Paralympic" derives from the Greek preposition "Para" (beside or alongside) and the word "Olympic." Its meaning suggests that the Paralympics are the parallel

The author has nothing to disclose.
Department of Health and Physical Education, Mount Royal University, 4825 Mount Royal Gate, Southwest, Calgary T4C1H4, Canada
E-mail address: dlegg@mtroyal.ca

Phys Med Rehabil Clin N Am 29 (2018) 417–425
https://doi.org/10.1016/j.pmr.2018.01.008
1047-9651/18/© 2018 Elsevier Inc. All rights reserved.

games to the Olympics and illustrates how the 2 movements exist side by side. Para sport, meanwhile, refers to all sport for athletes with physical disability but not necessarily at the international level. Persons with a disability or impairment are far from a homogenous group, so it should not be surprising that the sport system for this demographic is also diverse, and Para sport and Paralympic sport is far from all-encompassing for all disabilities.

Persons with an intellectual disability, for instance, typically participate in sport overseen by Special Olympics (http://www.specialolympics.org/). These Games were initiated in the 1960s, with the first official event held in Chicago in 1968. The most recent Special Olympics World Winter Games, meanwhile, were held in Austria with 2600 athletes from 105 nations competing in 9 Olympic-type sports. The next Special Olympic World Summer Games will be held in Abu Dhabi, United Arab Emirates, in March 2019. What complicates an understanding of disability sport and Para sport is that there are also athletes with intellectual disability who compete in the Paralympic Games (discussed later).

Persons who are deaf or hearing impaired compete in the Deaflympics overseen by the International Committee of Sports for the Deaf (http://www.ciss.org/). Deaf sport has a history dating back to 1888, when the first club was formed in Berlin. Deaf sport was also one of the founding organizations of the Paralympic movement. Soon thereafter, the organizations separated. The 2017 edition of the Summer Deaflympics took place in Samsun, Turkey, with 3148 athletes from 97 countries competing in 21 sports. As discussed previously, to complicate an understanding of disability sport, there are also many examples of where athletes with deafness or hearing impairment compete in able-bodied or Para sport.

Disability sport or sport for athletes with impairments thus includes the Special Olympics, Deaflympics, and Para sport or Paralympic sport, which is the focal point hereon.

PARA SPORT

Para sport, as previously discussed, had its genesis with World War II. Returning war veterans with spinal injuries benefitted from improved evacuation techniques and the invention of penicillin, which meant that their life spans were similar to able-bodied peers. Perhaps as a result of the newly extended life spans and a desire to assist in the return to normalcy for injured veterans, the focus on rehabilitation took on greater urgency. The example most often referenced was at Stoke Mandeville Hospital, northeast of London, with other lesser known examples occurring in the United States, Canada, and Australia. In 1944, the Stoke Mandeville Hospital opened a spinal injuries center under the leadership of Dr Ludwig Guttmann, where he held several sport-related activities that took place under the guise of rehabilitation. On July 29, 1948, Guttmann hosted a small archery competition, which by no coincidence was held on the same day as the opening ceremony of the London 1948 Olympic Games. Four years later, several veterans from the Netherlands visited the hospital and competed in the first International Stoke Mandeville Games. In 1960, and under the leadership of Guttmann, these Games were moved to Rome, which was also hosting that year's edition of the Summer Olympic Games. The Rome Games, then called the 9th International Stoke Mandeville Games, eventually became known as the first Paralympic Games. Here, just over 400 athletes from 23 countries participated in a variety of wheelchair sports. Athletes with other disabilities, meanwhile, joined the Games in the 1970s. The 1960 Games in Rome also began the process of disability sport leaders attempting to host a parallel Games in the same city as the Olympic organizers. The International Stoke Mandeville Games, meanwhile, continued to be held in the United Kingdom on an annual basis or in other locations to match the Olympic Games until the 1990s, when they had their name changes to World Wheelchair Games and then to the International Wheelchair & Amputee Sports Federation World Games.

Para sport is thus a comparatively newer and relatively smaller fish in a very big pond. People with disabilities, like most minority groups, have also historically sought for ways to be more included in the broader society. For these 2 reasons, perhaps, Para sport, since its inception, has been influenced, affected, and intricately linked by a desire to be included into the larger and more dominant able-bodied sport culture and system. As 1 example, Dr Robert Jackson, founding President of the Canadian Wheelchair Sports Association (1967), believed that sport for athletes with a disability was a medium for achieving inclusion into society.[2] Jackson hoped that society would recognize that if a person with paraplegia could "race a mile in seven minutes, or lift 472 pounds in a bench press, then the same individual could also work a full eight-hour day."[2]

After the competition held in Rome, Guttmann made an attempt to move the Games to coincide with the Olympic Games. In 1968 both Games were held in Tokyo and in 1972 the Olympics were held in Munich while the Paralympic Games were held in Heidelberg, Germany. In 1976, Montreal hosted the Olympic Games while Toronto hosted the Paralympic Games, which were called at that time the Toronto-lympiad for the Physically Disabled. This name was chosen versus the International Stoke Mandeville Games because 1976 was the first time the Games officially included athletes with disabilities other than those related to spinal cord injuries, including those with amputations and visual impairment/blindness. Athletes with cerebral palsy, meanwhile, competed for the first time in 1980. The first Winter Games were held in 1976 in Sweden with subsequent Games held in cities and countries different from Olympic Games until 1992, when both Games were held in Albertville, France.

In 1980 and 1984, the Paralympic Games went through a difficult period due to hosting challenges. Moscow declined the opportunity to host Paralympic Games in 1980 when they held the Olympic Games, and Paralympic competitions were instead held in the Netherlands. In 1984, Los Angeles hosted the Olympic Games with the Paralympic Games originally planned for the University of Illinois. Financing for these Games did not occur as planned and the University forfeited their hosting responsibilities. Paralympic leaders scrambled to locate a new site and the result was a split Games, with wheelchair events at the Stoke Mandeville Hospital and other disability events in New York City.

THE MODERN PARALYMPIC GAMES

The trajectory of the Paralympic Games then took a sharp and dramatic turn in 1988 when the Olympic Games were held in Seoul, South Korea. Here, the local organizing committee committed to hosting both Olympic Games and Paralympic Games consecutively using the same venues and athletes' villag, and having comparable opening and closing ceremonies. This set a precedent that has now been followed in every Summer Games and Winter Games since and thus the 1988 Games are sometimes referred to as the birth of the modern Paralympic Games. Now, every bid city for an Olympic Games must also bid to host the Paralympic Games, with the current agreement between the International Olympic Committee (IOC) and International Paralympic Committee (IPC) lasting until 2032.

The Games in Seoul were also significant in that this was a time when the grassroots movement of Paralympic leaders was spurred on to create a democratically elected international governing body. In 1987, disability sport leaders met in Arnhem, the Netherlands, to discuss options for governance models. A year later they reconvened in Seoul during the Games agreeing to meet again in 1989 in Düsseldorf, Germany. Here the IPC was officially created and for 10 years operated primarily as a volunteer-driven organization. In 1999, the IPC hired professional staff and opened its headquarters in Bonn, Germany, where it remains today.

Returning to the history of the Games, in 1992, 2 Paralympic Games were held in Spain, coinciding with the Olympic Games in Barcelona. Events for athletes with an intellectual disability were organized for the first time and held in Madrid. The Paralympic Games for those with a physical disability, meanwhile, competed in Barcelona. Events for athletes with an intellectual impairment (II) were then merged into the larger Paralympic Games in 1996 and 2000. At the Sydney Games, in 2000, it was discovered that members of Spain's II basketball team did not have the requisite intellectual disability and, as a result, the entire movement was banned from participating in future Paralympic Games until the classification system was rebuilt. This took 12 years, with the return of athletes with II not occurring until London in 2012 (**Table 1**).

INTERNATIONAL PARALYMPIC COMMITTEE AND INTERNATIONAL OLYMPIC COMMITTEE RELATIONSHIP

It was also at the Sydney Games that discussions between IPC President Dr Robert Steadward and IOC President Juan Antonio Samaranch focused on both Games being held in the same cities, a practice, as alluded to previously, that was eventually formalized. The official agreement was signed in 2001 confirming that the "Paralympic Games [would] always take place shortly after the Olympic Games, using the same sporting venues and facilities."[3(p388)] The 2008 Olympic Games and Paralympic Games in Beijing were thus the first to fall under this agreement because those in 2004 and 2006 had already been awarded.[4] The 2001 agreement covered items, such as the requirement for a common organizing committee with responsibility to organize both Games in the same host city and that the Paralympic Games be organized according to similar principles and standards as the Olympic Games. Further amendments to this agreement were made in 2006, 2012, and most recently 2016, resulting in the extension of the agreement to 2032.[5]

From a practical perspective, the evolving merger between the IOC and the IPC was also evident through several alterations made by host organizing committees. At the 2010 Vancouver Olympic Games and Paralympic Winter Games, for instance, the word, *Paralympic*, was added to the official name of the host Olympic Organizing Committee. As well, a joint marketing agreement was created with the host National Paralympic Committee and a member from the Canadian Paralympic Committee named as 1 of the Vancouver Organizing Committee (VANOC) board of directors. Other new initiatives at the 2010 Games included the creation of a separate countdown clock for the Paralympic Games and flying both Olympic and Paralympic flags side-by-side at the Olympic/Paralympic Village, the competition venues, as well as other official and Games support venues.[6–9] At the 2012 Games in London, the local organizing committee's logos for both Games used the same background and colors with the only difference that the 5 Olympic rings and the 3 Paralympic agitos being exchanged within the common logo.[9] London's local host organizing committee also intentionally created 2 companion mascots, Wenlock and Mandeville, whose

Table 1
Locations of past and future Paralympic Games

Year	Summer Paralympic Games Host(s)	Winter Paralympic Games Host(s)	Location of Olympic Games
1960	Rome		Rome
1964	Tokyo		Tokyo
1968	Tel Aviv		Mexico City
1972	Heidelberg, Germany		Munich
1976	Toronto	Örnsköldsvik, Sweden	Montreal; Innsbruck, Austria
1980	Arnhem, the Netherlands	Geilo, Norway	Moscow; Lake Placid, US
1984	Stoke Mandeville, England; New York City	Innsbruck, Austria	Los Angeles; Sarajevo, Bosnia and Herzegovina
1988	Seoul	Innsbruck, Austria	Seoul; Calgary, Canada
1992	Barcelona and Madrid	Tignes, France, and Albertville, France	Barcelona; Albertville, France
1994		Lillehammer, Norway	Lillehammer, Norway
1996	Atlanta		Atlanta
1998		Nagano, Japan	Nagano, Japan
2000	Sydney		Sydney
2002		Salt Lake City, USA	Salt Lake City, USA
2004	Athens		Athens
2006		Turin, Italy	Turin, Italy
2008	Beijing		Beijing
2010		Vancouver	Vancouver
2012	London		London
2014		Sochi, Russia	Sochi, Russia
2016	Rio de Janeiro		Rio de Janeiro
2018		Pyeongchang, South Korea	Pyeongchang, South Korea
2020	Tokyo		Tokyo
2022		Beijing	Beijing
2024	Paris		Paris
2026		?	?
2028	Los Angeles		Los Angeles

names celebrated the English towns that were the epicenters of British Olympic and Paralympic heritage.[10]

The evolving relationship between the IOC and IPC has thus placed the IPC into a strange balancing act.[8] In some respects, the IPC is seen as a multisport international federation similar in scope and manner to what the IOC expects from other able-bodied international federations. The IPC is also international governing body for the world's second largest multisport event. It might be suggested, therefore, that the current relationship between the IPC and IOC is somewhat perilous, which may also be due to the relationships and politics between the IPC and IOC. The IPC's decision, for instance, to ban the Russian Paralympic Team was in stark contrast to the IOC's decision to leave this decision to international sport federations at the 2016 Olympic and Paralympic Games.[11] The IOC, however, reversed this decision for the 2018

Games and banned the Russian team. A second example is IPC President Sir Philip Craven's negative comments about the IOC President, Thomas Bach, which were recorded through a media ruse and then shared publically.[12]

In present day and future Games, the 2018 Winter games will be held in Pyeongchang, South Korea; 2020 Summer Games in Tokyo; and the 2022 Winter Games in Beijing. Bid cities for the 2026 Winter Games, meanwhile, may include Calgary, Canada; Sion, Switzerland; and Sapporo, Japan.

GAMES LEGACY

The trajectory of the Games and movement has thus been rapid, growing from the first Games in 1960 with just over 400 athletes to the most recent Games in Rio de Janeiro with more than 4000 athletes. With this growth have come significant challenges as well as opportunities, perhaps most importantly the legacy left once the Games have ended. Understanding these legacies, however, is difficult because research pertaining to them has only just started.

The challenge of understanding legacy is also true within an Olympic context because recognition of the importance of legacy only started, arguably, in 2002 when the Olympic Studies Centre in Barcelona organized an international symposium on the Legacy of the Olympic Games, 1984–2000.[13(p2)] Gratton and Preuss[14(p1923)] noted that the conference "attempted to define legacy, but the participants found that there were several meanings of the concept, and some of the contributions highlighted the convenience of using other expressions and concepts that could mean different things in different languages and cultures."

Gilbert and Legg[15] recognized this confusion in assessing the Paralympic Games legacy and in their attempts to better understand the term, *legacy*, they noted that it likely means "something handed down or received from an ancestor or predecessor,"[16] "a birthright or heritage,"[17] "a form of bequeath," or literally "that which is left behind."[18] Gilbert and Legg[15] for their purposes choose "that which is left behind" as the definitive open-ended meaning, in part because it was broad enough to cover most aspects of legacy as displayed in the academic narratives by investigators, such as Cashman and collegues,[19,20] Chappelet,[13] Gratton and Preuss,[14] and Girginov and Hills.[21]

Using this understanding, it seems that the hope, although not always the reality, for many major sporting events is to leave behind something positive that is worth the expense of hosting the Games. Legacies and impacts of major Games, such as the Olympic Games and Paralympic Games, are thus diverse in their breadth, depth, and levels of understanding and impact. Specific examples of these legacies are many. With the London 2012 Paralympic Games hailed as the first to have sold out venues, future bid cities may have seen the economic handicapitalism benefits. More specifically, the London 2012 Paralympic Games sold 2.72 million tickets, making it the third biggest sporting event behind the Olympics and the FIFA World Cup. Meanwhile, the United Kingdom's Channel 4 gained 11.2 million viewers during its broadcast of the Paralympic opening ceremony—the channel's biggest audience in a decade.[22] Other legacies include improved accessibility for persons with impairment, with specific examples, portions of the Great Wall of China north of Beijing; the Acropolis in Athens; and transit systems in Rio de Janeiro and London. Brittain and Beacom,[23] meanwhile, presented the opposite perspective, suggesting that, contrary to popular claims, 4 years after hosting the Summer Olympics in London there has been little improvement in the daily lives of those with disabilities.

The IPC has also made reference to positive legacies emanating from hosting the Games in Sochi, Russia. Although difficult to measure regarding impact, according to the IPC, "the introduction of a new law drafted in Russia's State Duma on 28th October, 2008 that assured the status of the Olympic and Paralympic Winter Games and announced the introduction of IOC and IPC standards to Russia's national legal system. This new law, introduced in light of their successful bid for the Olympic and Paralympic Winter Games in Sochi in 2014 was expected to greatly increase the awareness of disability sport within Russia and benefit the 11 million Russians currently living with a disability."[24]

At the most recent Paralympic Games in Rio de Janeiro, during the closing ceremonies, Sir Phillip Craven also made clear his hope for the lasting legacy and impact of the Games. Sir Phillip Craven noted, "Paralympians, your exceptional performances focused the world on your sensational abilities. People were in awe at what you could do and forgot about what they believed you could not. You showed to the world that with a positive attitude the human body, and above all the human heart and mind, knows no limits and absolutely anything is possible. You defied expectations, rewrote the record books and turned ill-found pity into pride. You are now heroes and role models for a new generation of sports fans from all over the world." Whether the athletes were able to inspire others was truly achieved, however, remains to be seen.

The Tokyo 2020 Paralympic Games, meanwhile, have identified 5 pillars for the hoped-for legacy and impact of their Games. These include sport and health, urban planning and sustainability, culture and education, economy and technology, and recovery from recent disasters. One study, perhaps of interest to those in the medical community, is an attempt to create a theoretic framework for medical and health legacies. Along with colleagues from Japan and Switzerland, the authors are trying to ascertain how host cities and countries can have medical and/or health care for Paralympians lead to impacts for the public health care system and, furthermore, promote public health by using the knowledge and know-how obtained through the athletes' training and medical care. Another focus has been on accessibility with changes already having taken place in Japan, including the passing of the Universal Design 2020 Action Plan and the publication of Tokyo 2020's own accessibility guidelines.

The 2018 Winter Paralympics Games in Pyeongchang also have great potential to provide lasting impact and legacy. In his presentation at a recent legacy conference in South Korea, Dr Martin Block[1] suggested there were 5 areas that the Korean community could capitalize on to ensure that the Games' legacy is positive, including enlisting Paralympic athletes to travel to communities and schools and discuss and promote disability sports, bringing together community sports providers, such as football and skiing clubs, for workshops on how to include athletes with disabilities in their programs either through inclusive or separate programs. Block also suggested expanding the already strong top-down Paralympics program in South Korea to local communities and special schools to identify, educate, and recruit potential future athletes with disabilities, continuing to highlight Paralympic programs through local and national media, and creating school-based programs and materials to promote positive images of disability and disability sports to children without disabilities across South Korea. All these could then hopefully capitalize on prior research demonstrating a positive impact of hosting Paralympic Games on youth with disabilities in the host country.[25] Creating a mechanism to systematically identify and train future Paralympians has also been identified as a critical factor in maintaining a strong Paralympics program,[26] and[27] taking advantage of the exposure of the Winter Paralympic Games across South Korea and the celebrity of South Korean Paralympians could be used to continue to improve Paralympic sport in South Korea. Finally, research has shown that hosting Paralympic Games can have a positive impact on those who view the games.[28] With the momentum and excitement of the Pyeongchang Games, South

Korea could thus have a unique opportunity to expand their already strong Paralympic program and perhaps leave a long-lasting and positive legacy for the host country.

The challenge with all these examples is assessing if the benefits actually pan out and if the IPC is truly achieving its' vision "To enable Para athletes to achieve sporting excellence and inspire and excite the world."

What is clear is that a great deal has changed since the Games were first held in Rome in 1960. What will happen in the future is unknown but most likely will be heavily influenced by societal changes and the influence of stakeholders, such as the medical community. The future of Para sport is bright and the authors look forward to being part of its growth and evolution.

REFERENCES

1. Block M. Legacies of hosting the 2018 Paralympic Games, Presentation at the 2017 Olympic Legacy Conference, Pyeongchang, June 14, 2017.
2. Legg D. Strategy formation in the Canadian Wheelchair Sports Association (1967-1997) [Doctoral dissertation]. Edmonton (Canada): University of Alberta; 2000.
3. Purdue D, David Purdue EJ. An (In)convenient Truce? Paralympic stakeholders' reflections on the Olympic–Paralympic relationship. Sport Social Issues 2013; 37(3):1–19.
4. Brittain I, Legg D, Wolff E. 'Paralympian' – discrimination or a necessary form of differentiation?. In: Kilvington D, Price J, editors. Sport and discrimination. Routledge; 2017. Chapter 11. p. 153–66.
5. International Olympic Committee. 2016. IOC and IPC sign long-term agreement supporting the Paralympic movement. Available at: https://www.olympic.org/news/ioc-and-ipc-sign-long-term-agreement-supporting-the-paralympic-movement. Accessed November 28, 2017.
6. Coward D, Legg D. Vancouver 2010. In: Legg D, Gilbert K, editors. Paralympic legacies. Champaign (IL): Commonground Publishing; 2011. p. 131–42.
7. International Paralympic Committee. 2012. IOC and IPC Extend Co-operation Agreement Until 2020. (2012, August 5). Available at: http://www.paralympic.org/news/ioc-and-ipc-extend-co-operation-agreement until-2020. Accessed November 29, 2013
8. Legg D. Development of the IPC and Relations with the IOC and other stakeholders. In: Brittain I, Beacom A, editors. Palgrave handbook of Paralympic studies. Basingstoke, United Kingdom: Palgrave Macmillan; 2017.
9. Legg D, Steadward R. The history of the paralympic games, in paralympic legacies. In: Legg D, Gilbert K, editors. Champaign (IL): Commonground Publishing; 2011. p. 13–20.
10. Polley M. The British Olympics: Britain's Olympic heritage 1612 – 2012. London: English Heritage; 2011.
11. Associated Press, 2016.
12. Pavitt, M. 2016. IPC President allegedly criticizes Bach after falling victim to prank phone call, Available at: http://www.insidethegames.biz/articles/1042444/ipc-president-allegedly-criticises-bach-after-falling-victim-to-prank-phone-call. Accessed November 28, 2017.
13. Chappelet JL. Olympic environmental concerns as a legacy of the winter games. Int J Hist Sport 2008;25(14):1884–902.
14. Gratton C, Preuss H. Maximizing Olympic impacts by building up legacies. Int J Hist Sport 2008;25(14):1922–38.

15. Gilbert K, Legg D. Conceptualizing legacy, in Paralympic legacies, in Paralympic legacies. In: Legg D, Gilbert K, editors. Champaign (IL): Commonground Publishing; 2011. p. 3–12.
16. Macquarie dictionary. 4th edition. Australia: Macmillan Publishers; 2006.
17. Free-on-line Dictionary. 2010. Available at: http://www.thefreedictionary.com/. Accessed September 12, 2010.
18. Merriam Webster Dictionary, 2009.
19. Cashman R. The bitter-sweet awakening: the legacy of the Sydney 2000 Olympic games. Sydney: Walla Walla Press; 2003.
20. Cashman R, Kennett C, de Morgas M, et al, editors. What is Olympic legacy? The legacy of the Olympic games, 1984-2002. Lausanne, Switzerland: Olympic Museum; 2003. p. 31–42. IOC document.
21. Girginov V, Hills L. A sustainable sports legacy: creating a link between the London Olympics and sports participation. Int J Hist Sport 2008;25(14):2091–116.
22. Heilpern W. 2016. Why the Olympics and Paralympics are still separate events. Available at: http://uk.businessinsider.com/why-the-olympics-and-paralympics-are-separate-events-2016-8. Accessed November 28, 2017.
23. Brittain I, Beacom A. Leveraging the London 2012 Paralympic Games. J Sport Social Issues 2016;40(6):499–521.
24. International Paralympic Committee. 2014. Sochi 2014 setting Russia up for post-Games legacy, Available at: https://www.paralympic.org/news/sochi-2014-setting-russia-post-games-legacy. Accessed August 15, 2017.
25. Coates J, Vickerman PB. Paralympic legacy: exploring the impact of the games on the perceptions of young people with disabilities. Adapted Phys Activity Q 2016;33(4):338–57.
26. Hutzler Y, Higgs C, Legg D. Improving Paralympic development programs: athlete and institutional pathways and organizational quality indicators. Adapted Phys Activity Q 2016;33(4):305–10.
27. Legg D, Higgs C. How countries identify, recruit, and prepare future athletes for the Paralympics: case study - Canada. Palaestra 2016;30(3):23–30.
28. Ferrara K, Burns J, Mills H. Public attitudes toward people with intellectual disabilities after viewing Olympic or Paralympic performance. Adapted Phys Activ Q 2015;32(1):19–33.

Moving?

Make sure your subscription moves with you!

To notify us of your new address, find your **Clinics Account Number** (located on your mailing label above your name), and contact customer service at:

Email: journalscustomerservice-usa@elsevier.com

800-654-2452 (subscribers in the U.S. & Canada)
314-447-8871 (subscribers outside of the U.S. & Canada)

Fax number: 314-447-8029

Elsevier Health Sciences Division
Subscription Customer Service
3251 Riverport Lane
Maryland Heights, MO 63043

*To ensure uninterrupted delivery of your subscription, please notify us at least 4 weeks in advance of move.

Printed and bound by CPI Group (UK) Ltd, Croydon, CR0 4YY

03/10/2024

01040393-0008